DERMATOLOGY - LABORATORY AND CLINICAL RESEARCH

MELANIN: BIOSYNTHESIS, FUNCTIONS AND HEALTH EFFECTS

DERMATOLOGY - LABORATORY AND CLINICAL RESEARCH

Additional books in this series can be found on Nova's website
under the Series tab.

Additional E-books in this series can be found on Nova's website
under the E-book tab.

CELL BIOLOGY RESEARCH PROGRESS

Additional books in this series can be found on Nova's website
under the Series tab.

Additional E-books in this series can be found on Nova's website
under the E-book tab.

DERMATOLOGY - LABORATORY AND CLINICAL RESEARCH

MELANIN: BIOSYNTHESIS, FUNCTIONS AND HEALTH EFFECTS

XIAO-PENG MA
AND
XIAO-XIAO SUN
EDITORS

Nova Science Publishers, Inc.
New York

Library of Congress Cataloging-in-Publication Data

Melanin : biosynthesis, functions and health effects / editors, Xiao-Peng Ma and Xiao-Xiao Sun.
p. ; cm.
Includes bibliographical references and index.
ISBN 978-1-62100-991-7 (hardcover)
I. Ma, Xiao-Peng. II. Sun, Xiao-Xiao.
[DNLM: 1. Melanins--biosynthesis. 2. Skin Pigmentation. QU 110]

612.7'927--dc23
2011042412

Published by Nova Science Publishers, Inc. ✝ New York

Contents

Preface

Human melanin is synthesized in melanosomes located in melanocytes of the skin, hair, eyes, and leptomeninges. Melanin not only determines skin color, but also protects the skin from UV damage by absorbing UV light. In this book, the authors present current research in the study of the biosynthesis, functions and health effects of melanin. Topics include melanogenesis and natural hypopigmentation agents; fungal melanins; the coat color genes that regulate eumelanin and pheomelanin synthesis in melanocytes; the role of melanin production in gaeumannomyces graminis infection of cereal plants and the occurrence and function of melanic pigmentation in ectothermic vertebrates.

Chapter I - Human melanin is synthesized in melanosomes located in melanocytes of the skin, hair, eyes, ears, and leptomeninges. Melanin not only determines skin color, but also protects the skin from UV damage by absorbing UV light. Congenital pigmentary disorders that result in skin and hair depigmentation, such as Hermenksky Pudluk Syndrome, Chediak Higashi Syndrome, and Griscelli Syndrome are due to various gene mutations that cause defects in melanin synthesis. Excessive production of melanin, which occurs in response to UV-induced DNA damage, inflammation, or other skin injuries, however, can result in skin hyperpigmentation including freckles, melasma, solar lentigo, age spots, and post-inflammatory hyperpigmentation. In this article the authors review the synthesis of melanin, the signaling pathways related to the regulation of melanogenesis, the factors influencing melanogenesis and various pigmentation disorders, as well as the effectiveness of various natural products at reducing hyperpigmentation.

Chapter II - Melanins are hydrophobic polymers of high molecular weight, formed by oxidative polymerization of phenolic and indolic compounds, produced by organisms in all Kingdoms. They are typically black or dark brown in color and their molecular structures are diverse. Several fungi can produce melanins and the functions of this pigment enhance microbial survival under diverse unfavorable environmental and host conditions. The major melanin type encountered among fungi is the 1,8-dihydroxynaphthalene (DHN) melanin that is synthesized from acetyl-coenzyme A via the polyketide pathway. This melanin is generated by several human pathogenic fungi, such as *Fonsecaea pedrosoi*, *Exophialla dermatitidis*, *Aspergillus fumigatus*, *Histoplasma capsulatum* and *Sporothrix schenckii*. It is also present in phytopathogenic fungi such as *Colletotrichum* spp., *Magnaporte orizae* and *Ascochyta rabiei*. In addition to DHN melanin, fungi can also produce melanin via dihydroxyphenylalanine (DOPA), in which tyrosinases or laccases hydroxylate tyrosine via DOPA to dopaquinone that then auto-oxidizes and polymerizes, resulting in a polyphenolic heteropolymer of black color known as eumelanin. *Cryptococcus neoformans* is the best known fungus to produce this type of melanin, but other fungi such as *Candida albicans*, *Paracoccidioides brasiliensis* and *S. schenckii* can also produce eumelanin. A type of soluble fungal melanin is produced from L-tyrosine through *p*-hydroxyphenylpyruvate and homogentisic acid. This pigment is called pyomelanin and it is similar to alkaptomelanin produced by humans. *A. fumigatus*, *Madurella mycetomatis* and *Yarrowia lipolytica* are examples of fungi that can produce this type of pigment. Fungal melanins play an important role in the protection of fungi from several environmental stresses, such as desiccation, UV irradiation, heavy metals, temperature fluctuation and digestion by hydrolytic enzymes. Melanins also play a role in the virulence of a broad range of pathogenic fungi. These pigments protect the fungi from host defense mechanisms and antifungal agents. Although melanins challenge the immunological strategies of host defense, they are also targets for alternative antimicrobial strategies, by the use of antibodies against melanin or inhibitors of melanin synthesis.

Chapter III - In mice, eumelanin and pheomelanin synthesis is regulated by numerous coat color genes. Eumelanin and pheomelanin contents were measured in cultured melanocytes and in the epidermis/dermis and hairs of C57BL/10JHir (B10) and its congenic mice carrying the coat color genes. Eumelanin contents in agouti and dilute melanocytes are similar to black melanocytes, whereas the contents in brown, pink-eyed dilution, slaty and ruby-eye 2^d melanocytes are reduced to one third~one thirthieth. In contrast, pheomelanin contents in agouti, dilute, slaty and ruby-eye 2^d melanocytes are similar to its content in black melanocytes, whereas the content in brown melanocytes is increased. Eumelanin and pheomelanin contents in cultured epidermal melanocytes correlate well with those in skin and hair of the congenic mice, except that agouti melanocytes do not synthesize pheomelanin in culture, the pink-eyed dilution allele does not affect pheomelanin content in hairs, and the ruby-eye 2^d allele increases pheomelanin content in hairs. These results suggest that eumelanin and pheomelanin synthesis in melanocytes is regulated by numerous coat color genes in a complicated manner.

Chapter IV - *Gaeumannomyces graminis* var. *graminis* (*Ggg*) is an ascomycete that causes black sheath rot disease of rice (*Oryza sativa* L.) and take-all root rot of several turfgrass species. *G. g.* var. *graminis* synthesizes melanin and deposits it in hyphal cell walls. The authors' research indicates that the nature of the association between *Ggg* and plant root is parasitic, but can change to pathogenic and ultimately terminate as saprophytic. Melanin plays several roles during fungal growth and throughout infection and colonization of plant roots. First, hyphal morphology (diameter, shape and melanin concentration) appears to change as the fungus invades and colonizes the tissues of the root. Second, melanin appears to be a determinant of fungal pathogenicity. Wild-type isolates of *Ggg* were pathogenic, and colonized plants showed more severe symptoms of infection while isolates lacking melanin were able to ectotrophically colonize and penetrate roots as a parasite, but no macroscopic symptoms of take-all were observed to indicate pathogenicity.

Chapter V - In mice models of pigment anomalies, over 800 phenotypic alleles are known. This indicates that skin color is distinctly regulated by more than 800 genes. This requires several steps; (i) distribution of melanoblasts into skin in embryo, (ii) construction of melanosomes in melanocytes, (iii) production of melanin granules in melanosomes, (iv) translocation of melanosomes from perinuclear to peripheral region in melanocytes, (v) transfer of melanosomes from melanocytes to keratinocytes and (vi) translocation of transferred melanin granules from a peripheral to a supranuclear region in keratinocytes. The damage in each step induces pigment anomalies. The authors summarize biogenesis and function of melanin granules with pigment anomalies; piebaldism and Waadenburg syndrome caused by inadequate distribution of melanoblasts in embryo; Hermansky-Pudlak syndrome, Chediak-Higashi syndrome, and oculocutaneous albinism type 2 and 4 by improper biogenesis of melanosomes and melanin granules; and Griscelli syndrome by inappropriate intercellular translocation of melanosomes. Aberrant intercellular transfer of melanin granules is shown in a case of pediatric erythema dyschromicum perstans (ashy dermatosis). Aberrant translocation inside keratinocytes is present in Dowling-Degos disease. Unregulated melanogenesis is present in disorders affected in KITLG-KIT signaling and RAS-MAPK signaling. The loss or decreased enzymatic function in melanogenesis induces oculocutaneous albinism types 1 and 3. Pheomelanin-dominant production is present in red hair color phenotypes showing fair skin, poor tanning ability and elevated risk of freckles, malignant melanoma, basal cell carcinoma and squamous cell carcinoma. This section will provide the current findings to recognize the function and the health effect of melanin granules as well as the pathogenesis of pigmentation-associated disorders.

Chapter VI - Optical properties of synthetic and natural eumelanin are presented and compared, in order to investigate the structural organization of eumelanin, which is related to the function of this biopolymer. Synthetic eumelanin is produced by oxidation of tyrosine with hydrogen peroxide, whereas natural eumelanin is extracted from *Sepia Officinalis* and from *Rana Esculenta*. Vibrational spectroscopy techniques (as Raman scattering and infrared absorption) show that both types of biopolymer include chemical functional groups characteristic of the monomeric units of eumelanin, although natural eumelanin includes also protein-related groups, proportionally to the protein content. X-ray diffraction spectra are in agreement with the hypothesis that eumelanin monomers assembly themselves and form protomolecules consisting of stacked layers (distant 3 – 4 Å each other) of indolic sheets. Absorption measurements, characterized by a monotonic increase of optical density from near-IR to UV range, support the model that eumelanin consists of a distribution of aggregates of oligomeric structures having different size and chemical composition. The estimated values of the optical gap indicate that the natural eumelanins are characterized by a larger structural disorder than the synthetic one. Fluorescence spectra confirm that the biopolymer consists of ensembles of chemically distinct oligomer systems, which can be selectively excited. This result is also supported by Dynamic Light Scattering measurements, which permit to visualize the distribution of particles size. In fact, the nanoaggregate systems of natural eumelanin have a larger size than those of synthetic eumelanin. This might be related to the biological functions of such a biopolymer, particularly as far as photoprotective action is concerned.

Chapter VII - Ectotherms have specialized chromatophores whose pigments are responsible for the different colors of the epidermis. Melanocytes are one type of chromatophore that produce and store melanin in organelles called melanosomes. In ectotherms, cells containing melanin pigments occur in several organs and tissues. These cells are found in the capsule and stroma of the organs, giving it a dark coloration. The function of visceral pigment cells is poorly known, but melanomacrophages are known to perform phagocytosis in hematopoietic organs and also act against bacteria, due to melanin. In addition, the distribution of visceral melanocytes varies with physiological factors, such as age, nutritional status; and also environmental one, such as temperature and photoperiod. On the other hand, the pigmentation in some organs seems to be conservative, and may help in phylogenetic reconstructions.

Chapter VIII - Melanocytes produce melanin that determines the skin color. Skin color can be mildly manipulated by use of fairness creams with skin lightening/ whitening ingredients. Some of skin lightening ingredients are harmful to skin and health due to their deleterious effects. Yet the 'quest for fairness' is global and that puts the research on safe skin lightening products as one of the pinnacles in the billion dollar cosmetic industry. Tyrosine is the precursor in the sequels of biochemical pathways that lead to the formation of melanin pigment. Tyrosinase is the key enzyme that mediates two steps in the biochemical conversion of tyrosine to melanin. Hence most skin lightening ingredients exhibit their mode of action by tyrosinase inhibition. Melanocytes are dendritic cells and they are involved in the transfer of melanosomes to the keratinocytes. This process is aided by the dendrites in the melanocytes. Any qualitative and or quantitative changes to the dendrites in the melanocytes would effect the transfer and thereby the melanization of the skin. Besides understanding the tyrosinase modulating activity, it is also necessary to study the effect of the skin lightening agents on the dendrites in the melanocytes. The extracts of several plants such as bearberry, cranberry, mulberry or blueberry are used in the skin lightening formulations. The authors studied the tyrosinase inhibitory effects of the extracts of *Hemidesmus indicus*, *Decalepis hamiltonii*, *Raphanus sativus* var. *longipinnatus* (white), *Raphanus sativus* var. *sativus* (Red), *Curcuma zedoaria* and *Aloe vera* individually and in different permutation combinations. Tyrosinase inhibition assay, melanocyte cell culture assay, measurement of dendrite length and number of melanocytes were used as methods to evaluate the efficacy of the extract combinations. Tyrosinase activity was assayed spectrophotometrically by following the oxidation of DOPA to dopachrome at 475 nm. B16F10 murine melanoma cells were cultured in Eagles minimal essential medium with supplements. The extracts treated melanocytes were examined under microscope, the number and relative length of dendrites in each melanocyte were recorded at random and statistically compared with untreated control. The polyherbal extract combinations of *Curcuma zedoaria*, *Aloe vera* and *Decalepis hamiltonii* was found to be effective in inhibiting the melanin synthesis and may also have a suggestive role in preventing the melanin transfer to the keratinocytes thereby could bring about the desired skin lightening benefit.

In: Melanin: Biosynthesis, Functions and Health Effects
Editors: Xiao-Peng Ma and Xiao-Xiao Sun
ISBN: 978-1-62100-991-7

Chapter I

Melanogenesis and Natural Hypopigmentation Agents

H. M. Chiang, H. W. Chen, Y. H. Huang, S. Y. Chan, C. C. Chen, W. C. Wu and K. C. Wen*

Department of Cosmeceutics,
China Medical University,
Taichung, Taiwan

Abstract

Human melanin is synthesized in melanosomes located in melanocytes of the skin, hair, eyes, ears, and leptomeninges. Melanin not only determines skin color, but also protects the skin from UV damage by absorbing UV light. Congenital pigmentary disorders that result in skin and hair depigmentation, such as Hermenksky Pudluk Syndrome, Chediak Higashi Syndrome, and Griscelli Syndrome are due to various gene mutations that cause defects in melanin synthesis. Excessive production of melanin, which occurs in response to UV-induced DNA damage, inflammation, or other skin injuries, however, can result in skin hyperpigmentation including freckles, melasma, solar lentigo, age spots, and post-inflammatory hyperpigmentation. In this article we review the synthesis of melanin, the signaling pathways related to the regulation of melanogenesis, the factors influencing melanogenesis and various pigmentation disorders, as well as the effectiveness of various natural products at reducing hyperpigmentation.

* Correspondence to: Professor Kuo-Ching Wen. Department of Cosmeceutics. China Medical University. Taichung, Taiwan 404. E-mail: kcwen0520@mail.cmu.edu.tw. Telephone: 886-4-22053366 ext. 5302. Fax: 886-4-22078083.

Abbreviations

ACTH, adrenocorticotropin melanocyte stimulating hormone;
AHA, α-hydroxy acids;
ASP, agouti signaling protein;
ATP, adenosine 5'-triphosphate;
BBI, Bowman Birk inhibitor;
bFGF, basic fibroblast growth factor;
BHAs, β-hydroxy acids;
cAMP, cyclic AMP;
CRE, cAMP response element;
CREB, cAMP-response element binding protein;
CRH, corticotropin-releasing hormone;
DCT, TRP2,DOPAchrome tautomerase;
DHI, 5,6-dihydroxyindole;
DHICA, 5,6-dihydroxyindole-2-carboxylic acid;
DKK 1, dickkopf-related protein 1;
DPPH, 1,1-diphenyl-2-picryl-hydrazyl;
ECE, ET converting enzyme;
ERK2, extracellular signal-regulated kinase 2;
ET-1, endothelin-1;
ETBR, endothelin B receptor;
FOXD3, forkhead-box transcription factor D3;
GM-CSF, granulocyte-macrophage colony-stimulating factor;
GSK3β, glycogen synthase kinase-3β;
HGF, hepatocyte growth factor;
HPS, Hermansky-Pudlak syndrome;
HQ, hydroquinone;
IL, interleukin;
ITF2, immunoglobulin transcription factor-2;
L-DOPA, 3,4-dihydroxyphenylalanine;
LEF-1, lymphoid-enhancing factor-1;
LIF, leukemia inhibitory factor;
LT, leukotrienes;
MAP kinase, mitogen-activated protein kinase;
MC1R, melanocortin 1 receptor;
MITF, microphthalmia-associated transcription factor;
MOPB, methylophiopogonanone B;
NGF, nerve growth factor;
NHKC, normal human keratinocytes;
NHMC, normal human melanocytes;
NO, nitric oxide;
NRG, neuregulin;
PAR-2, protease activated receptor 2;
PAX3, paired box 3;

PGs, Prostaglandins;
PIAS3, protein inhibitor of activated STAT3;
PKA, protein kinase A;
PKC, protein kinase C;
PLA2, phospholipase A2;
POMC, pro-opiomelanocortin;
ROS, reactive oxygen species;
RSK, ribosomal S6 kinase;
SA, salicylic acid;
SCCE, stratum corneum chemotrypic enzyme;
SCF, Stem cell factor;
SEM, skin equivalent model;
SOX, Sry-related HMG box;
STAT3, signal transducer and activator of transcription 3;
STI, soybean trypsin inhibitor;
TGF-β1, transforming growth factor-β1;
TNF-α, tumor necrosis factor α;
TPA, 12-*O*-tetradecanoylphorbol-13-acetate;
TRP1, tyrosinase-related protein 1;
UV, ultraviolet;
α-MSH, α-melanocyte-stimulating hormone;

Introduction

Variations in human skin, hair, and eye color are due to the type, amount, stage, and distribution of melanin[1]. Melanin, one of the most widely distributed pigments, is a heterogeneous polyphenol-like biopolymer with a complex structure and color varying from yellow to black[2]. More than 150 genes regulate and contribute to skin pigmentation[3, 4]. In addition to contributing to the color of skin and hair, melanin also protects skin from physical (such as ultraviolet (UV) irradiation damage), chemical (such as environmental pollutants, heavy metals, and oxidative stress), and biochemical (such as bacteria) challenges[5, 6]. Overexposure to solar UV irradiation can result in photoaging, mutagenesis, and photocarcinogenesis in human skin[7, 8].

The incidence of skin cancer is increasing at a rate of 3% to 4% per year, and the mortality rate associated with skin cancer (melanoma) is increasing more rapidly than the mortality rate associated with any other cancer[9]. Melanocytes transfer melanosomes through their dendrites to surrounding kerotinocytes where they form melanin caps. This accumulation of melanin plays a protective role against UV irradiation by absorbing and transforming UV energy into harmless heat. Melanin can also scavenge toxic xenobiotics and reactive oxygen species (ROS) as well as bind to drugs, thereby protecting human skin against chemical and biochemical challenges[5, 6, 10-12]. However, excessive production of melanin and its accumulation in the skin can cause pigmentation disorders, including melasma, solar lentigo, and post-inflammatory hyperpigmentation[13]. Overproduction of melanin is not only a dermatological issue but also poses esthetic problems, especially among patients in Asian cultures.

In this article we review the synthesis of melanin, the signaling pathways related to the regulation of melanogenesis, the factors influencing melanogenesis and various pigmentation disorders, as well as the effectiveness of various natural products at reducing hyperpigmentation.

Melanosynthesis

Variations in dermal pigmentation depend on the number, size, composition, and distribution of melanocytes as well as the activity of melanogenic enzymes.

Melanin synthesis by melanocytes within membrane-bound organelles (melanosomes) and their transfer to keratinocytes within the epidermal melanin unit determines cutaneous pigmentation.

Melanin synthesis is characterized by an increased number of melanocytes in the basal layer of the epidermis, the size, maturation, and number of melanosomes, the production of melanin, the dendricity of melanocytes, the transfer of melanosomes from melanocytes to keratinocytes, the proliferation of keratinocytes, and the thickening of the epidermis and stratum corneum.

Melanocytes and Melanosomes

Melanin is synthesized in melanocytes, which are localized at the basal layer of the epidermis.

Each melanocyte is functionally related to underlying fibroblasts in the dermis and to keratinocytes in the epidermis. Each melanocyte transfers pigment-containing melanosomes via dendritic melanocytes to approximately 36 basal and suprabasal keratinocytes – the so-called epidermal melanin unit[3, 14, 15] (Figure 1).

This inter-cell cross-talk regulates the function and phenotype of human skin[16]. Protease-activated receptor 2 (PAR-2) plays an important role in melanosomal transfer[17, 18]. PAR-2, a G protein-coupled receptor, mediates the phagocytosis of melanosomes in a Rho-dependent manner[19]. The amount and type of melanin produced and transferred to the keratinocytes with subsequent incorporation, aggregation, and degradation influences skin complexion coloration[20]. Melanoblasts, melanocyte precursor cells, are derived from the neural crest and migrate to target sites such as dermis and eyes[21]. Melanoblasts differentiate into melanocytes when they reach their destination and start to produce melanosomes, the organized elliptic membrane-bound organelles where melanin is synthesized. Melanin synthesis starts with the exportation of structural proteins from the endoplasmic reticulum to the cytosol, where they fuse with melanosome-specific regulatory glycoproteins that have been released in coated vesicles from the Golgi apparatus. Melanin synthesis ensues subsequent to the sorting and trafficking of these proteins to melanosomes[22, 23]. Melanosomes are divided into four maturation stages according to their structure and to the type and amount of melanin produced[24, 25]. 'Early' melanosomes (stages I and II) present with little or no pigment, while 'late' melanosomes (stages III and IV) present with some to complete pigment. Stage I melanosomes are spherical vacuoles lacking tyrosinase activity and internal structural components. Stage II melanosomes are elongated, fibrillar organelles containing tyrosinase and little melanin[26, 27]. After stage II, melanin synthesis starts. Stage III melanosomes have uniformly deposited pigment on the internal fibrils. Mature melanosomes (stage IV) are either elliptical or ellipsoidal in shape, are electron-opaque due to complete melanization, and have minimal tyrosinase activity. Highly pigmented melanocytes are rich in Stage IV melanosomes which are transferred by melanocyte dentrites to keratinocytes [16].

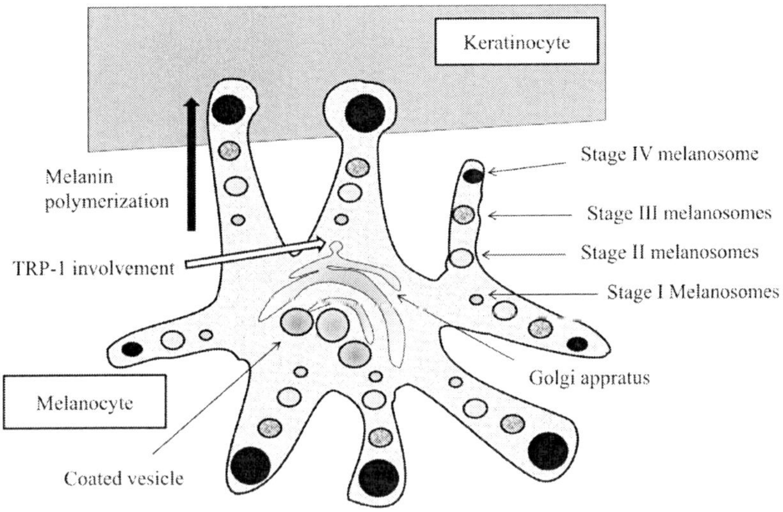

Figure 1. Melanosome transfer.

The trafficking of sorting vesicles to their target organelles is controlled by two classes of microtubule-associated motor proteins – kinesins and cytoplasmic dyneins[28]. Kinesins power plus-end-directed microtubule-based motility, while cytoplasmic dyneins drive minus-end-directed motility [29, 30]. Dyneins and kinesins also play roles in retrograde and in anterograde transport of melanosomes [31-34], whereas dyneins and spectrin dominate the movement of early melanosomes [35].

The methods of melanosome transfer from melanocytes to keratinocytes include cytophagocytosis of melanocyte dendrite tips[36, 37] and exocytosis of melanosomes into the extracellular space and their subsequent uptake by phagocytosis into keratinocytes[38, 39], either by filopodia-mediated melanosome transfer[40-42] or the filopodial-phagocytosis model[43]. Rab, melanophilin, and myosin Va have been shown to be involved in the movement of melanosomes[37, 44].

Melanin Biosynthesis

Melanins are polymorphous, multifunctional biopolymers. The major types of melanins include eumelanin, pheomelanin, a combination of eumelanin and pheomelanin (mixed melanin), and neuromelanin (Figure 2). Eumelanin is a blackish-brown heterogeneors polymer consisting of 5,6-dihydroxyindole (DHI) and 5,6-dihydroxyindole-2-carboxylic acid (DHICA). Pheomelanin is yellowish-red in color and consists of sulfur-containing benzothiazine derivatives[2, 45].

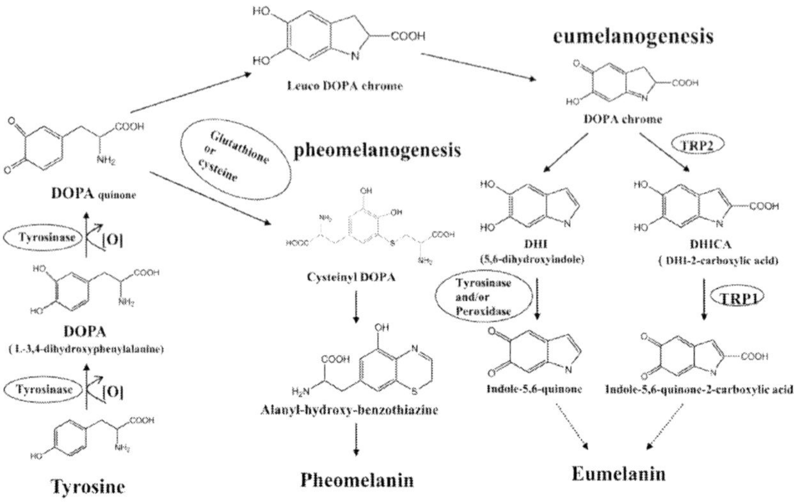

Figure 2. Pathway of melanin biosynthesis.

Neuromelanin is produced in dopaminergic neurons of the human substantia nigra, the dorsal motor nucleus of the vagus nerve, and the median raphe nucleus of the pons. Neuromelanin has the capacity to chelate redox-active metals such as Cu, Mn, and Cr as well as toxic metals such as Cd, Hg, and Pb to avoid neuron degeneration[46]. If the level of neuromelanin decreases, dopamine synthesis may be diminished, resulting in diseases associated with neuronal degradation. Massive loss of dopamine-producing pigmented neurons in the substantia nigra has been found in patients with Parkinson's disease[47].

The biosynthetic pathway governing melanin formation is well established[48-52] (Figure 2). Synthesis of melanin starts with the conversion of the amino acid L-tyrosine to dopaquinone by tyrosinase, a copper-containing glycosylated type I membrane-bound glycoprotein that catalyzes the rate-limiting step of melanin biosynthesis[53, 54]. Tyrosinase is synthesized by melanosomal ribosomes on the rough endoplasmic reticulum[55]. The enzyme is glycosylated en route to and within the Golgi apparatus, and subsequently delivered to melanosomes via coated vesicles[55, 56]. Tyrosinase is the most common target for therapeutic agents intended to alleviate hyperpigmentation[57-59]. Tyrosinase catalyzes two distinct oxidation reactions. First, tyrosinase catalyzes the oxidation of monophenol (L-tyrosine) to o-diphenol (3,4-dihydroxyphenylalanine, L-DOPA (monophenolase activity)). Second, L-DOPA is oxidized to o-quinone (dopaquinone) (diphenolase activity). Tyrosinase gene transcription has been shown to correlate with the differentiation of lysosomes and/or peroxisomes into melanosomes[60, 61]. Tyrosinase-related protein 1 (TPR-1) and DOPAchrome tautomerase (DCT, also known as TRP-2) subsequently metabolize dopaquinone into eumelanin through a process referred to as eumelanogenesis. Dopaquinone is transferred to DHI via multiple processes including decarbxylation, oxidation, and polymerization and DOPAchrome is converted to DHICA. Pheomelanogenesis refers to the process through which dopaquinones conjugate with thiol-containing cysteines or glutathiones to form pheomelanin. As mentioned above, dopaquinone plays pivotal roles both in eumelanogenesis and pheomelanogenesis[16]. Eumelanogenesis involves the activation of tyrosinase, TRP-1, and TRP-2 whereas the synthesis of pheomelanin only requires the activation of tyrosinase[16, 62]. Following the synthesis of those pigments, melanin-containing melanosomes are transferred to neighboring keratinocytes. However, without successful transfer of melanosomes to keratinocytes, the skin can appear essentially unpigmented[63].

Factors Regulating Melanin Biosynthesis

UV radiation from the sun stimulates melanin synthesis in skin. After UV exposure, melanocytes increase their expression of pro-opiomelanocortin (POMC, the precursor of α-MSH) and its receptor melanocortin 1 receptor (MC1R), tyrosinase, TRP-1, protein kinase C (PKC), and other signaling factors[64-66] (Figure 3). Upon exposure to UV irradiation, fibroblasts release the above-mentioned cytokines, growth factors, and inflammatory factors, which then stimulate melanin production and/or stimulate melanin transfer. UV also stimulates the production of endothelin-1 (ET-1) and POMC in keratinocytes, factors that then act in a paracrine manner to stimulate melanocyte function[67, 68]. Other keratinocyte-derived factors that regulate the proliferation and/or differentiation of melanocytes include α-MSH, adrenocorticotropin melanocyte stimulating hormone (ACTH), basic fibroblast growth factor (bFGF), nerve growth factor (NGF), endothelins, granulocyte-macrophage colony-stimulating factor (GM-CSF), steel factor, leukemia inhibitory factor (LIF), and hepatocyte growth factor (HGF)[69]. Melanocytes have been shown to increase the production of intracellular nitric oxide (NO), which in turn triggers signal transduction cascades to initiate melanogenesis[70, 71] through the enzyme tyrosinase. In addition, human melanocyte proliferation requires cross-talk between several signaling pathways including the cAMP/PKA, PKC, and tyrosine kinase pathways; therefore, the mechanisms by which various factors increase skin pigmentation are closely inter-related[52, 72-75].

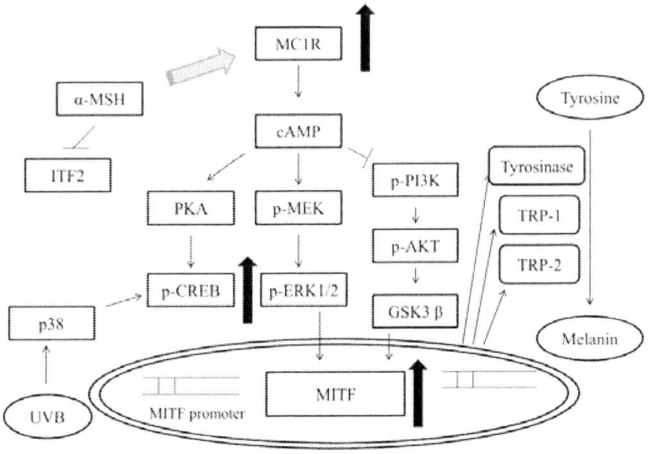

Figure 3. Factors regulating melanin biosynthesis.

UV radiation has been shown to influence melanogenesis through a paracrine regulation process involving keratinocytes[52, 76](Figure 3). Both autocrine and paracrine cytokine networks are involved in UV-induced upregulation of melanogenesis[77]. α-MSH is a major mediator of the response of melanocytes to UV[78]. The POMC gene is activated in the pituitary gland but POMC-derived peptides are also generated in keratinocytes and melanocytes[79, 80]. The POMC gene encodes a large precursor protein, which is then enzymatically cleaved to form several different peptides including α-MSH, ACTH, melanocortin, and β-endorphin[80]. The binding of α-MSH and ACTH to MC1R on the melanocyte membrane[81] activates intracellular adenylate cyclase through G proteins, which then catalyze the conversion of adenosine triphosphate to cyclic AMP (cAMP)[82]. cAMP exerts its function through protein kinase A (PKA)[83]. The intracellular elevation of cAMP increases the protein expression of microphthalmia-associated transcription factor (MITF), tyrosinase, and TRP-2, but not tyrosinase or TRP-2 mRNAs[84]. PKA promotes the activation of the cAMP-response element binding protein (CREB) that binds to the cAMP response element (CRE) that is present in the M promoter of the MITF gene[85, 86]. MITF is a transcription factor with a basic helix-loop-helix-leucine zipper motif. MITF regulates melanocyte cellular differentiation and the transcription of melanogenic enzymes such as tyrosinase, TRP-1, and TRP-2 and the transcription of melanosome structural proteins including MART-1 and Pmel17[87-90]. Pmel17 is a structural matrix protein and an amyloid protein required for the generation of the internal fibril[91]. The promoter sequences of tyrosinase, TRP-1, and TRP-2 share a highly conserved motif known as the M-box, which contributes to their melanocyte-specific expression[92, 93](Figure 4). TRP-1 promoter activity is up regulated by paired box 3 (PAX3)[94]. The M-box (AGTCATGTGCT) is an extended E-box (ACATGTGA) and is necessary for promoter up-regulation by MITF[16, 95]. The E-box is more important than the M-box in promoting the transcription factor MITF[96](Figure 4). MITF is exclusively expressed in melanocytes. It binds to the M-box promoter elements of tyrosinase and modulates TRP-1 and TRP-2, resulting in hyperpigmentation[97-99]. In addition to the process of melanization, MITF also regulates melanocyte proliferation, differentiation, development, apoptosis, and survival[100-102].

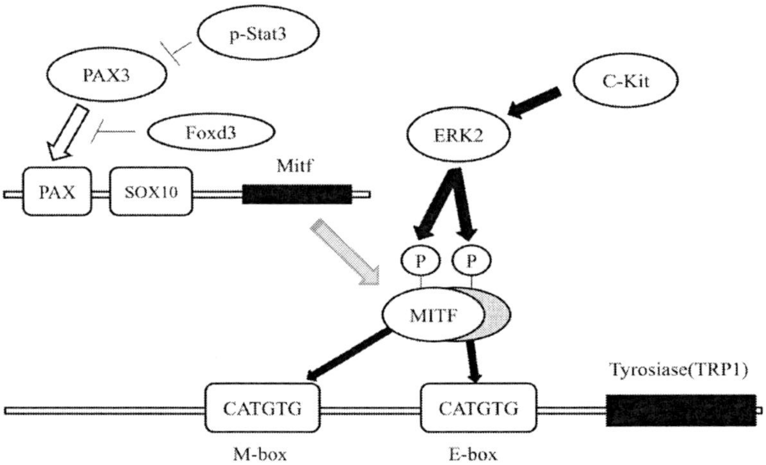

Figure 4. Tyrosinase gene expression.

A transient increase in MITF leads to the up-regulation of tyrosinase, TRP-1, and TRP-2[103] as well as to increased dendricity[88]. Many transcription factors including Sry-related HMG box (SOX) 9 and 10, PAX3, signal transducer and activator of transcription 3 (STAT3), protein inhibitor of activated STAT3 (PIAS3), lymphoid-enhancing factor-1 (LEF-1), immunoglobulin transcription factor-2 (ITF2), and forkhead-box transcription factor D3 (FOXD3) are able to modulate the expression and/or transcriptional activity of MITF in vivo[104] (Figure 4). The transcription factor SOX9 may play an important role in UVB-induced melanocyte differentiation and pigmentation through MITF regulation[105]. SOX10 regulates the expression of MITF and TRP-2. SOX10 has been demonstrated to activate the TRP-2 promoter-reporter construct and to work in synergy with MITF[106, 107]. PAX3 binds to the MITF gene promoter to regulate MITF expression[108]. In addition, PAX3 has been shown to act in synergy with SOX10 to up regulate the expression of MITF[109]. The transcriptional activity of MITF is regulated through the interaction between STAT3 and PIAS3. LEF-1, a transcription factor involved in the Wnt signal transduction pathway, initiates and facilitates MITF expression, while ITF2 and FOXD3 down regulate MITF expression[104, 110-112].

The transcriptional activity of MITF is regulated by phosphorylation of tyrosinase residues on extracellular signal-regulated kinase 2 (ERK2) following signals from c-kit (tyrosinase-type receptor) and then by phosphorylation of the 73rd serine residue in the N terminal domain of MITF[113] (Figure 4). The tyrosinase gene and TRP-1 promoter zones share a CATGTG motif. When MITF is activated, binding to the formed dimmers serves to regulate the expression of the tyrosinase gene TRP-1. MITF is also regulated at the transcriptional level by interleukin-6 (IL-6) and the Wnt signaling pathway and it is post-transcriptionally regulated by phosphorylation via ribosomal S6 kinase (RSK), glycogen synthase kinase-3β (GSK3β), p38 stress signaling, and the mitogen-activated protein kinase (MAP kinase) pathways[89, 90, 98, 114-116](Figure3). α-MSH also stimulates p38 MAP kinase, which in turn phosphorylates upstream transcription factors that bind to the tyrosine promoter[52].

Human placental lipid upregulates p38 activation and subsequent tyrosinase expression, thereby promoting melanogenesis[117]. Down-regulation of p38 expression leads to an increase in expression of biomarkers associated with differentiation such as tyrosinase and tyrosinase-related proteins.

The mechanism involved in the p38-mediated regulation of melanogenesis is the ubiquitin–proteasome pathway, through which melanogenic enzymes are degraded[118]. In addition, inhibition of ERK and AKT signaling via MITF up-regulation plays a key role in inducing hyperpigmentation[119]. ERK activation results in phosphorylation of MITF and its subsequent ubiquitination and degradation[120]. Sphingosine-1-phosphate, C2-ceramide, and sphingosylphosphorylcholine activate ERK and may play important roles in the inhibition of melanogenesis[120-122].

Transforming growth factor-β1 (TGF-β1) inhibits melanogenesis by mediating the down-regulation of MITF promoter activity as well as by reducing the production of tyrosinase, TRP-1, TRP-2, and MITF protein levels. In addition, TGF-β1 inhibits the expression of PAX 3, which in turn inhibits melanogenesis[123]. It has been reported that TGF-β1 influences the ERK pathway and down regulates MITF and the production of melanogenic enzymes[115, 124, 125].

The agouti signaling protein (ASP) can down regulate MITF gene expression and compete with α-MSH in binding to MC1R, causing inhibition of α-MSH signaling on the MC1R receptor. ASP modulates the frequency, rate, and extent of eumelanin and pheomelanin generation[4].

Studies have demonstrated that high levels of ASP are associated with yellow-pigmented bands in mouse hair because ASP inhibits α-MSH binding to MC1R [16]. Thus, MC1R and its ligands, α-MSH and ASIP, regulate the switch between eumelanin and pheomelanin synthesis in melanocytes[79, 126].

UVB exposure activates the transcription factor p53, which in turn induces the expression of POMC. Expression of that α-MSH precursor leads to the secretion of α-MSH and the up-regulation of melanogenesis via MC1R in keratinocytes[127, 128]. In addition, p53 directly stimulates the expression of the genes encoding tyrosinase and TRP1 in melanocytes[129]. UVB also induces the expression of corticotropin-releasing hormone (CRH) in melanocytes, which is mediated by the CREB–PKA signaling pathway with consequent stimulation of POMC expression through the CRH-R1 receptor. The POMC gene has been shown to be p53-responsive following UV irradiation[130].

Kichina et al. demonstrated that stable transfection of wild-type p53 into pigmented melanoma cells leads to overexpression of wild-type p53 and a decrease in tyrosinase mRNA levels and tyrosinase activity[131].

Khlgatian et al. have shown that UV irradiation results in increased p53-dependent tyrosinase mRNA levels in melanoma cells and that p53 is required for the thymidine dinucleotide-induced increase in tyrosinase function in mouse epidermis[132]. They also reported that tanning is part of a p53-mediated adaptive response of mammalian skin to UV-induced DNA damage[132].

Other hormones, such as steroids and sex hormones, can influence pigmentation[79, 127, 133], and it has been reported that cholesterol is capable of increasing the expression of MITF and its target genes in melanocytes through the up-regulation of the CREB protein[134]. Two fibroblast-derived paracrine factors, namely dickkopf-related protein 1 (DKK1) and neuregulin-1 (NRG1), regulate melanogenesis. DKK1 is a factor secreted by fibroblasts. DKK1 has been shown to suppress growth of melanocytes, strongly inhibit melanin production, and inhibit binding of Wnt proteins to their receptors, which results in down-regulation of melanogenesis[102, 135].

In addition, DKK1 suppresses melanocyte growth and function by inhibiting the Wnt/b-catenin signaling pathway[136, 137]. DKK1 has also been shown to regulate the expression of PAR-2[137].

Pigmentary Disorders

Hyperpigmentation disorders are characterized by the overproduction of melanin and include melasma, postinflammatory hyperpigmentation, freckles, moles, chloasma, age spots, and lentigines[138-140]. Hypopigmentation disorders are characterized by the underproduction of melanin and include disorders such as oculocutaneous albinism, Hermansky–Pudlak syndrome, Griscelli syndrome, Chediak-Higashi syndrome, and Waardenburg syndrome.

Oculocutaneous albinism is an inherited autosomal recessive disorder characterized by deficiency or complete absence of melanin[61]. At least 10 types of oculocutaneous albinism exist. Patients with the disorder present with hypopigmention of the skin, hair, and eyes as well as reduced visual acuity with nystagmus and photophobia. Furthermore, in these patients there is often complete lack of tyrosinase activity[141, 142].

Oculocutaneous albinism type 2, which is characterized by a congenital reduction or absence of melanin pigment in the skin, hair, and eyes, is the most common type and the incidence is highest in black Africans[16].

Hermansky-Pudlak syndrome (HPS) is a genetically heterogeneous group of related autosomal recessive conditions. It is divided into eight types according to the HPS genes that carry mutations[143].

Defects in proteins encoded by these genes can affect the biogenesis or function of intracellular organelles such as melanocytes and retinal pigment epithelial cells. HPS is also associated with lung disease, inflammatory bowel disease, renal disease, and bleeding problems due to platelet dysfunction[16].

Griscelli syndrome is an autosomal recessive disorder characterized by pigmentary dilution of the skin and the accumulation of large and abnormal end-stage melanosomes in the center of melanocytes[144].

It may be caused by defects in the formation of the Rab27a–Mlph–MyoVa protein complex in melanocytes, an important protein that connects melanosomes to the actin network[144]. Chediak-Higashi syndrome is an autosomal recessive disorder similar to oculocutaneous albinism[145].

Patients with this syndrome are susceptible to infection because they lack natural killer cell function and are at risk for developing lymphofollicular malignancy and peripheral neuropathies[146, 147].

Mutations in the human homolog of the MITF gene are associated with auditory and pigmentary abnormalities in patients with Waardenburg syndrome type IIA[109, 148, 149]. Mutations in the PAX3 gene are associated with Waardenburg syndrome type I, while SOX 10 mutations are characteristic of Waardenburg syndrome type IV[4, 51].

Mechanisms of Depigmentation

Studies on the processes of cellular melanogenesis and the response of pigment-producing cells to UV radiation have been instrumental in promoting the development of depigmenting agents[57, 58, 114, 150, 151].

The mechanisms of action by which biological and chemical agents cause hypopigmentation include (i) tyrosinase inhibition, maturation, and enhancement of its degradation; (ii) inhibition of tyrosinase mRNA transcription; (iii) inhibition of MAP kinases, TRP-1, TRP-2, and MITF; (iv) downregulation of MC1R activity; (v) interference with melanosome maturation and transfer; and (vi) melanocyte loss and desquamation[57, 114, 150-153].

Tyrosinase inhibition is the most common approach to achieve skin hypopigmentation as this enzyme catalyses the rate-limiting step of pigmentation[114, 152]. Tyrosinase inhibitors can be classified as competitive, uncompetitive, mixed type, and non-competitive inhibitors[57, 154].

Tyrosinase can be inhibited at the transcriptional and post-transcriptional levels by inhibiting tyrosinase mRNA transcription and disrupting tyrosinase glycosylation by using competitive or non-competitive inhibitors to attenuate the catalytic activity of tyrosinase, by accelerating tyrosinase degradation, and by modulating tyrosinase stability[155, 156].

Natural Hypopigmentation Agents

Hydroquinone, ascorbic acid, and retinoic acid have been shown to be effective skin-whitening agents; however, they are associated with harmful side effects, thereby limiting their clinical use[155]. Compounds derived from natural products, on the other hand, have been shown to be as effective as chemical-based products at reducing hyperpigmentation. Some natural skin-depigmenting products have been reported to directly effect melanogenesis; enhance tyrosinase degradation; interfere with melanosome maturation and its transfer; inhibit inflammation-induced melanogenesis; and accelerate skin desquamation[51, 154, 157-159].

Effect on Melanogenesis

As shown in Table 1, whitening agents derived from natural products can be divided into three groups: phenols, polyphenols, and others [58]. Table 1 also presents the plants from which the compounds are derived, the mode of action including tyrosinase inhibition, other enzyme inhibition (OEI (TRP1 and TRP2), melanin inhibition (MI), and other mechanisms of action, as well as the IC_{50} values of said compounds. The mechanisms of tyrosinase inhibition can be evaluated by measuring enzyme inhibition kinetics using Lineweaver-Burk plots with varying concentrations of L-DOPA as the substrate. Moraceae, Anacardiaceae, Chloranthaceae, Ericaceae, Lamiaceae, Sapindaceae, and Fabaceae are rich in phenols and polyphenols that have anti-melanogenesis activity. Most studies used B16 melanoma cells as a model to investigate the mechanism of action governing melanin inhibition. Some of the studies used mouse melan-a or mel-ab melanocyte cultures or normal human melanocytes (NHMC) as experimental models.

Data from studies that involved the use of NHMC cells are probably more reliable because those cells mimic the response to stimuli seen *in vivo*. Human melanocyte proliferation and enhancement of melanin synthesis require cross-talk between several cytokines and hormones that are released from keratinocytes. Co-cultures of melanocytes and keratinocytes from mouse[160, 161] or human skin[162] also more closely mimic the response seen *in vivo*.

Table 1. Whitening ingredients from natural sources effect on melanogenesis

Compounds (phenol, polyphenols, others)	Source	Mode of action				Refs.
		TI	OEI (TRP-1, TRP-2)	other	MI	
Phenols						
Anacardic acid, 6-[8(Z),11(Z),14-pentadecatrienyl]-salicylic acid, 5-[8(Z),11(Z),14-pentadecatrienyl] resorcinol	*Anacardium occidentale* cashew fruit (Anacardiaceae)	Yes (c)				[249]
10'(Z)-heptadecenylhydroquinone [HQ17(1)]	*Rhus succedanea* (Anacardiaceae)	Yes IC_{50}= 37 μM			Yes IC_{50}= 40 μM	[250]
2-hydroxy-4-methoxybenzaldehyde	*Rhus vulgaris* Meikle Sclerocarya caffra Sond (Anacardiaceae) *Mondia whitei* (Hook) Skeels (Asclepiadaceae)	Yes (m) IC_{50}=0.03 mM				[251]
3,4-Dihydroxyacetophenone	Ilex pubescens (Aquifoliaceae)	Yes IC_{50}= 10 μM		Reduction of TYR and MITF protein level	Yes	[252]
p-Coumaric acid	*Panax ginseng* (Araliaceae)	Yes (m) IC_{50}= 3.65 mM				[253]

Table 1. (Continued)

Compounds (phenol, polyphenols, others)	Source	Mode of action	Refs.			Refs.
		TI	OEI (TRP-1, TRP-2)	other	MI	
p-Coumaric acid	*Sasa quelpaertensis* (Gramineae)	Yes (c)		Reduction of TYR protein level	Yes	[254]
2',4',6'-trihydroxydihydrochalcone	*Greyia flanaganii* (Greyiaceae)	Yes IC_{50}= 69.15 µM				[255]
protocatechuic aldehyde	*Salvia miltiorrhiza* (Lamiaceae)	Yes (c) IC_{50}=19.92 µM				[256]
protocatechualdehyde	*Phellinus linteus* (Hymenochaetaceae)	Yes (c)				[257]
protocatechuic acid methyl ester	Black Rice Bran	Yes IC_{50}= 0.28 µM				[258]
phloroglucinol (1), eckstolonol (2), eckol (3), hlorofucofuroeckol A (4), ieckol (5)	*Ecklonia stolonifera.* brown alga extracts (Laminariaceae)	Yes [(1) and (2), -- (c)] (1) IC_{50}= 92.8 µg/mL (2) IC_{50}= 126 µg/mL Yes [(3) , (4) and (5) -- (n)] (3) IC_{50}=33.2 µg/mL (4) IC_{50}=177 µg/mL (5) IC_{50}=2.16 µg/mL			Yes	[259]
Phloroglucinol, dieckol, eckol,	*Ecklonia cava* (Lessoniaceae)	Yes Dieckol (88.9% of TYR at 50 µM)		Reduction of UV-B induced cell damages	Yes	[260]

Compounds (phenol, polyphenols, others)	Source	Mode of action	Refs.			Refs.
		TI	OEI (TRP-1, TRP-2)	other	MI	
7-phloroeckol	*Ecklonia cava* (Lessoniaceae)	Yes (nc) IC_{50} =0.85 μM			Yes	[261]
cinnamaldehyde(1), 2-methoxy cinnamaldehyde (2) cinnamic acid (3) O-coumaric acid (4) , icariside DC (5), dihydromelilotoside (6), dihydromelilotoside (7)	*Cinnamomum cassia* (Lauraceae)	Yes (1) IC_{50}=0.52 ±0.03 mM, (2) IC_{50}=0.42 ±0.02 mM, (3) IC_{50}=0.41 ±0.01 mM, (4) IC_{50}=0.67 ±0.03 mM, (5) IC_{50}=0.71 ±0.03 mM, (6) IC_{50}=0.57 ±0.01 mM, (7) IC_{50}=0.63 ±0.02 mM				[262]
Mulberroside F (moracin M-6, 39-di-O-β-D-glucopyranoside)	*Morus alba* leaves (Moraceae)	Yes TYR (mushroom) IC_{50}=0.29 μg/mL ; TYR (mammalian) IC_{50}=68.3 μg/mL		Superoxide Scavenging Activity	Yes (30.6% of MI at 1 mg/mL)	[263]
4-Substituted resorcinols	*Artocarpus incises* (Moraceae)	Yes (c)				[264]

Table 1. (Continued)

Compounds (phenol, polyphenols, others)	Source	Mode of action	Refs.			Refs.
		TI	OEI (TRP-1, TRP-2)	other	MI	
Macelignan	*Myristica fragrans* (Myristicaceae)	Yes IC_{50}=30 μM	TRP-1 TRP-2	Reduction of TYR, TRP-1 and TRP-2 protein level	Yes IC_{50}=13 μM	[265]
Americanin A (1), 3,3'-bisdemethylpinoresinol (2)	*Morinda citrifolia* seeds (Rubiaceae)	Yes (1) IC_{50} =2.7 mM (2) IC_{50} =0.3 mM		SOD-like activity		[266]
3-caffeoylquinic acid 4-caffeolyquinic acid 5-caffeoylquinic acid 5-feruloylquinic acid 3,4-dicaffeoylquinic acid 3,5-dicaffeoylquinic acid 4,5-dicaffoylquinic acid	green coffee beans (Rubiaceae)	Yes				[267]
3,4-dihydroxycinnamic acid (1), 4-Hydroxy-3-methoxycinnamic acid (2)	*Pulsatilla cernua* (Ranunculaceae)	Yes (nc) (1) IC_{50}=0.97 mM (2) IC_{50}=0.33 mM				[268]
4-acetonyl-3,5-dimethoxy-*p*-quinol (1), cis-*p*-coumaric acid (2), trans-*p*-coumaric acid (3), *p*-hydroxybenzoic acid (4), Vanillic acid (5)	*Synsepalum dulcificum* (Sapotaceae)	Yes (1) IC_{50}=208.1 μM, (2) IC_{50}=197.9 μM, (3) IC_{50}=168.7 μM, (4) IC_{50}=358.6 μM, (5) IC_{50}=174.4 μM				[269]

Compounds (phenol, polyphenols, others)	Source	Mode of action	Refs.			Refs.
		TI	OEI (TRP-1, TRP-2)	other	MI	
Compounds (phenol, polyphenols, others)	Source	Mode of action	Refs.			Refs.
		TI	OEI (TRP-1, TRP-2)	other	MI	
Cardamonin	*Alpinia katsumadai Hayata* (Zingiberaceae)	Yes		MITF	Yes	[270]
Isopanduratin A (1) , 4-hydroxypanduratin A (2)	*Kaempferia pandurata.* (Zingiberaceae)	Yes (1) IC_{50}=10.5 μM (2) IC_{50}>30 μM		Reduction of TYR protein level	Yes (1) IC_{50}= 10.64 μM (2) IC_{50}= 23.25 μM	[271]
Curcumin, yakuchinone A, yakuchinone B, eugenol ferulic acid	Chouji Syzygium aromaticum (Myrtaceae) and Yakuchi Alpinia oxyphylla (Zingiberaceae)	Yes (c) (Curcumin and yakuchinone B)				[272]
polyphenols						
1,2,3,4,6-penta-O-galloyl-â-D-glucose	*Galla rhois* (Anacardiaceae)	Yes (nc)				[273]
2,3,4,6-tetra-O-galloyl-D-glucopyranose (1), 1,2,3,6-tetra-O-galloyl-beta-D-glucopyranose (2), 1,2,3,4,6-penta-O-galloyl-beta-D-glucopyranose (3)	*Rhus chinensis* (Anacardiaceae)	Yes (nc) (1) IC_{50} = 54 μM, (2) IC_{50} = 30 μM, (3) IC_{50} = 15 μM			Yes	[274]

Table 1. (Continued)

Compounds (phenol, polyphenols, others)	Source	Mode of action	Refs.			Refs.
		TI	OEI (TRP-1, TRP-2)	other	MI	
Tannic acid	*Rhus javanica leaves (Anacardiaceae)*	Yes (c) IC50= 22 μM				[275]
Icariside I (1), Icariside II (2), Icaritin (3)	*Epimedium grandiflorum* (Berberidaceae)				Yes (1) IC_{50}= 49.04 μM, (2) IC_{50}= 10.53 μM, (3) IC_{50}= 11.13 μM	[276]
Xanthohumol	*Humulus lupulus* L. (Cannabaceae)	Yes	Reduction of TRP-1 and TRP-2 mRNA level	Reduction of cAMP, MITF protein and its mRNA expression and TYR protein expression	Yes	[277]
GB-2 (biflavanones)	*Garcinia kola*Seed (Clusiaceae)	Yes IC_{50} = 582 μM				[278]
GS contained 2 biflavonoids; 2R,3S-5,7,4',5'',7'',3''',4'''-heptahydroxy-flavanone[3-8''] flavone (1), 5,7,4',5'',7'',3''',4'''-heptahydroxy[3-8''] biflavanone (2)	*Garcinia subelliptica* (Clusiaceae)	Yes (1) IC_{50} = 2.5 μM (2) IC_{50} = 26 μM				[279]

Compounds (phenol, polyphenols, others)	Source	Mode of action	Refs.			Refs.
		TI	OEI (TRP-1, TRP-2)	other	MI	
3 flavonols: Quercetin (1), Kaempferol (2), Morin (3), 2 flavones: Luteolin (4), Luteolin 7-*O*-glucoside (5)	*Heterotheca inuloides* (Asteraceae)	3 favonols-(c) (1) $ID_{50} = 0.07$ mM (2) $ID_{50} = 0.23$ mM (3) $ID_{50} = 2.32$ mM 2 flavones-(n) (1) $ID_{50} = 0.19$ mM (2) $ID_{50} = 0.50$ mM				[280]
Luteolin		Yes		Inhibition of adenyl cyclase activity	Yes	[281]
N-feruloylserotonin (1), N-(*p*-coumaroyl)serotonin (2), acacetin (3)	*Carthamus tinctorius* L. (Asteraceae)	Yes (1) $IC_{50} = 0.023$ mM (2) $IC_{50} = 0.074$ mM (3) $IC_{50} = 0.779$ mM			Yes (1) $IC_{50} = 0.191$ mM (2) $IC_{50} = 0.245$ mM (3) $IC_{50} > 20$ mM	[282]
Inulavosin	*Inula nervosa (Asteraceae)*			Mistargeting of tyrosinase to lysosomes	Yes	[283]

Table 1. (Continued)

Compounds (phenol, polyphenols, others)	Source	Mode of action	Refs.			Refs.
		TI	OEI (TRP-1, TRP-2)	other	MI	
Anastatin A (1), Isosilybin A (2), Isosilybin B (3), Luteolin (4), Quercetin (5), (+)-Dehydrodiconiferyl alcohol (6), (+)-Balanophonin (7), 3,4-Dihydroxybenzaldehyde (8)	*Anastatica hierochuntica* (Cruciferae)			Isosilybin A (2) and Isosilybin B (3) inhibit the mRNA expression of TRP-2.	Yes (1) IC_{50} = 16 µM, (2) IC_{50} = 10 µM, (3) IC_{50} = 6.1 µM, (4) IC_{50} = 14 µM, (5) IC_{50} = 15 µM, (6) IC_{50} = 16 µM (7) IC_{50} = 15 µM (8) IC_{50} = 17 µM	[284]
Silymarin	*Silybum marianum* (milk thistle) (Asteraceae)	Yes		Reduction of TYR protein levels	Yes IC_{50}= 28.2 µg/mL	[285]
5,2',4'-trihydroxy-2'',2''-dimethylchromene-(6,7:5'',6'')-flavanone	*Dalea elegans* (Fabaceae)	Yes [(m) L-tyrosine IC_{50}= 0.26 µM] [(nc) L-DOPA IC_{50}= 18.61 µM]				[286]
Kuraridin (1), Kurarinone (2), Norkurarinol (3)	*Sophora flavescens (Fabaceae)*	Yes (1) IC50= 1.1 µM (2) IC50= 1.3 µM (3) IC50= 2.1 µM				[287]

Compounds (phenol, polyphenols, others)	Source	Mode of action	Refs.			Refs.
		TI	OEI (TRP-1, TRP-2)	other	MI	
Sophoraflavanone G (1), Kurarinone (2) Kurarinol (3)	*Sophora flavescens* (Fabaceae)	Yes (1) nc- IC_{50} = 4.7 μM, (2) nc- IC_{50} = 2.2 μM (3) c- IC_{50} = 0.1 μM				[288]
Sophoraflavanone G (1), Kuraridin (2), Kurarinone (3)	*Sophora flavescens* (Fabaceae)	Yes (1) IC_{50} = 6.6 μM (2) IC_{50} = 0.6 μM (3) IC_{50} = 6.2 μM				[289]
Kurarinone (1) Kushnol F (2)	*Sophora flavescens* (Fabaceae)	Yes (1)-nc (1) IC_{50} = 4.6 μg/mL (2) IC_{50} = 9.0 μg/mL				[290]
Kurarinol (1), Kuraridinol (2)	*Sophora flavescens* (Fabaceae)	Yes (1,2)-nc (1) IC_{50} =8.60±0.51 μM (2) IC_{50} =0.88±0.06 μM			Yes (1) IC_{50}=29 μM, (2) IC_{50}=17 μM	[291]
5,2',4'-trihydroxy-2'',2''-dimethylchromene-(6,7:5'',6'')-flavanone	*Dalea elegans* (Fabaceae)	Yes [(m) L-tyrosine IC_{50}= 0.26 μM] [(nc) L-DOPA IC_{50}= 18.61 μM]				[286]
Kuraridin (1), Kurarinone (2), Norkurarinol (3)	*Sophora flavescens* (Fabaceae)	Yes (1) IC_{50}= 1.1 μM (2) IC_{50}= 1.3 μM (3) IC_{50}= 2.1 μM				[287]
N-Feruloyl-N′-cis-feruloyl-putrescine	*Sophora japonica* (Fabaceae)	Yes (m) IC_{50} = 85.0 μM				[292]

Table 1. (Continued)

Compounds (phenol, polyphenols, others)	Source	Mode of action	Refs.			Refs.
		TI	OEI (TRP-1, TRP-2)	other	MI	
Dalbergioidin	*Lespedeza cyrtobotrya* (Fabaceae)	Yes (nc) IC_{50}=20 µM			Yes IC_{50}=27 µM	[293]
Haginin A	*Lespedeza cyrtobotrya* (Fabaceae)	Yes (nc) IC_{50}=5.0 µM	TRP-1 protein level	Reduction of TYR, and MITF protein level, Induction of ERK and Akt/PKB protein level	Yes Melan-a cells IC_{50}= 3.3 µM ; HEMn cells IC_{50} = 2.7 µM	[294]
Glycyrrhisoflavone (1), Glyasperin C (2)	*Glycyrrhiza uralensis* (Fabaceae)	Yes (2) IC_{50} = 0.13 µg/mL			Yes (1) 63.73 ± 6.8 % inhibition at 5 µg/mL (2) 17.65 ± 8.8 % at 5 µg/mL	[295]
Licuraside (1), Isoliquiritin(2), Licochalcone A (3)	*Glycyrrhiza uralensis* (1-2) *Glycyrrhiza inflate* (3) (Fabaceae)	Yes 1, 2 and 3 (c) (1) IC_{50} =0.072 mM (2) IC_{50} =0.038 mM (3) IC_{50} =0.0258 mM				[296]

Compounds (phenol, polyphenols, others)	Source	Mode of action	Refs.			Refs.
		TI	OEI (TRP-1, TRP-2)	other	MI	
Calycosin	*Astragalus membranaceus* (Fabaceae)	Yes IC_{50} = 38.4 μM			Yes IC_{50} = 40 μM	[297]
Butin	*Spatholobus suberectus* (Fabaceae)	Yes IC_{50} = 35.9 μM	Reduction of TRP-1 and TRP-2 protein and mRNA level	Reduction of TYR protein and mRNA level	Yes 29.26% at 100 μM	[298]
Gallocatechin (1), Epi-gallocatechin gallate(2), Quercitrin (3)	*Distylium racemosum* (Hamamelidaceae)	Yes (1) IC_{50} = 4.8 μg/ mL, (2) IC_{50} = 30.2 μg/ mL, (3) IC_{50} = 37.7 μg/ mL				[299]
Quercetin(1) Tiliroside (2)	*Marrubium velutinum* and *Marrubium cylleneum* (Lamiaceae)	Yes Yes 100% inhibition (1) 49.67 ± 1.16 mM (2) 30.19 ± 9.60 mM				[300]
Kaempferol	*Crocus sativus* L. (Iridaceae)	Yes (c) ID_{50} =0.23 mM				[301]
Bibenzyl xyloside-1 (1), Bibenzyl xyloside-2 (2), Bibenzyl xyloside-3 (3)	*Chlorophytum arundinaceum* (Liliaceae)	Yes (1) IC_{50} =1.6 μM (2) IC_{50} =0.43 μM (1) IC_{50} =0.73 μM				[302]

Table 1. (Continued)

Compounds (phenol, polyphenols, others)	Source	Mode of action	Refs.			Refs.
		TI	OEI (TRP-1, TRP-2)	other	MI	
Resveratrol (1), Oxyresveratrol (2)	*Veratrum patulum* (Liliaceae)	Yes (1) $IC_{50} = 43.5\ \mu M$ (2) $IC_{50} = 1.2\ \mu M$				[303]
2"- O-Feruloylaloesin, aloesin	Aloe extracts Aole vera (Liliaceae)	Yes (n)				[304]
Aloesin		Yes		in vitro pigmented skin equivalent model	Yes	[305]
Artocarpfuranol(1), dihydromorin (2), steppogenin (3), norartocarpetin (4), artocarpanone (5), artocarpesin (6), isoartocarpesin (7)	*Artocarpus heterophyllus* (Moraceae)	Yes (1) $IC_{50} = 47.93\ \mu M$ (2) $IC_{50} = 10.34\ \mu M$ (3) $IC_{50} = 0.57\ \mu M$ (4) $IC_{50} = 0.46\ \mu M$ (5) $IC_{50} = 1.54\ \mu M$ (6) $IC_{50} = 0.52\ \mu M$ (7) $IC_{50} = 0.66\ \mu M$				[306]
Norartocarpetin (1), Resveratrol (2)	*Artocarpus gomezianus* (Moraceae)	Yes				[307)
3-prenyl luteolin	*Artocarpus heterophyllus* (Moraceae)	Yes $IC_{50} = 76.3\ \mu M$			Yes $IC_{50} = 57.6\ \mu M$	[308]

Compounds (phenol, polyphenols, others)	Source	Mode of action	Refs.			Refs.
		TI	OEI (TRP-1, TRP-2)	other	MI	
1,3-diphenylpropanes: kazinol C (1), kazinol F (2), broussonin C (3), kazinol S (4)	*Broussonetia kazinoki.* (Moraceae)	Yes (c) (1) IC_{50} = 15.5 µM (2) IC_{50} = 0.96 µM (3) IC_{50} = 0.43 µM (4) IC_{50} = 17.9 µM				[309]
chlorophorin	*Chlorophora excelsa* (Moraceae)	Yes (c) IC_{50} = 1.3 µM				[310]
4-[(2''*E*)-7''-hydroxy-3'',7'' -dimethyloct-2'' -enyl]-2' ,3,4',5-tetrahydroxy-*trans*-stilbene	*Chlorophora excelsa* (Moraceae)	Yes (c) IC_{50} = 96 µM				[310]
(±)2,3-cis-dihydromorin (1), 2,3-trans-dihydromorin (2), Oxyresveratrol (3)	*Cudrania cochinchinensis* (Moraceae)	Yes (1) IC_{50} = 31.1 µM (2) IC_{50} = 21.1 µM (3) IC_{50} = 2.33 µM				[311]
2,4,2',4'-Tetrahydroxy-3-(3-methyl-2-butenyl)-chalcone	Morus nigra (Moraceae)	Yes (c) IC_{50} =0.95 µM			Yes	[312]
Oxyresveratrol	*Morus alba* L. (Moraceae)	Yes (nc) IC_{50} = 1 µM				[313]
Polyphenols: Compound 1,5,9	*Morus lhou* (Moraceae)	Yes (c) (1) IC_{50} = 1.3 µM (5) IC_{50} = 1.2 µM (9) IC_{50} = 7.4 µM				[314]
Betulinic acid	Morus alba L. and Morus rotundiloba K. (Moraceae)	Yes				[315]

Table 1. (Continued)

Compounds (phenol, polyphenols, others)	Source	Mode of action	Refs.			Refs.
		TI	OEI (TRP-1, TRP-2)	other	MI	
Crude extract (C-AP) Anthocyanins: cyanidin-3-alpha-O-rhamnoside (1), pelargonidin-3-alpha-O-rhamnoside (2)	*Malpighia emarginata.* acerola fruit (Malpighiaceae)	Yes (C-AP) $IC_{50=}15$ µg/mL, (1) (2) – (nc) (1) IC_{50}=40 µM, (2) IC_{50}=19.1 µM			Yes (data no shown)	[316]
2R,3S-5,7,4',5",7",3"',4"'-heptahydroxy- flavanone[3-8"] flavone, and 5,7,4',5",7",3"',4"'-heptahydroxy[3-8"] biflavanone	*Hibiscus tiliaceus* (Malvaceae)	Yes				[279]
Globulusin A (1), Eucaglobulin (2)	*Eucalyptus globules* (Myrtaceae)				Yes	[194]
Kaempferol (1), quercetin (2), mudanpioside B (3), benzoyl-oxypaeoniflorin (4), mudanpioside H (5), pentagalloyl-β-D-glucose (6)	*Paeonia suffruticosa* (Paeoniaceae)	Yes (1) to (5) --(c) (1) IC_{50} = 0.12 µM (2) IC_{50} = 0.11 µM (3) IC_{50} = 0.37 µM (4) IC_{50} = 0.45 µM (5) IC_{50} = 0.32 µM (6) -- (nc) (6) IC_{50} = 0.06 µM				[317]

Compounds (phenol, polyphenols, others)	Source	Mode of action	Refs.			Refs.
		TI	OEI (TRP-1, TRP-2)	other	MI	
2,3-dihydro-4',4'''-di-O-methylamentoflavone	*Podocarpus macrophyllus var. macrophyllus* (Podocarpaceae)	Yes IC_{50}=0.10 mM	Reduction of TRP-2 mRNA		Yes	[318]
Anthraquinones	*Polygonum cuspidatum* (Polygonaceae)	Yes				[319]
(2R,3R)-(+)-taxifolin	*Polygonum hydropiper* L. (Benitade) (Polygonaceae)	Yes IC_{50}=0.24 mM				[320]
3,4-Dihydroxycinnamic acid (1), 4-hydroxy-3-methoxycinnamic acid (2)	*Pulsatilla cernua* (Ranunculaceae)	Yes (nc) (1) IC_{50} = 0.97 mM (2) IC_{50} = 0.33 mM				[268]
Quercetin	*Rosa canina* L. (Rosaceae)	Yes			Yes Reducing melanin content to 64% at 10 μM, 34.5% at 20 μM, 17.5% at 17.7% at 40 μM	[321]
3,3'-Bisdemethylpinoresinol (1), Quercetin (2)	*Morinda citrifolia* (Rubiaceae)	Yes (1) IC_{50} = 0.3 mM, (2) IC_{50} = 0.1 mM				[266]

Table 1. (Continued)

Compounds (phenol, polyphenols, others)	Source	Mode of action	Refs.			Refs.
		TI	OEI (TRP-1, TRP-2)	other	MI	
Nobiletin	Peel of *Citrus* fruit (Rutaceae)	Yes IC_{50}=46.2 μM				[322]
Betulin, Lupeol, Soyacerebroside I	*Guioa villosa* (Sapindaceae)	Yes				[323]
(+)-*epi*-Syringaresinol (1), *N*-cis-Feruloyltyramine (2)	*Synsepalum dulcificum* (Sapotaceae)	Yes (1) IC_{50}=200 μM, (2) IC_{50}=215.5 μM				[269]
Acetone extract, epigallocatechin gallate (1), Procyanidin B_1(2)	*Sideroxylon inerme* (Sapotaceae)	Yes Acetone extract IC_{50}=63 μg/mL, (1)IC_{50}=30 μg/mL (2)$IC_{50}>$200 μg/mL			yes	[324]
Negundin A (1), Negundin B (2), 6-hydroxy-4-(4-hydroxy-3-methoxy)-3-hydroxymethyl-7-methoxy-3,4-dihydro-2-naphthaledehyde (3), Vitrofolal E (4), (+)-lyoniresinol (5), (+)-lyoniresinol-3α-O-β-D-glucoside (6), (+)-(−)-pinoresinol (7), (+)-diasyringaresinol (8)	*Vitex negundo Linn.* (Verbenaceae)	Yes (1) IC_{50} = 10.06 μM (2) IC_{50} = 6.72 μM (3) IC_{50} = 7.81 μM (4) IC_{50} = 9.76 μM (5) IC_{50} = 3.21 μM (6) IC_{50} = NA (7) IC_{50} = 15.13 μM (8) IC_{50} = 5.61 μM				[325]

Compounds (phenol, polyphenols, others)	Source	Mode of action	Refs.			Refs.
		TI	OEI (TRP-1, TRP-2)	other	MI	
isopanduratin A (1), 4-hydroxypanduratin A (2)	*Kaempferia pandurata* (Zingiberaceae)	Yes (1) IC_{50}=10.5 μM (2) IC_{50} > 30 μM			Yes (1) IC_{50} = 10.64 μM, (2)IC_{50} = 23.25 μM	[271]
Gentol	*Gnetum* genus (Zingiberaceae)	Yes IC_{50}=4.5 μM			Yes	[326]
(-)-epigallocatechin gallate (EGCG) (1) (-)-gallocatechin 3-0-gallate (GCG) (2) (-)-epicatechin gallate (ECG) (3)	Green tea	Yes (c) (1) IC_{50} = 34.10 μM (2) IC_{50} = 17.34 μM (3) IC_{50} = 34.58 μM				[327]
1,2,3,6-Tetra-Ogalloyl-b-D-glucose (1), 1,2,3,4,6-Penta-O-galloyl-b-D-glucose, (2) 2,3,4,6-Tetra-O-galloyl-D-glucose (3)	10 Chinese Galls	Yes (nc) (1) IC_{50}=30 μM (2) IC_{50}=15 μM (3) IC_{50}=54 μM			Yes	[274]
N,N′-dicoumaroyl-putrescine (DCP), N,N′-diferuloyl-putrescine (DFP)	Corn bran	yes (DCP) IC_{50}=181.73 μM (DFP) IC_{50}=291.3 μM			Yes (DCP) IC_{50} =3169.5 μM (DFP) IC_{50} =733.64 μM	[328]

Table 1. (Continued)

Compounds (phenol, polyphenols, others)	Source	Mode of action	Refs.			Refs.
		TI	OEI (TRP-1, TRP-2)	other	MI	
7,8,4'-Trihydroxyisoflavone (1), 7,3',4'-Trihydroxyisoflavone (2), Genistein (3)	Korean fermented soybean paste (Doenjang)	Yes (1) IC_{50} = 11.21 ± 0.8 μM (2) IC_{50} = 5.23 ±0.6 μM			Yes (1) IC_{50} = 12.23±0.7 μM (2) IC_{50} = 7.83 ±0.7 μM (3) IC_{50}= 57.83 ±0.5 μM	[329]
5,7-dihydroxyflavone (chrysin)	propolis			Blocking adenylyl cyclase activity	Yes (51.6% at10 μM, 40.90% at 100μM)	[330]
Others						
Eextract	*Salicornia herbacea* (Amaranthaceae)	Yes			Yes	[331]
70% Acetone extract	*Rhus chinensis* (Anacardiaceae)	Yes IC_{50}= 22 μg/mL			Yes	[274]
Isoimperatorin Imperatorin	*Angelica dahurica* (Apiaceae)	Yes		Reduction of TYR mRNA levels	Yes	[332]
Anisic acid	*Pimpinella anisum* (Apiaceae)	Yes (u) IC_{50}=0.68 mM				[268]

Compounds (phenol, polyphenols, others)	Source	Mode of action	Refs.			Refs.
		TI	OEI (TRP-1, TRP-2)	other	MI	
Anisaldehyde	*Pimpinella anisum* (Apiaceae)	Yes (nc) IC_{50}=0.38 mM				[268]
Cumic acid (1), Cuminaldehyde (2)	*Cuminum cyminum* (Apiaceae)	Yes (nc) (1) IC_{50} = 0.26 mM (2) IC_{50} = 0.05 mM				[333]
ethanolic extract	Areca catechu (Arecaceae)	Yes IC_{50} = 0.48 mg/mL			Yes	[334]
	Lichen species: *Graphina glaucorufa, Graphina multistriata, Graphina salacinilabiata, Graphis assamensis, Graphis nakanishiana, Phaeographopsis indica*	Yes				[335]
(2Z,8Z)-Matricaria acid methyl ester	*Erigeron breviscapus* (Asteraceae)	Yes			Yes IC_{50}=25.4 μM	[336]
selina-4(14),7(1)-dien-8-one	*Atractylodis Rhizoma Alba.* (Asteraceae)	Yes	TRP-1, TRP-2		yes	[337]
Extract	*Lepidium apetalum* (Brassicaceae)	Yes		Reduction of TYR mRNA and MITF protein level	yes	[338]

Table 1. (Continued)

Compounds (phenol, polyphenols, others)	Source	Mode of action	Refs.			Refs.
		TI	OEI (TRP-1, TRP-2)	other	MI	
2 germacrane-type sesquiterpenes	*Chloranthus henryi* (Chloranthaceae)	Yes IC_{50}=325 μM and 269 μM				[339]
Tianmushanol (1), 8-O-methyltianmushanol (2)	*Chloranthus tianmushanensis* (Chloranthaceae)	Yes (1) IC_{50}=358 ±3 μM (2) IC_{50}=312 ±3 μM				[340]
3β,21,22,23-tetrahydroxycycloart-24(31),25(26)-diene	*Amberboa ramosa* (Asteraceae)	Yes IC_{50}=1.32 μM				[341]
1β-Hydroxy arbusculin A (1), costunolide (2), reynosin (3)	*Saussurea lappa* Clarke (Asteraceae)				Yes (1) IC_{50} = 11 μg/mL, (2) IC_{50} = 3.0 μg/mL (3) IC_{50} = 2.5 μg/mL	[342]
methanolic extract fraction	*Arbutus andrachne* L. (Ericaceae)	Yes IC_{50}=1000 mg/mL				[343]
Esculetin	*Euphorbia lathyris* L. (Euphorbiaceae)	Yes(c) IC_{50}= 43 μM				[344]
three steroids: stigmast-5-ene-3 beta,26-diol (1), stigmast-5-ene-3-ol (2), campesterol (3)	*Trifolium balansae* (Fabaceae)	Yes (1) stronger than (2) and (3) (1) IC_{50} =2.39 μM				[345]

Compounds (phenol, polyphenols, others)	Source	Mode of action	Refs.			Refs.
		TI	OEI (TRP-1, TRP-2)	other	MI	
	Stryphnodendron barbatimao, *Entada africana* *Prosopis africana* (Fabaceae) *Cariniana brasiliensis*, (Lecythidaceae) *Portulaca pilosa*, (Portulacaceae)	Yes				[346]
Trifolirhizin	*Sophora flavescens* (Fabaceae)	Yes IC_{50} =506.77±4.49 μM			Yes (3) IC50 = 36 μM	[291]
methyl gallate	*Distylium racemosum* branches (Hamamelidaceae)	Yes IC_{50} = 40.5 μg/ mL				[299]
5-hydroxymethyl-2-furaldehyde	*Phellinus linteus* (Hymenochaetaceae)	Yes (nc) IC_{50} = 90.8 μg/mL				[257]
crocusatin-K	*Crocus sativus* (Iridaceae)	Yes IC_{50}= 260 μM				[347]
Trans-cinnamaldehyde	*Cinnamomum cassia* (Lauraceae)	Yes (c)				[348]
linderanolide B and subamolide A	*Cinnamomum subavenium* (Lauraceae)	Yes			Yes	[349]
Extract	*Portulaca pilosa* (Lecythidaceae)	Yes				[346]

Table 1. (Continued)

Compounds (phenol, polyphenols, others)	Source	Mode of action	Refs.			Refs.
		TI	OEI (TRP-1, TRP-2)	other	MI	
(-)-N-formylanonaine	Michelia alba D.C. (Magnolianceae)	Yes IC_{50}= 74.3 µM		DPPH, reducing power, and chelating metal ions.	yes	[350]
1',3'-dilinolenoyl-2'-linoleoylglycerol	*Flammulina velutipes* (Marasmiaceae)	Yes IC_{50} =16.1 ± 0.5µg/mL				[351]
ethanolic extract of mulberry twigs (EEMT), ethanolic extract of mulberry root bark (EEMR)	*Morus alba* (Moraceae)	Yes				[352]
A series of α,β-unsaturated aldehydes	*Olea europaea* L. (Oleaceae)	Yes(n)		their ability to form a Schiff base with a primary amino group in the enzyme		[353]
(2E)-alkenal (C 7)	*Oliva olea* L. (Oleaceae)	Yes (nc)				[353]
acetonic extract	*Osmanthus fragrans* (Oleaceae)	Yes (u) IC_{50}= 2.314 mg/mL			Yes	[354]
methanol extract	Lichen species: *Usnea ghattensis* (Parmeliaceae)	Yes IC_{50}= 8.5 µg/mL				[355]

Compounds (phenol, polyphenols, others)	Source	Mode of action	Refs.			Refs.
		TI	OEI (TRP-1, TRP-2)	other	MI	
methanol extract	Lichen species: *Arthothelium awasthii* (Parmeliaceae)	Yes IC_{50}= 17.8 μg/mL				[355]
Sesamol (3,4-methylenedioxyphenol)	*Sesamum indicum* L. (Pedaliaceae)	Yes(c) IC_{50} = 1.9 μM			Yes 63% decreased in 100 mg/mL	[356]
5-(Hydroxymethyl)-2-furfural	*Dictyophora indusiata* (Phallaceae)	Yes (nc) ID_{50}=0.98 mM				[357]
piperlonguminine	*Piper longum* (Piperaceae)	Yes		Reduction of TYR mRNA, and MITF protein level, phosphorylates CREB	Yes	[358]
geranic acid	*Cymbopogon citrates* (Poaceae)	Yes IC_{50}=0.14 mM (trans) IC_{50}=2.3 mM (cis)				[359]
Extract	*Coccoloba uvifera* (Polygonaceae)	Yes IC_{50}= 68.84 μg/ml				[360]
Ethanol extract and distilled water extract	*Ganoderma lucidum* (Polyporaceace)	Yes IC_{50} =0.32 mg/mL				[361]
Dichloromethane fraction	*Cimicifuga heracleifolia* (Ranunculaceae)	Yes	TRP1	Phosphorylates MEK, ERK1/2 and Akt, MITF	Yes	[362]

Table 1. (Continued)

Compounds (phenol, polyphenols, others)	Source	Mode of action	Refs.			Refs.
		TI	OEI (TRP-1, TRP-2)	other	MI	
50% ethanolic extract	*Citrus hassaku* (Rutaceae)	Yes IC_{50}=4.7 mg/mL			Yes	[363]
Extract	*Dimocarpus longan* (Sapindaceae)	Yes IC_{50}= 2.9–3.2 mg/mL				[364]
1-O-methyl-fructofuranose	*Schisandra chinensis* (Turcz.) Baill (Schisandraceae)	Yes		via activation of MEK/ERK and PI3K/Akt signaling pathway and subsequent MITF downregulation.	Yes	[365]
ethanol extract, water extract, adenosine (1), Ethyl-*α*-D-glucopyranoside (2)	*Stichopus japonicas* (Stichopodidae)	Yes (m) ethanol extract 0.49–0.61 mg/mL, water extract 1.80–1.99 mg/mL, (1) IC_{50}= 0.13 mg /mL, (2) IC_{50}=0.19 mg /mL				[366]
hirsein A, hirsein B	*Thymelaea hirsuta* (Thymelaeaceae)	Yes	TRP1, TRP2	Decrease PKC activity, MITF, TRP1, TRP2,	Yes	[367]
Metallothionein (protein)	*Aspergillus niger* (Trichocomaceae)	Yes (m)				[368]

Compounds (phenol, polyphenols, others)	Source	Mode of action	Refs.			Refs.
		TI	OEI (TRP-1, TRP-2)	other	MI	
9-Hydroxy-4-methoxypsoraln	*Angelica dahurica* (Umbelliferae)	Yes (nc) IC_{50}=2.0 μg/mL				[369]
Alpinia galanga extract	*Alpinia galanga* Rhizome (Zingiberaceae)	Yes IC_{30}=18.5 μg/mL			Yes	[370]
Extract	*Curcuma aromatica* Rhizome (Zingiberaceae)	Yes IC_{30}=8.9 μg/mL			Yes	[370]
partial purification	*Curcuma longa* (Zingiberaceae)	Yes	TRP	Phosphorylates MEK, ERK1/2 and Akt, MITF, and TRP-2 protein level	Yes	[371]
triacylglycerols; triolein (1), trilinolein (2)	Sake lees	Yes (nc) TI 2 > 1 (1) IC_{50}=30 μM (2) IC_{50}=8.4 μM				[372]
aqueous extracts	green asparagus	Yes (m) IC_{50}= 1.21 mg/mL		radical scavenging, chelating activities and protected liposome against oxidative damage.		[373]
rsolic acid		Yes		Tyrosinase mRNA and protein	Yes	[374]

Table 1. (Continued)

Compounds (phenol, polyphenols, others)	Source	Mode of action	Refs.			Refs.
		TI	OEI (TRP-1, TRP-2)	other	MI	
San-bai-tang	San-bai-tang	Yes IC_{50}= 215.6 ± 10.3 μg/mL	TRP1, TRP2	MITF	Yes IC_{50}= 254.8 ± 14.5 μg/mL	[375]

TI: tyrosinase inhibiton, (c) competitive (u) uncompetitive (nc) noncompetitive and (m) mixed mode, OEI: other enzyme inhibition, MI: melanin inhibition, TRP-1: tyrosinase related protein-1, TRP-2: tyrosinase related protein-2, PKC: protein kinase C, MITF: microphthalmia-associated transcription factor.

The brownish guinea pig (GP) model is commonly used to study the effects of skin-whitening agents on reducing hyperpigmentation induced by UV or exposure to exogenous α-MSH (Table 1). In human studies, the activities of skin-whitening agents are normally investigated by evaluating skin color changes using a Chromameter or a Mexameter or by histochemical investigations of DOPA positive cells [163, 164]. Beginning in September 2009, the Commission of the European Communities established a prohibition to test finished cosmetic products and cosmetic ingredients on animals (European Commission - Consumer Affairs). Commercially available skin equivalent models (SEMs), a keratinocyte and melanocyte co-culture system [165], and MatTek's MelanoDerm™ (MatTek Corporation), a human three dimensional skin-like tissue structure, are useful *in vitro* models for evaluating the ability of cosmetic and pharmaceutical agents to modulate skin pigmentation. A common vertebrate model organism that is used for whitening studies is the zebrafish, which has been [165, 166] proved to be a useful model for demonstrating the *in vivo* toxicity of whitening agents.

Enhancing Tyrosinase Degradation

Fatty acids are ubiquitous components of cell membranes and serve as a biological energy source. They also play important roles in intracellular signaling and as precursors for ligands that bind to nuclear receptors[152, 167-169]. Fatty acids act as intrinsic factors that modulate the proteasomal degradation of membrane glycoproteins such as tyrosinase. In addition, they regulate the selective degradation of melanogenic enzymes through the ubiquitin-proteasome pathway[170]. Ando et al. found that fatty acids regulate the ubiquitination of tyrosinase and are responsible for modulating the proteasomal degradation of the enzyme[170] and that they had remarkable regulatory effects on melanogenesis in cultured B16F10 murine melanoma cells by modulating proteolytic degradation of tyrosinase[171]. Physiological doses of oleic acid and linoleic acid have been shown to increase the proteolytic activity of 20S proteasomes in rat skeletal muscle [172].

Interference with Melanosome Maturation and Transfer

Table 2 presents the natural products that have been shown to interfere with melanosome maturation and transfer.

Soybean Extract

Protease-activated receptors (PARs) are a subfamily of related G protein-coupled trans-membrane receptors that are proteolytically activated by serine proteases (including trypsin or mast cell tryptase). PAR-2 is expressed in keratinocytes but not in melanocytes.

Stimulation of this receptor enhances the rate of phagocytosis of keratinocytes, which in turn leads to increased melanin transfer[173]. Soybean contains small serine proteases, such as Bowman Birk inhibitor (BBI) and soybean trypsin inhibitor (STI, Kunitz-type trypsin inhibitor), that have been shown to inhibit the PAR-2 pathway in keratinocytes.

Interference with the PAR-2 pathway was shown to induce depigmentation by reducing the phagocytosis of melanosomes by keratinocytes, thereby diminishing melanin transfer [17, 174-176]. Interestingly, only unpasteurised soybean milk exhibits this activity.

Table 2. Whitening agents from natural sources interference with melanosome maturation and transfer

Source	Compounds	Mode of action			Refs.
		maturation	transfer	others	
Soybean extract	Bowman Birk inhibitor (BBI), soybean trypsin inhibitor (STI)		yes		[175]
Achillea millefolium, Yarrow	Centaureidin	Yes	Yes	Inhibition of melanogenesis and reduction the amount of tyrosinase.	[177, 179]
Ophiopogon japonicus	Methylophiopogonanone B	Yes	Yes		[179]
Root of vegetable and yeast	Niacinamide		Yes		[162, 180-182]
	Lectins and Neoglycoproteins		Yes		[162, 376, 377]

Centaureidin

Centaureidin (5,7,3'-trihydroxy-3,6,4'-trimethoxyflavone), a flavone from yarrow, has been shown to reduce melanosome transfer and melanocyte dentrite outgrowth[177]. Centaureidin either directly or indirectly activates Rho, a small GTP-binding protein that acts as a master regulator of dendrite formation. Ito et al. reported that activation of Rho in cells exposed to centaureidin resulted in dendrite retraction and reduced melanocyte trafficking of melanin to keratinocytes[178]. In addition, Saeki et al. found that centaureidin inhibited melanogenesis and reduced the total amount of tyrosinase, but not TRP-1[177].

Methylophiopogonanone B (5,7-Dihydroxy-6,8-Dimethyl-3-(4-Methoxybenzyl)Chroman-4-One, MOPB)

Studies have shown that MOPB-induced activation of Rho causes reversible dendrite retraction, microtubule disorganization, and tubule depolymerization, which in turn leads to reduced melanosome transfer. The effect MOPB has on melanogenesis, however, is not the same as the effect centaureidin has on melanin synthesis. Ito et al. showed that MOPB did not influence melanin synthesis or the expression of melanogenic enzymes[179].

Niacinamide

Niacinamide (nicotinamide; 3-pyridinecarboxamide), the amide form of vitamin B_3, is a biologically active form of niacin found in many root vegetables as well as in yeast. Studies have shown that niacinamide down regulates melanogenesis via inhibiting the transfer of melanosomes from melanocytes to keratinocytes[162, 180]. Other studies have reported that niacinamide is a tyrosinase inhibitor[181, 182].

Lectins and Neoglycoproteins

Cellular recognition between melanocytes and keratinocytes is an important process in melanosome transfer. Lectins and neoglycoproteins are glycosylated residues on melanocyte and keratinocyte membranes that play inhibitory roles in the process of receptor-mediated endocytosis, a process that facilitates melanosome transfer[63]. Specifically, plasma membrane lectins and their glycoconjugates are thought to interrupt melanocyte and keratinocyte contact and interaction by binding to their specific plasma membrane receptors, resulting in inhibition of melanosome transfer[183]. This inhibition is reversible and has been shown to be enhanced in the presence of niacinamide[162].

Inhibition of Inflammation-Induced Melanogenesis

Some mediators produced by keratinocytes after exposure to primary inflammatory stimuli or UV exposure, such as interleukin-1α (IL-1α), tumor necrosis factor α (TNF-α), ET-1, and Stem cell factor (SCF) are able to promote melanogenesis. ET-1 shows a unique behavior in exerting stimulatory effects both on DNA synthesis and melanization in human melanocytes[65, 184-186]. Activation of epidermal ETs is determined by the enzymatic cleavage of inactive prepolypeptides by an endopeptidase termed ET converting enzyme (ECE), which is regulated by the primary inflammatory cytokine IL-1α[187]. The SCF expressed in keratinocytes is involved in melanocyte growth and the synthesis, migration, and maintenance of melanin. UV exposure stimulates the overexpression of SCF, which binds to its receptor, c-kit, resulting in enhanced melanogenesis[188]. Arachidonate-derived chemical mediators, namely the cysteinyl leukotrienes (LTC) LTC4 and LTD4, and thromboxanes, such as TXB2, are released from membrane phospholipids by phospholipase A2 (PLA2). Leukotrienes not only significantly up-regulate tyrosinase, but also enhance the transfer of melanosomes to keratinocytes. These results suggest that PLA2 itself triggers melanin synthesis following UV irradiation or inflammation, thereby resulting in hyperpigmentation[52, 189]. Prostaglandins (PGs) synthesized from arachidonic acid by cyclooxygenase are responsible for regulating cellular growth, differentiation, and apoptosis. In the skin, PGs (especially PGE2, PGF2α) are produced and rapidly released by keratinocytes after exposure to UV irradiation, resulting in hyperpigmentation[190]. Therefore, anti-inflammatory compounds could be useful for the prevention or treatment of post-inflammatory hyperpigmentation.

Table 3 lists some natural products that have been shown to be effective treatments for inflammation-induced hyperpigmentation. Topical application of *Matricaria chamomilla* extract has been shown to inhibit UVB-induced pigmentation by supprerssing ET-1-induced DNA synthesis. The extract, however, did not affect IL-α-induced ET-1 production or tyrosinase activation[184].

Table 3. Whitening agents from natural sources inhibiting on inflammation-induced melanogenesis

Source	Compounds	Mode of action	Refs.
Matricaria chamomilla	*Matricaria chamomilla* extract	Antagonist for ET-receptor (*in vitro* and *in vivo*)	[184]
Sanguisorba officinalis L.		Suppression of endothelin-converting enzyme-1α (*in vitro* and *in vivo*)	[191]
Althaea officinalis L.	roots extract	Inhibits both the secretion and action of ET-1 (*in vitro*)	[192]
sea algae	fucoxanthin	Suppression of prostaglandin (PGE2) synthesis and melanoge stimulant receptors (neurotrophin, PGE2 and α-MSH). (*p.o.*)	[193]
Fenugreek seed (Trigonella foenum-graecum L.)	steroidal saponins	Inhibition of TNF-α and melanogenesis (*in vitro*)	[195]
Eucalyptus globulus	Globulusin A and eucaglobulin	Anti-inflammatory and anti-melanogenesis activity (*in vitro*) 改小寫	[194]
Azadirachta indica seed	nimolicinol	Inhibition of melanogenesis (*in vitro*) and TPA-induced inflammation (*in vivo*)	[378]
Guava (Psidium guajava L.)	leaves extract	Suppression of skin inflammation and melanogenesis (*p.o.*)	[196]
anti-melanogenesis may due to antioxidant activity			
glabridin	superoxide anion productions and cyclooxygenase activities	Inhibition of UVB-induced pigmentation and erythema (*in vivo*), inhibition of superoxide anion productions and cyclooxygenase activities (*in vitro*)	[379]
	luteolin	Inhibiting adenyl cyclase induced by MSH, anti-oxidant activity in DPPH, NBT/XO and intracellular ROS and xanthine oxidase (*in vitro*)	[281]
pine bark	Pycnogenol (catechin, epicatechin and epicatechin-4-(2-hydroxyethyl)thio ether)	Inhibition of tyrosinase and melanin biosynthesis, suppressing ·O2, NO·, ONOO−, and ·OH in (*in vitro*)	[380]
Ecklonia cava (brown alga)	Phlorotannins (dieckol)	Inhibition of tyrosinase activity and reduction of intracellular ROS induced by UV-B radiation (*in vitro*)	[381]
Ishige okamurae (marine algae)	diphlorethohydroxy carmalol	Inhibition of tyrosinase activity and reduction of intracellular ROS induced by UV-B radiation (*in vitro*)	[382]
ginger	[6]-Gingerol	Decreasing ROS level and suppressing TYR activity (*in vitro*)	[383]

Hachiya et al. reported that a 50% ethanol extract of *Sanguisorba officinalis* root inhibited UVB-induced pigmentation of brownish guinea pig skin. The results of their study suggest that the mechanism governing the inhibition of ET-1 production in human keratinocytes is via the suppression of endothelin-converting enzyme-1α[191]. Kobayashi et al. reported that a 45% 1,3-butylene glycol extract of *Althaea officinalis* roots inhibited both the secretion of ET-1 from normal human keratinocytes (NHKC) and the action of ET-1 on NHMC, mainly by suppressing ET-1-induced calcium mobilization. They found that binding of ET-1 to the endothelin B receptor (ETBR) on the cell surface of NHMC induced the mobilization of intracellular calcium [192]. Fucoxanthin, a carotenoid derived from edible sea algae, exhibited anti-pigmentary activity when applied either topically or orally in an animal model of UVB-induced melanogenesis. This effect of fucoxanthin may be due to suppression of PGE2 synthesis and melanogenic stimulant receptors (neurotrophin, PGE2 and MC1R) [193, 194].

Globulusin A and eucaglobulin, monoterpene glycosides isolated from *Eucalyptus globules,* not only have DPPH free radical scavenging activity, thereby inhibiting phorbol myristate acetate-induced expression of tumor-necrosis factor-α and interleukin-1β, but also inhibit melanogenesis *in vitro*.[194] In addition, a methanolic extract and its steroidal saponins, 26-*O*-*β*-*D*-glucopyranosyl-(25*R*)-furost-5(6)-en-3*β*,22*β*,26-triol-3-*O*-*α*-*L*-rhamnopyranosyl-(1″→ 2′)-*O*-[*β*-*D*-glucopyranosyl-(1‴ → 6′)-*O*]-*β*-*D*-glucopyranoside, minutoside B, and pseudoprotodioscin isolated from Fenugreek seed (*Trigonella foenum-graecum* L. Fabaceae) inhibited the production of phorbol-12-myristate-13-acetate-induced inflammatory cytokines, namely TNF-*α* and melanogenesis *in vitro*[195]. Guava leaf extracts have been shown to suppress UVB-induced skin inflammation. Takashi et al. found that the skin color of guinea pigs that had been exposed to UVB irradiation followed by treatment with guava extract (p.o.) became lighter as a result of the tyrosinase inhibitory activity of guava leaf extract[196]. Nimolicinol, a limonoid isolated from *Azadirachta indica* seeds, shows inhibitory effects both on melanogenesis in B16 melanoma cells and on 12-*O*-tetradecanoylphorbol-13-acetate (TPA)-induced inflammation in mice.

Many studies have found that compounds with potent free radical scavenging activities inhibit tyrosinase expression. Some of the most potent compounds with free radical scavenging ability and tyrosinase inhibiting activity include glabridin, diarylheptanoids and phenolic compounds from *Acer nikoense*; luteolin and pycnogenol from pine bark; phlorotannins from *Ecklonia cava*; diphlorethohydroxycarmalol from *Ishige okamurae*; and [6]-gingerol from ginger (Table 3).

Accelerating Skin Desquamation

Desmosomes, which are classified as a molecular complex of cell adhesion proteins consisting of desmoglein and desmocollin, are mainly responsible for the adhesion between epidermal cells. As the cells move upward from the basal layers to the stratum corneum, the desmosome attachments become weaker. This weakening action is accelerated by enzymes, namely the stratum corneum chemotrypic enzyme (SCCE) and Cathepsin D, by breaking the bonds of the desmosomes, resulting in the sloughing off of cells. Keratinization refers to the turnover of the stratum corneum and begins at the basal layer and gradually moves upward to the stratum corneum corneocytes. This desquamation process normally takes about four weeks and is normally more efficient in younger skin. The process stimulates the growth of newer cells at a deeper level; however, in skin of advanced age, the intercellular desmosomes become glue-like in their ability to cement cells together. As a result, cell sloughing becomes more difficult, which leads to a thicker skin with a dull appearance. The stratum corneum has a pH of 7 at the bottom layer and a pH ranging from 4.5-5.4 at the surface[(197)]. The optimal pH for SCCE and Cathepsin D activity in the final desquamation stage *ranges from 4 to 6,* which explains why those enzymes are most active at the surface of the stratum corneum[198-200].

The capability of a compound to accelerate the turnover of epidermal layers and/or disperse melanin pigment can result in skin lightening. Depigmenting agents lighten the skin by stimulating the removal of pigmented keratinocytes[155, 201]. Pigmented spots, such as freckles or actinic lentigines, melasma spots, and post-inflammatory hypermelanosis macules may be removed by the peeling of corneocytes and epidermal keratinocytes.

Chemical Exfoliants and Their Mode of Action

(1) α-Hydroxyacids

α-Hydroxyacids (AHA, i.e. lactic acid, glycolic acid, and malic acid) are weak organic acids found in fruits, plants, and milk[202]. Studies on cell cohesion and skin pH changes indicate that keratin bonds may became weaker at low pH values. AHA solution is activated under low pH conditions and may dissolve the desmosome protein linkages causing a burst in skin exfoliation. AHAs have also been used to successfully treat pigmentary lesions such as solar lentigenes, lesions caused by melasma, and post-inflammatory hyperpigmentation macules. AHAs promote exfoliation by decreasing corneocyte cohesion and by stimulating dermal cell growth in the basal layer at low concentrations, while at higher concentrations AHAs promote epidermolysis and dispersal of basal layer melanin. The accelerated desquamation of the stratum corneum by AHAs is complemented by a direct inhibition of tyrosinase, without influencing mRNA or protein expression[201-203]. Lactic acid can be isolated from sour milk[201]. Glycolic acid can be isolated from natural sources, such as sugarcane, sugar beets, pineapple, cantaloupe, and unripe grapes. Both glycolic acid and lactic acid affect the skin layers in the same manner as described above. Furthermore, additional beneficial effects unique to lactic acid include an increase in dermal glycosaminoglycans (GAGs-natural moisturizers) and ceramides (epidermal barrier lipids), and improved water barrier properties. Glycolic acid stimulates collagen synthesis in a manner similar to that of lactic acid[204]. Yamamoto et al. studied the histological differences between patients who received a six-week treatment of topical AHA, glycolic acid, lactic acid, or citric acid as treatment for photo-aged skin and found that patients who had received AHA showed increased epidermal thickness, decreased melanin deposition, and up-regulated collegen levels relative to patients who received topical glycolic acid, lactic acid, or citric acid[205]. In addition, the authors found that AHA treatment not only decreased melanin deposition, but also resulted in the remodeling of the epidermis and the acceleration of desquamation[205]. The Cosmetic Ingredient Review, a panel endorsed by the Esthetics Manufacturers and Distributors Alliance of the American Beauty Association suggests that consumers should not use glycolic acid or lactic acid products with concentrations exceeding 10% or at a pH of 3.5; for professional use, the limits are extended to 30% and the lowest advisable pH value is 3.0.

(2) β-hydroxyacids (BHAs)

Salicylic acid (SA) is a β-hydroxyacid (BHA) found in willow bark and sweet birch. It is also a phytohormone that acts similar to hormones that regulate cell growth and differentiation. SA functions as a desquamating agent by penetrating and dissolving the intercellular matrix of the stratum corneum[114, 202]. Unlike lactic acid, salicylic acid does not hydrate the skin and does not help to normalize epidermal anatomy or physiology. Salicylic acid, which is primarily a keratolytic agent, dissolves the stratum corneum layer by layer from the outside in, resulting in a thinning of the stratum corneum. The effect of salicylic acid on hyperpigmentation inhibition has been demonstrated in a number of studies, but only at very high concentrations (50%). SA is more lipophilic than AHAs, enabling it to penetrate sebaceous substances in the hair follicles and exfoliate the pores. The water solubility of AHAs is lower than that of SA. Since SA has a much stronger comedolytic effect than AHAs, it can be used in acne therapy.

(3) Retinol

Retinol (Vitamin A) is a potent skin exfoliant and antiaging agent. Retinol has been shown to improve the visible signs of photoaging as well as normal chronological aging when used on a daily basis. Studies have shown that retinol slows down collagen degradation in skin that has been chronically exposed to sunlight. In addition, retinol has been demonstrated to inhibit enzymes that are responsible for the degradation of collagen, such as collagenase[206].

(4) Liquiritin

Liquiritin, a flavonoid glycoside derived from liquorice, significantly reduces hyperpigmentation in patients with bilateral and symmetrical idiopathic epidermal melasma[207]. Zhu et al. found that a 20% liquiritin cream was effective at inducing skin lightening by dispersing melanin in a clinical trial involving patients with melasma [208]. The proposed mechanisms involve melanin dispersion by means of the pyran ring of its flavonoidal nucleus and acceleration of epidermal renewal.

Whitening Agents Verified by Clinical Trials

Whitening agents derived from natural products that have been tested in clinical trials are listed in Table 4 and described below:

Arbutin and its Derivatives

The compound 4-hydroxyanisole has been shown to act as an alternative substrate for tyrosinase both *in vivo* and *in vitro*[209]. However, 4-hydroxyanisole and other phenolic compounds have the potential to generate toxic quinone products and have, therefore, been used in various studies to evaluate the toxic effects mediated by tyrosinase in melanoma cells[210, 211].

Hydroquinone (HQ) was widely used as an effective skin-whitening agent before it was banned by the US Food and Drug Administration in 2006 because animal studies in South Africa, the United Kingdom, and the USA revealed that HQ was a potential carcinogen and was associated with an increased incidence of ochronosis._HQ is defined as a drug since its cancer-causing properties have not yet been proved in humans. Other phenolic compounds that have been used to evaluate the toxic effects mediated by tyrosinase include arbutin, kojic acid and ascorbic acid derivatives (Table 4).

Table 4. The effect of whitening agents have been verified by clinical trials

Compounds	Indication of clinical trials	Refs.
3% Arbutin	Treating hyperpigmentary disorders, such as melasma	[212]
3% Deoxyarbutin	Acceleration of the fading of UV-induced tan	[384]
1% Kojic acid	Treating hyperpigmentary disorders, such as melasma, post-inflammatory hyperpigmentation, age spots, and freckles	[216]
10% Magnesium L-ascorbic acid 2-phosphate	Effective for reducing melasma and age spots	[220]
SLM (skin lightening moisturizer containing 3% magnesium ascorbyl phosphate	Reduction of hyperpigmented spots on the face	[385]
0.3% Rucinol	Treating hyperpigmentary disorders, such as melasma	[222]
0.5% Ellagic acid	Effective for treating UVB-induced hyperpigmentation of the skin	[224]
Ellagic Acid (200 mg, 100 mg/oral administration)	Inhibitory effect on a slight pigmentation in the human skin caused by UV irradiation	[386]
Ellagic acid	Melasma	[387]
0.5% Chamomilla extract	Effective for treating UVB-induced hyperpigmentation of the skin	[225, 226]
0.5% 5,5'-Dipropyl-biphenyl-2,2'-diol	Effective for treating UVB-induced hyperpigmentation of the skin	[228]
0.5% 5,5'-Dipropyl-biphenyl-2,2'-diol	Effective in treating hyperpigmentary disorders, such as melasma and senile lentigo	[229]
2 % Rhododendrol	Effective for treating UVB-induced hyperpigmentation of the skin	[153]
20% Azelaic acid	Melasma	[115]
Tranexamic acid	Treating melasma	[388]
3% adenosine Monophosphate Disodium Salt	Effective for treating hyperpigmentary disorders, such as melasma	[239]
4% N-acetyl-4-S-cysteaminylphenol (4-S-CAP)	Melasma	[240]
0.1% Linoleic acid	Effective for treating melasma and to lighten UVB-induced hyperpigmentation of the skin	[241-243]
5 % Glycolic acid	Whitening	[244]
10% Glycolic acid	Melasma	[245]
Lactic acid, full strength (92%; pH 3.5),	Peeling agent in the treatment of melasma	[246]
8% Glycolic acid and 8% lactic acid	Hypopigmentation	[247]
30% Salicylic acid peels	Skin whitening	[248]

Arbutin is a glycosylated form of HQ that is present in bearberry extracts but it can also be synthesized from HQ by glucosidation. Its principal modes of action are competitive inhibition of tyrosinase and TRP-1 activity, inhibition of UV-induced formation and elongation of melanocyte dendritic processes and inhibition of production of $\cdot O_2^-$ and $\cdot OH$. It has been shown that a 3% arbutin-containing formulation is effective for treating hyperpigmentary disorders, such as melasma[212]. A combination therapy comprising a YAG laser and 7% α-arbutin solution has been shown to be an effective and well-tolerated treatment for refractory melasma [213]. Deoxyarbutin inhibits tyrosine hydroxylase and DOPA oxidase activities of tyrosinase. In vitro studies have demonstrated that the inhibition constant (Ki) of mushroom-derived tyrosinase is 350-fold lower than the Ki of arbutin. In a human clinical trial, topical treatment with Deoxyarbutin for 12 weeks resulted in a significant reduction in overall skin lightness in a population of light-skinned individuals and a slight reduction in overall skin lightness and improvement in solar lentigines in a population of darkskinned individuals[214, 215].

Kojic Acid

Kojic acid is a γ-pyrone compound produced during the fermentation of aspergillus species, penicillium species and filiform bacteria. Kojic acid exerts a slow-binding inhibition of tyrosinase activity, mainly by chelating copper, and inhibits the polymerization of DHI and DHICA. In a clinical trial, Mishima et al. showed that a 1% kojic acid-containing formulation was effective at treating melasma, post-inflammatory hyperpigmentation, age spots and freckles[216]. In 2003, however, the Japanese Ministry of Health, Labor and Welfare notified suppliers of kojic acid to delay manufacture or import of the product because of concerns about possible carcinogenic effects in animals [217]. However, in 2005, kojic acid was deemed to be a safe cosmetic ingredient and continues to be used as a skin-lightening quasi-drug [218].

Ascorbic Acid and its Derivatives

Ascorbic acid is highly unstable when exposed to heat or highly acidic conditions; derivatives of ascorbic acid, however, are much more stable. Some of the more commonly administered ascorbic acid derivatives include magnesium ascorbyl phosphate, ascorbyl glucoside, sodium ascorbyl phosphate and 3-O-ethyl ascorbic acid. Ascorbic acid is a potent reducer of DOPA quinone and melanin.

It has been reported that ascorbyl glucoside releases ascorbic acid gradually through hydrolysis due to the action of α-glucosidase in living organisms[219].

In a clinical trial, Kameyama et al. found that a 10% magnesium ascorbyl phosphate-containing formulation was shown to be effective at reducing the number of melasma patches and age spots[220]. In another clinical trial, Miyai et al. found that a 2% ascorbyl glucoside-containing cream was effective at accelerating the disappearance of UVB-induced hyperpigmentation[221].

Rucinol

Rucinol (4-n-butylresorcinol) has been reported to be an inhibitor of tyrosinase and TRP1 activity. Katagiri et al. found that a 0.3% Rucinol®-containing lotion was effective at alleviating UV-induced pigmentation and melasma patches[222].

Potassium Methoxysalicylate

Hideya et al. found that potassium methoxysalicylate inhibits melanin synthesis via a mechanism involving competitive inhibition of tyrosinase activity.

This mechanism is similar to the mechanisms governing the modes of action of arbutin and Rucinol[153].

Ellagic Acid

Ellagic acid, a polyphenolic compound, is found in strawberries, apples and a variety of plants.

Shimogaki et al. demonstrated that ellagic acid is a potent antioxidant and that it inhibits tyrosinase activity through copper chelation[223]. Kamide et al. showed that application of 0.5% ellagic acid-containing cream was effective for treating UVB-induced hyperpigmentation and melasma patches[224].

Chamomilla Extract

Chamomilla extract is a crude plant extract.

It inhibits melanin synthesis by binding to endothelin receptors and by inducing the synthesis of inositol triphosphate. Ichihashi et al. demonstrated that a 0.5% chamomilla extract-containing cream was effective at treating UVB-induced hyperpigmentation in humans[225, 226].

5,5′-Dipropyl-Biphenyl-2,2′-Diol (Magnolignan®)

5,5'-Dipropyl-biphenyl-2,2'-diol is a biphenyl compound isolated from *Magnolia heptapeta.*

It has been shown to inhibit melanin synthesis by interfering with the process of tyrosinase maturation[227]. Takeda et al. found that a 0.5% Magnolignan®-containing formulation was effective at treating melasma, senile lentigo and UVB-induced hyperpigmentation in humans[228, 229].

Rhododendrol (4-(4-Hydroxyphenyl)-2-Butanol)

Rhododendrol is a phenolic compound derived from White Birch and Nikko Maple. Rhododendrol inhibits melanin synthesis through competitive inhibition of tyrosinase activity.

In 2010, Kanebo Cosmetics Inc. obtained approval from the Japanese Ministry of Health, Labor and Welfare to use Rhododendrol as a whitening agent[153].

Azelaic Acid

Azelaic acid is a naturally occurring saturated nine-carbon dicarboxylic acid. Its use originated from the finding that Pityrosporum species can oxidize unsaturated fatty acids to dicarboxylic acids, which competitively inhibit tyrosinase. Azelaic acid was initially developed as a topical drug for the treatment of acne. However, because of its effect on tyrosinase, it has also been used to treat melasma, lentigo maligna and other hyperpigmention disorders[230, 231]. In addition, azelaic acid has been shown to be effective at treating postinflammatory hyperpigmentation due to acne by inhibiting the production of free radicals[232, 233]. In the USA, 20% azelaic acid is only indicated for treatment of acne, although it has off-label use for hyperpigmentation. However, studies have found that 20% azelaic acid is equivalent to or better than 2% hydroquinone for the treatment of melasma[233, 234].

Tranexamic Acid and Tranexamic Acid Cetyl Ester Hydrochloride

Plasmin, a protease found in blood serum, not only enhances the intracellular release of arachidonic acid, a precursor of prostaglandins(235), but also elevates the levels of α-MSH[236]. Tranexamic acid has been shown to inhibit UV-induced plasmin activity in keratinocytes by preventing the binding of plasminogen to keratinocytes, which ultimately results in less free arachidonic acid and a diminished ability to produce PGs, thereby decreasing the activity of tyrosinase in melanocytes[189, 237]. Both arachidonic acid and α-MSH can activate melanin synthesis in melanocytes. Therefore, the anti-plasmin activity of tranexamic acid is thought to play a role in its topical effectiveness at treating melasma. The effect of tranexamic acid cetyl ester hydrochloride in treating hyperpigmentary disorders is due to its ability to inhibit UVB-induced inflammation, leading to the quiescence of active melanocytes. This mechanism is similar to the mechanisms of action of chamomilla extract and tranexamic acid.

Adenosine Monophosphate Disodium Salt

Adenosine is the building block of adenosine 5'-triphosphate (ATP), the main intracellular source of energy. Since energy is essential for cell proliferation and maturation, supporting ATP levels with topical adenosine safely accelerates epidermal turnover[238]. Adenosine monophosphate has the potency to increase the amount of intracellular glucose uptake, which is necessary for the biosynthesis of adenosine triphosphate. Therefore, adenosine monophosphate disodium salt accelerates epidermal turnover by elevating intracellular energy metabolism, which leads to the excretion of melanin from the skin. A clinical trial found that topical administration of a 3% adenosine monophosphate disodium salt-containing formulation was effective at treating hyperpigmentary disorders, such as melasma[239].

N-Acetyl-4-S-Cysteaminylphenol

N-acetyl-4-S-cysteaminylphenol is a tyrosinase substrate, and, on exposure to tyrosinase, it forms a melanin-like pigment. The depigmentation effect of *N*-acetyl-4-S-cysteaminylphenol is associated with a decrease in the number of functioning melanocytes and in the number of melanosomes transferred to keratinocytes. A 4% N-acetyl-4-S-cysteaminylphenol emulsion (O/W) was shown to be effective for treating melasma[240].

Linoleic Acid

Linoleic acid accelerates tyrosinase degradation, resulting in the down-regulation of melanin synthesis. In clinical trials, topical application of a 0.1% linoleic acid-containing liposomal formulation alleviated melasma symptoms[241] and UVB-induced hyperpigmentation of the skin[242, 243].

AHAs and BHAs

Many clinical studies on the effectiveness of AHAs such as glycolic acid and lactic acid as peeling agents for accelerating skin desquamation have been conducted in patients with pigmentation disorders. For example, a 5% glycolic acid topical cream was shown to improve skin texture and photoaging-induced discoloration[244]. In addition, a 10% glycolic acid lotion has been reported to be effective at improving symptoms of melasma [245]. Furthermore, a 92% lactic acid (pH 3.5) formulation has been shown to be effective at treating melasma[246]. A combination of 8% glycolic acid and 8% lactic acid creams has been shown to be modestly useful in ameliorating mottled hyperpigmentation, sallowness, and roughness due to chronic cutaneous photodamage[247].A clinical trial showed that 30% salicylic acid in absolute ethanol was effective at treating acne and postinflammatory hyperpigmentation[248].

Conclusion

In this article we have reviewed the synthesis of melanin, the signaling pathways related to the regulation of melanogenesis, the factors influencing melanogenesis and various pigmentation disorders, as well as the effectiveness of various natural products at reducing hyperpigmentation. An important issue regarding crude extracts or fractions from natural products used in cosmetics is the standardization of cultivation, harvesting, collecting, storage and extraction processes of the plants. Isolation of the active components from natural products for skin-whitening formulations will clarify the effect and mechanism on hypopigmentation. In addition, multi-functional formulations may increase the efficacy of skin-whitening products.

References

[1] Spritz, R. A. & Hearing, V. J. Jr. (1994). Genetic disorders of pigmentation. *Advances in human genetics, 22,* 1-45.

[2] Prota, G. (1992). *Melanins and Melanogenesis*. New York, Academic.

[3] Bennett, D. C. & Lamoreux, M. L. (2003). The color loci of mice--a genetic century. *Pigment Cell Melanoma Res., 16,* 333-344.

[4] Yamaguchi, Y. & Hearing, V, J. (2009). Physiological factors that regulate skin pigmentation. *Biofactors, 35,* 193-199.

[5] Frenk, E. (1995) Treatment of melasma with depigmenting agents. *In: Melasma: New Approaches to Treatment (London, Martin Dunitz)*, 9-15.

[6] Hamilton, A. J. & Gomez, B. L. (2002). Melanins in fungal pathogens. *J. Med. Microbiol., 53,* 189-191.

[7] Honigsmann, H. (2002). Erythema and pigmentation. *Photodermatol. Photoimmunol. Photomed., 18*, 75-81.

[8] Garcia-Borron, J. C. (2008). SOX9 and the tanning response: something new under the sun. *Pigment Cell Melanoma Res., 21,* 3-4.

[9] Howe, H. L., Chen, V. W., Hotes, J. L., Wu, X. C., Correa, N. C. & Fulton, J. P. (2001). Cancer in North America, 1994-1998. *North American Association of Central Cancer Registries, 1: Incidence.*

[10] Perluigi, M., De Marco, F., Foppoli, C., Coccia, R., Blarzino, C., Marcante, M. L. & Cini, C. (2003). Tyrosinase protects human melanocytes from ROS-generating compounds. *Biochem. Biophys. Res. Commun., 305,* 250-256.

[11] Herrling, T., Jung, K & Fuchs, J. (2008). The role of melanin as protector against free radicals in skin and its role as free radical indicator in hair. *Spectroc. Acta Pt. A-Molec. Biomolec. Spectr., 69,* 1429-1435.

[12] Ortonne, J. P. (2002). Photoprotective properties of skin melanin. *Br. J. Dermatol., 61,* 7-10.

[13] Hearing, V. J. Jr. (1987). Mammalian monophenol monooxygenase (tyrosinase): purification, properties, and reactions catalyzed. *Methods Enzymol, 142*, 154-165.

[14] Raposo, G. & Marks, M. S. (2007). Melanosomes--dark organelles enlighten endosomal membrane transport. *Nat. Rev. Mol. Cell Biol., 8,* 786-797.

[15] Jiménez-Cervantes, C., Solano, F., Kobayashi, T., Urabe, K., Hearing, V. J., Lozano, J. A. & García-Borrón, J. C. (1994). A new enzymatic function in the melanogenic pathway. The 5,6-dihydroxyindole-2-carboxylic acid oxidase activity of tyrosinase-related protein-1 (TRP1). *J. Biol. Chem., 269,* 17993-18000.

[16] Kondo, T., Hearing, V. J. (2011). Update on the regulation of mammalian melanocyte function and skin pigmentation. *Expert. Rev. Dermat., 6,* 97-108.

[17] Seiberg, M., Paine, C., Sharlow, E., Andrade-Gordon, P., Costanzo, M., Eisinger, M. & Shapiro, S. S. (2000). Inhibition of melanosome transfer results in skin lightening. *J. Dermatol., 115,* 162-167.

[18] Seiberg, M. (2001). Keratinocyte-melanocyte interactions during melanosome transfer. *Pigment Cell Melanoma Res.,14,* 236-242.

[19] Scott, G., Leopardi, S., Parker, L., Babiarz, L., Seiberg, M. & Han, R. (2003). The proteinase-activated receptor-2 mediates phagocytosis in a Rho-dependent manner in human keratinocytes. *J. Invest. Dermatol., 121,* 529-541.

[20] Boissy, R. E. (2003). Melanosome transfer to and translocation in the keratinocyte. *Exp. Dermatol., 12,* 5-12.

[21] Nordlund, J. J., Boissy, R. E., Hearing, V. J., King, R. A., Oetting, W. S. & Ortonne, J. P. (2006). Chemistry of Melanins. *The Pigmentary System. Physiology and Pathophysiology (2nd Edition).* 282-310.

[22] Turner, W. A., Taylor, J. D. & Tchen, T. T. (1975). Melanosome formation in the goldfish: the role of multivesicular bodies. *J. Ultrastruct Res., 51,* 16-31.

[23] Boissy, R. H., Gahl, W., Nordlund, J. J., Boissy, R. E., Hearing, V. J., King, R. A., Oetting, W. S., Ortonne, J. P. (2006). Biogenesis of melanosomes., *In The Pigmentary System: Physiology and Pathophysiology, 2nd ed.* 155-170.

[24] Ozeki, H., Ito, S., Wakamatsu, K. & Hirobe, T. (1995). Chemical characterization of hair melanins in various coat-color mutants of mice. *J. Invest. Dermatol., 105,* 361-366.

[25] Lamoreux, M. L., Wakamatsu, K. & Ito, S. (2001). Interaction of major coat color gene functions in mice as studied by chemical analysis of eumelanin and pheomelanin. *Pigment Cell Melanoma Res., 14,* 23-31.

[26] Berson, J. F., Harper, D. C., Tenza, D., Raposo, G. & Marks, M. S. (2001). Pmel17 initiates premelanosome morphogenesis within multivesicular bodies. *Mol. Biol. Cell., 12,* 3451-3464.

[27] Kushimoto, T., Basrur, V., Valencia, J., Matsunaga, J., Vieira, W. D., Ferrans, V. J., Muller, J., Appella, E. & Hearing, V. J. (2001). A model for melanosome biogenesis based on the purification and analysis of early melanosomes. *Proc. Natl. Acad. Sci. U. S. A, 98,* 10698-10703.

[28] Watabe, H., Valencia, J. C., Pape, E. L., Yamaguchi, Y., Nakamura, M., Rouzaud, F., Hoashi, T., Kawa, Y., Mizoguchi, M. & Hearing, V. J. (2008). Involvement of dynein and spectrin with early melanosome transport and melanosomal protein trafficking. *J. Invest. Dermatol., 128,* 162-174.

[29] Vallee, R. B., Wall, J. S., Paschal, B. M. & Shpetner, H. S. . (1988). Microtubule-associated protein 1C from brain is a two-headed cytosolic dynein. *Nature, 32,* 561-563.

[30] Schnapp, B. J. & Reese, T. S. (1989). Dynein is the motor for retrograde axonal transport of organelles. *Proc. Natl. Acad. Sci. USA, 86,* 1548-1552.

[31] Byers, H. R., Yaar, M. Y., Eller, M. S., Jalbert, N. L. & Gilchrest, B. A., (2000). Role of cytoplasmic dynein in melanosome transport in human melanocytes. *J. Invest. Dermatol., 114,* 990-997.

[32] Hara, M., Yaar, M., Byers, H. R., Goukassian, D., Fine, R. E., Gonsalves, J. & Gilchrest, B. A. (2000). Kinesin participates in melanosomal movement along melanocyte dendrites. *J. Invest. Dermatol., 114,* 438-443.

[33] Vancoillie, G., Lambert, J., Haeghen, Y. V., Westbroek, W., Mulder, A., Koerten, H. K., Mommaas, A. M., Van, Oostveldt. P. & Naeyaert, J. M. (2000). Colocalization of dynactin subunits P150Glued and P50 with melanosomes in normal human melanocytes. *Pigment Cell Res., 13,* 449-457.

[34] Wu, M., Hemesath, T. J., Takemoto, C. M., Horstmann, M. A., Wells, A. G., Price, E. R., Fisher, D. Z. & Fisher, D. E. (2000). c-Kit triggers dual phosphorylations, which

couple activation and degradation of the essential melanocyte factor Mi. *Genes. Dev., 14,* 301-312.

[35] Watabe, H., Valencia., Le Pape, E., Yamaguchi, Y., Nakamura, M., Rouzaud, F., Hoashi, T., Kawa, Y., Mizoguchi, M. & Hearing, V. J. (2007). Involvement of dynein and spectrin with early melanosome transport and melanosomal protein trafficking. *J. Invest. Dermatol., 128,* 162-174.

[36] Seiberg, M., Paine, C., Sharlow, E., Andrade-Gordon, P., Costanzo, M., Eisinger, M. & Shapiro, S. S. (2000). Inhibition of melanosome transfer results in skin lightening. *J. Invest. Dermatol., 115,* 162-167.

[37] Van Den Bossche, K., Naeyaert, J. M. & Lambert, J. (2006). The quest for the mechanism of melanin transfer. *Traffic, 7,* 769-778.

[38] Marks, M. S. & Seabra, M. C. (2001). The melanosome: membrane dynamics in black and white. *Nat. Rev. Mol. Cell. Biol., 2,* 738-748.

[39] Virador, V. M., Muller, J., Wu, X., Abdel-Malek, Z. A., Yu, Z. X., Ferrans, V. J., Kobayashi, N., Wakamatsu, K., Ito, S., Hammer, J. A. & Hearing, V. J. (2002). Influence of alpha-melanocyte stimulating hormone and ultraviolet radiation on the transfer of melanosomes to keratinocytes. *FASEB. J., 16,* 105-107.

[40] Singh, S. K., Nizard, C., Kurfurst, R., Bonte, F., Schnebert, S. & Tobin, D. J. (2008). The silver locus product (Silv/gp100/Pmel17) as a new tool for the analysis of melanosome transfer in human melanocyte-keratinocyte co-culture. *Exp. Dermatol., 17,* 418-426.

[41] Scott, G., Leopardi, S., Printup, S. & Madden, B. C. (2002). Filopodia are conduits for melanosome transfer to keratinocytes. *J. Cell Sci., 115,* 1441-1451.

[42] Zhang, R. Z., Zhu, W. Y., Xia, M. Y. & Feng, Y. (2004). Morphology of cultured human epidermal melanocytes observed by atomic force microscopy. *Pigment Cell Res., 17,* 62-65.

[43] Singh, S. K., Kurfurst, R., Nizard, C., Schnebert, S., Perrier, E & Tobin, D. J. (2010). Melanin transfer in human skin cells is mediated by filopodia--a model for homotypic and heterotypic lysosome-related organelle transfer. *FASEB. J., 24,* 3756-3769.

[44] Kuroda, T. S. & Fukuda, M. (2004). Rab27A-binding protein Slp2-a is required for peripheral melanosome distribution and elongated cell shape in melanocytes. *Nat. Cell Biol., 6,* 1195-1203.

[45] Ito, S., Wakamatsu, K., & Ozeki, H. (2000). Chemical analysis of melanins and its application to the study of the regulation of melanogenesis. *Pigment Cell Res., 13 Suppl. 8,* 103-109.

[46] Zecca, L., Shima, T., Stroppolo, A., Goj, C., Battiston, G. A., Gerbasi, R., Sarna, T. & Swartz, H. M. (1996). Interaction of neuromelanin and iron in substantia nigra and other areas of human brain. *Neuroscience, 73,* 407-415.

[47] Grossman, M. (1999). Sentence processing in Parkinson's disease. *Brain Cogn., 40,* 387-413.

[48] Raper, H. S. (1928). The anaerobic oxidases. *Physiol. Rev., 8,* 245-282.

[49] Mason, H. S. (1948). The chemistry of melanin. III. Mechanism of the oxidation of trihydroxyphenylalanine by tyrosinase. *J. Biol. Chem., 172,* 83-99.

[50] Lerner, A. B., Fitzpatrick, T. B., Calkins, E. & Summerson, W. H. (1949). Mammalian tyrosinase-preparation and properties. *J. Biol. Chem., 178,* 185-190.

[51] Lin, J. Y., Fisher, D. E. (2007). Melanocyte biology and skin pigmentation. *Nature, 445,* 843-850.

[52] Costin, G. E., Hearing, V. J. (2007). Human skin pigmentation: melanocytes modulate skin color in response to stress. *FASEB. J., 21*, 976-994.

[53] Hearing, V. J. & Tsukamoto, K. (1991). Enzymatic control of pigmentation in mammals. *FASEB. J., 5,* 2902-2909.

[54] Cooksey, C. J., Garratt, P. J., Land, E. J., Pavel, S., Ramsden, C. A., Riley, P. A. & Smit, N. P. (1997). Evidence of the indirect formation of the catecholic intermediate substrate responsible for the autoactivation kinetics of tyrosinase. *J. Biol. Chem., 272,* 26226-26235.

[55] Halaban, R., Patton, R. S., Cheng, E., Svedine, S., Trombetta, E. S., Wahl, M. L., Ariyan, S. & Hebert, D. N. (2002). Abnormal acidification of melanoma cells induces tyrosinase retention in the early secretory pathway. *J. Biol. Chem., 277,* 14821-14828.

[56] Halaban, R., Cheng, E., Svedine, S., Aron, R. & Hebert, D. N. (2001). Proper folding and endoplasmic reticulum to golgi transport of tyrosinase are induced by its substrates, DOPA and tyrosinase. *Biol. Chem., 276,* 11933-11938.

[57] Chang, T. S. (2009). An updated review of tyrosinase inhibitors. *Int. J. Mol. Sci., 10,* 2440-2475.

[58] Lin, J. W., Chiang, H. M., Lin, Y. C. & Wen, K. C. (2008). Natural Products with Skin-Whitening Effects. *J. Food Drug Anal., 16,* 1-10.

[59] Chiang, H. M., Ko. Y. L., Shih, I. C. & Wen, K. C. (2011). Development of wine cake as a skin-whitening agent and humectant. *J. Food Drug Anal., 19,* 223-229.

[60] Ando, H., Itoh, A., Mishima, Y. & Ichihashi, M. (1995). Correlation between the number of melanosomes, tyrosinase mRNA levels, and tyrosinase activity in cultured murine melanoma cells in response to various melanogenesis regulatory agents. *J. Cell Physiol., 163,* 608-614.

[61] Oetting, W. S. (2000). The tyrosinase gene and oculocutaneous albinism type 1 (OCA1): a model for understanding the molecular biology of melanin formation. *Pigment Cell Res., 13*, 320-325.

[62] Costin, G. E., Valencia., Wakamatsu, K., Ito, S., Solano, F., Milac, A. L., Vieira, W. D., Yamaguchi, Y., Rouzaud, F., Petrescu, A. J., Lamoreux, M. L. & Hearing, V. J. (2005). Mutations in dopachrome tautomerase (Dct) affect eumelanin/pheomelanin synthesis, but do not affect intracellular trafficking of the mutant protein. *Biochem. J., 391,* 249-259.

[63] Minwalla, L., Zhao, Y., Cornelius, J., Babcock, G. F., Wickett, R. R., Le Poole, I. C. & Boissy, R. E. (2001). Inhibition of melanosome transfer from melanocytes to keratinocytes by lectins and neoglycoproteins in an in vitro model system. *Pigment. Cell Res., 14,* 185-194.

[64] Chakraborty, A. K., Funasaka, Y., Slominski, A., Ermak, G., Hwang, J., Pawelek, J. M. & Ichihashi, M. (1996). Production and release of proopiomelanocortin (POMC) derived peptides by human melanocytes and keratinocytes in culture: regulation by ultraviolet B., *Biochim. Biophys. Acta, 1313,* 130-138.

[65] Funasaka, Y., Chakraborty, A. K., Hayashi, Y., Komoto, M., Ohashi, A., Nagahama, M., Inoue, Y., Pawelek, J. & Ichihashi, M. (1998). Modulation of melanocyte-stimulating hormone receptor expression on normal human melanocytes: evidence for a

regulatory role of ultraviolet B, interleukin-1 alpha, interleukin-1 beta, endothelin-1 and tumor necrosis factor-alpha. Br. J. Dermatol., *139*, 216-224.
[66] Wakamatsu, K., Graham, A., Cook, D. & Thody, A. J. (1997). Characterisation of ACTH peptides in human skin and their activation of the melanocortin-1 receptor. *Pigment Cell Melanoma Res., 10*, 288-297.
[67] Tada, A., Suzuki, I., Im, S., Davis, M. B., Cornelius, J., Babcock, G., Nordlund, J. J. & Abdel-Malek, Z. A. (1998). Endothelin-1 is a paracrine growth factor that modulates melanogenesis on human melanocytes and participates in their responses to ultraviolet radiation. *Cell Growth Differ., 9*, 575-584.
[68] Abdel-Malek, Z., Scott, M. C., Suzuki, I., Tada, A., Im, S., Lamoreux, L., Ito, S., Barsh, G. & Hearing, V. J. (2000). The melanocortin-1 receptor is a key regulator of human cutaneous pigmentation. *Pigment Cell Melanoma Res., 13 Suppl. 8*, 156-162.
[69] Hirobe, T. (2005). Role of keratinocyte-derived factors involved in regulating the proliferation and differentiation of mammalian epidermal melanocytes. *Pigment Cell Melanoma Res., 18*, 2-12.
[70] Romero-Graillet, C., Aberdam, E., Biagoli, N., Massabni, W., Ortonne, J. P. & Ballotti, R. (1996). Ultraviolet B radiation acts through the nitric oxide and cGMP signal transduction pathway to stimulate melanogenesis in human melanocytes. *J. Biol. Chem., 271*, 28052-28056.
[71] Weller, R. (2003). Nitric oxide: a key mediator in cutaneous physiology. *Clin. Exp. Dermatol., 28*, 511-514.
[72] Abdel-Malek, Z. A., Swope, V. B., Amornsiripanitch, N. & Nordlund, J. J. (1987). *In vitro* modulation of proliferation and melanization of S91 melanoma cells by prostaglandins. *Cancer Res., 47*, 3141-3146.
[73] Hunt, G., Todd, C., Cresswell, J. E. & Thody, A. J. (1994). α-MSH and its analog Nle4Dphe7 α-MSH affect morphology, tyrosinase activity and melanogenesis in cultured human melanocytes. *J. Cell Sci., 107*, 205-211.
[74] Hara, M., Yaar, M. & Gilchrest, B. A. (1995). Endothelin-1 of keratinocyte origin is a mediator of melanocyte dendricity. *J. Invest. Dermatol., 105*, 744-748.
[75] Ancans, J., Flanagan, N., Hoogduijn, M. J. & Thody, A. J. (2003). P-locus is a target for the melanogenic effects of MC-1R signaling: a possible control point for facultative pigmentation. Ann.N. Y. Acad. Sci., *994*, 373-377.
[76] Hirobe, T. (2004). Role of keratinocyte-derived factors involved in regulating the proliferation and differentiation of mammalian epidermal melanocytes. *Pigment Cell Melanoma Res., 18*, 2-12.
[77] Masaki, H. (2003). The measuring method of tyrosinase activity and the evaluation method of whitening effect up-to-date. *Fragrance J., special issue 18*, 35-41.
[78] Kadekaro, A. L., Kavanagh, R., Kanto, H., Terzieva, S., Hauser, J., Kobayashi, N., Schwemberger, S., Cornelius, J., Babcock, G., Shertzer, H. G., Scott, G. & Abdel-Malek, Z. A. (2005). Alpha-melanocortin and endothelin-1 activate antiapoptotic pathways and reduce DNA damage in human melanocytes. *Cancer Res., 65*, 4292-4299.
[79] Slominski, A., Tobin, D, J., Shibahara, S. & Wortsman, J. (2004). Melanin pigmentation in mammalian skin and its hormonal regulation. *Physiol. Rev., 84*, 1155-1228

[80] Rousseau, K., Kauser, S., Pritchard, L. E., Warhurst, A., Oliver, R. L., Slominski, A., Wei, E. T., Thody, A. J., Tobin, D. J. & White, A. (2007). Proopiomelanocortin (POMC), the ACTH/melanocortin precursor, is secreted by human epidermal keratinocytes and melanocytes and stimulates melanogenesis. Faseb. J., *21,* 1844-1856.

[81] Cone, R. D., Lu, D., Koppula, S., Vage, D. I., Klungland, H., Boston, B., Chen, W., Orth, D. N., Pouton, C. & Kesterson, R. A. (1996). The melanocortin receptors: agonist, antagonist, and the hormonal control of pigmentation. *Recent. Prog. Horm. Res., 51*, 287-317.

[82] Im, S., Moro, O., Peng, F., Medrano, E. E., Cornelius, J., Babcock, G., Nordlund, J. J. & Abdel-Malek, Z. A. (1998). Activation of cyclic AMP pathway by α-melanotropin mediates the response of human melanocytes to ultraviolet B radiation. *Cancer Res., 58*, 47-54.

[83] Insel, P. A., Bourne, H. R., Coffino, P. & Tomkins, G. M. (1975). Cyclic AMP-dependent protein kinase: pivotal role in regulation of enzyme induction and growth. *Science, 190*, 896-898.

[84] Newton, R. A., Cook, A. L., Roberts, D. W., Leonard, J. H. & Sturm, R. A. (2007). Post-transcriptional regulation of melanin biosynthetic enzymes by cAMP and resveratrol in human melanocytes. *J. Invest. Dermatol., 127*, 2216-2227.

[85] Busca, R. & Ballotti, R. (2000). Cyclic AMP a key messenger in the regulation of skin pigmentation. *Pigment Cell Melanoma Res., 13*, 60-69.

[86] Tachibana, M. (2000). MITF: a stream flowing for pigment cells. *Pigment Cell Melanoma Res., 13*, 230-240.

[87] Shibahara, S., Takeda, K., Yasumoto, K., Udono, T., Watanabe, K., Saito, H. & Takahashi, K. (2001). Microphthalmia-associated transcription factor (MITF): Multiplicity in structure, function, and regulation. *J. Investig. Dermatol. Symp. Proc., 6*, 99-104.

[88] Tachibana, M., Takeda, K., Nobukuni, Y., Urabe, K., Long, J. E., Meyers, K., Aaronson, S. A., & Miki, T. (1996). Ectopic expression of MITF, a gene for Waardenburg syndrome type 2, converts fibroblasts to cells with melanocyte characteristics. Nature Genet., *14*, 50-54.

[89] Levy, C., Khaled, M. & Fisher, D. E. (2006). MITF: Master regulator of melanocyte development and melanoma oncogene. *Trends Mol. Med., 12*, 406-414.

[90] Ebanks, J. P., Wickett, R. R. & Boissy, R. E. (2009). Mechanisms Regulating Skin Pigmentation: The Rise and Fall of Complexion Coloration., *Int. J. Mol. Sci., 10*, 4066-4087.

[91] Theos, A. C., Truschel, S. T., Raposo, G. & Marks, M. S., (2005). The *Silver* locus product Pmel17/gp100/Silv/ME20: controversial in name and in function. *Pigment Cell Melanoma Res., 18*, 322-336.

[92] Yasumoto, K., Yokoyama, K.,Takahashi, K.,Tomita. Y. & Shibahara, S. (1997). Functional analysis of microphthalmia-associated transcription factor in pigment cell-specific transcription of the human tyrosinase family genes. *J. Biol. Chem., 272*, 503-509.

[93] Aksan, I. & Goding, C. R. (1998). Targeting the microphthalmia basic helix-loop-helix-leucine zipper transcription factor to a subset of E-box elements *in vitro* and *in vivo. Mol. Cell. Biol., 18*. 6930-6938.

[94] Galibert, M. D., Yavuzer, U., Dexter, T. J. & Goding, C. R., (1999). Pax3 and regulation of the melanocyte-specific tyrosinase-related protein-1 promoter. *J. Biol. Chem., 274*, 26894-26900.

[95] Bertolotto, C., Buscà, R., Abbe, P., Bille, K., Aberdam, E., Ortonne, J. P. & Ballotti, R. (1998). Different *cis*-acting elements are involved in the regulation of TRP1 and TRP2 promoter activities by cyclic AMP: pivotal role of M boxes (GTCATGTGCT) and of microphthalmia. *Mol. Cell. Biol., 18*, 694-702.

[96] Bentley, N. J., Eisen, T. & Goding, C. R. (1994). Melanocyte-specific expression of the human tyrosinase promoter: activation by the microphthalmia gene product and role of the initiator. *Mol. Cell. Biol., 14*, 7996-8006.

[97] Hemesath, T. J., Steingrímsson, E., McGill, G., Hansen, M. J., Vaught, J., Hodgkinson, C. A., Arnheiter, H., Copeland, N. G., Jenkins, N. A. & Fisher, D. E. (1994). microphthalmia, a critical factor in melanocyte development, defines a discrete transcription factor family. *Genes Dev., 8*, 2770-2780.

[98] Lin, C. B., Babiarz, L., Liebel, F., Roydon, P. E., Kizoulis, M., Gendimenico, G. J., Fisher, D. E. & Seiberg, M. (2002). Modulation of microphthalmia-associated transcription factor gene expression alters skin pigmentation., *J. Invest. Dermatol., 119*, 1330-1340.

[99] Yasumoto, K., Yokoyama, K., Shibata, K., Tomita, Y. & Shibahara, S. (1994). Microphthalmia-associated transcription factor as a regulator for melanocyte-specific transcription of the human tyrosinase gene. *Mol. Cell. Biol., 14*, 8058-8070.

[100] Moore, K. J. (1995). Insight into the microphthalmia gene. *Trends Genet., 11*, 442-448.

[101] Widlund, H. R. & Fisher, D. E. (2003). Microphthalamia-associated transcription factor: A critical regulator of pigment cell development and survival. *Oncogene, 22*, 3035-3041.

[102] Yamaguchi, Y., Brenner, M. & Hearing, V. J. (2007). The regulation of skin pigmentation. *J. Biol. Chem., 282*, 27557-27561.

[103] Kim, Y. J. & Uyama, H. (2005). Tyrosinase inhibitors from natural and synthetic sources: structure, inhibition mechanism and perspective for the future. *Cell Mol. Life Sci., 62*, 1707-1723.

[104] Wan, P., Hu, Y., & He, L. (2011). Regulation of melanocyte pivotal transcription factor MITF by some other transcription factors. *Mol. Cell Biochem., 354*, 241-246.

[105] Passeron, T., Valencia., Bertolotto, C., Hoashi, T., Le, P. E., Takahashi, K., Ballotti, R. & Hearing, V. J. (2007). SOX9 is a key player in ultraviolet B-induced melanocyte differentiation and pigmentation. *Proc. Natl. Acad. Sci. USA., 104*, 13984-13989.

[106] Jiao, Z., Mollaaghababa, R., Pavan, W. J., Antonellis, A., Green, E. D. & Hornyak, T. J. (2004). Direct interaction of Sox10 with the promoter of murine dopachrome tautomerase (DCT) and synergistic activation of DCT expression with MITF. *Pigment Cell Melanoma Res., 17*, 352-362.

[107] Ludwig, A., Rehberg, S. & Wegner, M. (2004). Melanocyte-specific expression of dopachrome tautomerase is dependent on synergistic gene activation by the Sox10 and MITF transcription factors. *FEBS Lett., 556*, 236-244.

[108] Watanabe, A., Takeda, K., Ploplis, B. & Tachibana, M. (1998). Epistatic relationship between Waardenburg syndrome genes MITF and PAX3. *Nat Genet., 18*, 283-286.

[109] Bondurand, N., Pingault, V., Goerich, D. E., Lemort, N., Sock, E., Le, C. C., Wegner, M. & Goossens, M. (2000). Interaction among SOX10, PAX3 and MITF, three genes altered in Waardenburg syndrome. *Hum. Mol. Genet., 9*, 1907-1917.

[110] Hearing, V. J. (2000). The melanosome: the perfect model for cellular responses to the environment. *Pigment Cell Melanoma Res., 13*, 23-34.

[111] Thomas, A. J. & Erickson, C. A. (2009). FOXD3 regulates the lineage switch between neural crest-derived glial cells and pigment cells by repressing MITF through a non-canonical mechanism. *Development, 136*, 1849-1858.

[112] Curran, K., Lister, J. A., Kunkel, G. R., Prendergast, A., Parichy, D. M. & Raible, D. W. (2010). Interplay between Foxd3 and Mitf regulates cell fate plasticity in the zebrafish neural crest. *Dev. Biol., 344*, 107-118.

[113] Hemesath, T. J., Price, E. R., Takemoto, C., Badalian, T. & Fisher D. E. (1998). MAP kinase links the transcription factor Microphthalmia to c-Kit signalling in melanocytes. *Nature., 391*, 298-301.

[114] Solano, F., Briganti, S., Picardo, M. & Ghanem, G. (2006). Hypopigmenting agents: an updated review on biological, chemical and clinical aspects. *Pigment Cell Melanoma Res., 19*, 550-571.

[115] Saha, B., Singh, S. K., Sarkar, C., Bera, R., Ratha, J., Tobin, D. J. & Bhadra, R. (2006). Activation of the Mitf promoter by lipid-stimulated activation of p38-stress signalling to CREB. *Pigment Cell Melanoma Res., 19*, 595-605.

[116] Kim, D. S., Park, S. H., Kwon, S. B., Na, J. I., Huh, C. H., & Park, K. C. (2007). Additive effects of heat and p38 MAPK inhibitor treatment on melanin synthesis. *Arch. Pharm. Res., 30*, 581-586.

[117] Singh, S. K., Sarkar, C., Mallick, S., Saha, B., Bera, R., & Bhadra, R. (2005). Human placental lipid induces melanogenesis through p38 MAPK in B16F10 mouse melanoma. *Pigment Cell Melanoma Res., 18*, 113-121.

[118] Bellei, B., Maresca, V., Flori, E., Pitisci, A., Larue, L. & Picardo, M. (2010). p38 regulates pigmentation via proteasomal degradation of tyrosinase. *J. Biol. Chem., 285*, 7288-7299

[119] Oka, M., Nagai, H., Ando, H., Matsumura, M., Araki, K., Ogawa, W., Miki, T., Sakaue, M., Tsukamoto, K., Konishi, H., Kikkawa, U. & Ichihashi, M. (2000). Regulation of melanogenesis through phosphatidylinositol 3-kinase-Akt pathway in human G361 melanoma cells. *J. Invest. Dermatol., 115*, 699-703.

[120] Kim, D. S., Park, S. H., Kwon, S. B., Park, E. S., Huh, C. H., Youn, S. W. & Park, K. C. (2006). Sphingosylphosphorylcholine-induced ERK activation inhibits melanin synthesis in human melanocytes. *Pigment Cell Res., 19,* 146-153.

[121] Kim, D. S., Hwang, E. S., Lee, J. E., Kim, S. Y., Kwon, S.B. & Park, K.C. (2003). Sphingosine-1-phosphate decreases melanin synthesis via sustained ERK activation and subsequent MITF degradation. *J. Cell Sci., 116,* 1699-1706.

[122] Kim, D. S., Kim, S. Y., Chung, J. H., Kim, K. H., Eun, H. C. & Park, K. C. (2002). Delayed ERK activation by ceramide reduces melanin synthesis in human melanocytes. *Cell. Signal., 14,* 779-785.

[123] Yang, G., Li, Y., Nishimura, E. K., Xin, H., Zhou, A., Guo, Y., Dong, L., Denning, M. F., Nickoloff, B.J. & Cui, R. (2008). Inhibition of PAX3 by TGF-β modulates melanocyte viability. *Mol. Cell. Biol., 32,* 554-563.

[124] Englaro, W., Bertolotto, C., Buscà, R., Brunet, A., Pagès, G., Ortonne, J. P. & Ballotti, R. (1998). Inhibition of the mitogen-activated protein kinase pathway triggers B16 melanoma cell differentiation. *J. Biol. Chem., 273,* 9966-9970.

[125] Kim, D. S., Park, S. H. & Park, K. C. (2004). Transforming growth factor-β1 decreases melanin synthesis via delayed extracellular signal-regulated kinase activation. *Int. J. Biochem., 36,* 1482-1491.

[126] Hida, T., Wakamatsu, K., Sviderskaya, E. V., Donkin, A. J., Montoliu, L., Lynn Lamoreux, M., Yu, B., Millhauser, G. L., Ito, S., Barsh, G. S., Jimbow, K. & Bennett, D. C. (2009). Agouti protein, mahogunin, and attractin in pheomelanogenesis and melanoblast-like alteration of melanocytes: a cAMP-independent pathway. *Pigment Cell Melanoma Res., 22,* 623-634.

[127] Slominski, A. & Wortsman, J. (2000). Neuroendocrinology of the skin., *Endocr. Rev., 21,* 457-487.

[128] Zbytek, B., Wortsman, J. & Slominski, A. (2006). Characterization of a ultraviolet B-induced corticotropin-releasing hormone-proopiomelanocortin system in human melanocytes. *Mol. Endocrinol., 20,* 2539-2547.

[129] Nylander, K., Bourdon, J. C., Bray, S. E., Gibbs, N. K., Kay, R., Hart, I. & Hall, P. A. (2000). Transcriptional activation of tyrosinase and TRP-1 by p53 links UV irradiation to the protective tanning response. *J. Pathol.,190,* 39-46.

[130] Cui, R., Widlund, H. R., Feige, E., Lin, J.Y., Wilensky, D.L., Igras, V.E., D'Orazio, J., Fung, C.Y., Schanbacher, C.F., Granter, S.R. & Fisher, D.E. (2007). Central role of p53 in the suntan response and pathologic hyperpigmentation. *Cell, 128,* 853-864.

[131] Kichina, J., Green, A. & Rauth, S. (1996). Tumor suppressor p53 down-regulates tissue-specific expression of tyrosinase gene in human melanoma cell lines. Pigment Cell Melanoma Res., *9,* 85-91.

[132] Khlgatian, M. K., Hadshiew, I. M., Asawanonda, P., Yaar, M., Eller, M. S., Fujita, M., Norris, D. A. & Gilchrest, B. A. (2002). Tyrosinase gene expression is regulated by p53. *J. Invest. Dermatol., 118,* 126-132.

[133] Tadokoro, T., Rouzaud, F., Itami, S., Hearing, V. J. & Yoshikawa, K. (2003). The inhibitory effect of androgen and sex-hormone-binding globulin on the intracellular cAMP level and tyrosinase activity of normal human melanocytes. Pigment Cell Melanoma Res., *16,* 190-197.

[134] Schallreuter, K. U., Hasse, S., Rokos, H., Chavan, B., Shalbaf, M., Spencer, J. D. & Wood, J. M. (2009). Cholesterol regulates melanogenesis in human epidermal melanocytes and melanoma cells. *Exp. Dermatol., 18,* 680-688.

[135] Glinka, A., Wu, W., Delius, H., Monaghan, A, P., Blumenstock, C. & Niehrs, C. (1998). Dickkopf-1 is a member of a new family of secreted proteins and functions in head induction. *Nature, 391,* 357-362.

[136] Yamaguchi, Y., Itami, S., Watabe, H., Yasumoto, K., Abdel-Malek, Z. A., Kubo, T., Rouzaud, F., Tanemura, A., Yoshikawa, K. & Hearing, V.J. (2004). Mesenchymal-epithelial interactions in the skin: increased expression of dickkopf1 by palmoplantar fibroblasts inhibits melanocyte growth and differentiation. *J. Cell Biol., 165,* 275-285.

[137] Yamaguchi, Y., Passeron, T., Hoashi, T., Watabe, H., Rouzaud, F., Yasumoto, K., Hara, T., Tohyama, C., Katayama, I., Miki, T. & Hearing, V.J. (2008). Dickkopf 1 (DKK1) regulates skin pigmentation and thickness by affecting Wnt/b-catenin signaling in keratinocytes. Faseb J., *22,* 1009-1020.

[138] Urabe, K. N., J.; Hori, Y., Nordlund, J. J., Boissy, R. E., Hearing, V. J., King, R. A., Oetting, W. S. & Ortonne, J. P. (1998). Mixed epidermal and dermal hypermelanoses. *The Pigmentary System: Physiology and Pathophysiology.* 909-913.

[139] Virador, V., Matsunaga, N., Matsunaga, J., Valencia, J., Oldham, R. J., Kameyama, K., Peck, G. L., Ferrans, V. J., Vieira, W. D., Abdel-Malek, Z. A. & Hearing, V. J. (2001). Production of melanocyte-specific antibodies to human melanosomal proteins: Expression patterns in normal human skin and in cutaneous pigmented lesions. Pigment Cell Melanoma Res., *14,* 289-297.

[140] Cullen, M. K., Norlund, J. J., Boissy, R. E., Hearing, V. J., Norlund, J. J., Boissy, R.E., Hearing, V.J., King, R.A. & Ortonne, J.P. (1998). Genetic epidermal syndromes: disorders characterized by lentigines. *The Pigmentary System: Physiology and Pathophysiology* 760-766.

[141] Tomita, Y. & Suzuki, T. (2004). Genetics of pigmentary disorders. *Am. J. Med. Genet. C., 131C,* 75-81.

[142] Boissy, R. E. & Nordlund, J. J. (1997). Molecular basis of congenital hypopigmentary disorders in humans: a review. Pigment Cell Melanoma Res., *10,* 12-24.

[143] Wei, M. L. (2006). Hermansky-Pudlak syndrome: a disease of protein trafficking and organelle function. Pigment Cell Melanoma Res., *19,* 19-42.

[144] Spritz, R. A., Chiang, P, W., Oiso, N. & Alkhateeb, A. (2003). Human and mouse disorders of pigmentation. *Curr. Opin. Genet. Dev., 13,* 284-289.

[145] Ménasché, G., Ho, C. H., Sanal, O., Feldmann, J., Tezcan, I., Ersoy, F., Houdusse, A., Fischer, A. & de Saint Basile, G. (2003). Griscelli syndrome restricted to hypopigmentation results from a melanophilin defect (GS3) or a MYO5AF-exon deletion (GS1). *J. Clin. Invest., 112,* 450-456.

[146] Huizing, M., Helip-Wooley, A., Westbroek, W., Gunay-Aygun, M., & Gahi, W. A. (2008). Disorders of lysosome-related organelle biogenesis: clinical and molecular genetics. *Annu. Rev. Genomics Hum. Genet., 9,* 359-386.

[147] Van Gele, M., Dynoodt, P. & Lambert, J. (2009). Griscelli syndrome: a model system to study vesicular trafficking. *Pigment Cell Melanoma Res., 22,* 268-282.

[148] Steingrímsson, E., Copeland, N. G. & Jenkins, N. A. (2004). Melanocytes and the microphthalmia transcription factor network. *Annu. Rev. Genet. 38,* 365-411.

[149] Takeda, K., & Shibahara, S. (2007). Transcriptional Regulation of Melanocyte Function. *The Pigmentary System: Physiology and Pathophysiology (2nd).* 242-260. Blackwell Publishing Ltd.

[150] Gillbro, J. M. & Olsson, M. J. (2011). The melanogenesis and mechanisms of skin-lightening agents- existing and new approaches. *Int. J. Cosmet. Sci., 33,* 210-221.

[151] Smit, N., Vicanova, J. & Pavel, S. (2009). The hunt for natural skin whitening agents. *Int. J. Mol. Sci., 10,* 5326-5349.

[152] Chiang, H. M., Lin, J. W., Hsiao, P. L., Tsai, S. Y., & Wen, K. C. (2011). Hydrolysates of citrus plants stimulate melanogenesis protecting against UV-induced dermal damage. *Phytother. Res., 25,* 569-576.

[153] Ando, H., Matsui, M. S., & Ichihashi, M. (2010). Quasi-drugs developed in Japan for the prevention or treatment of hyperpigmentary disorders. *Int. J. Mol. Sci., 11,* 2566-2575.

[154] Parvez, S., Kang, M., Chung, H. S. & Bae, H. (2007). Naturally occurring tyrosinase inhibitors: mechanism and applications in skin health, cosmetics and agriculture industries. *Phytother. Res., 21,* 805-816.

[155] Briganti, S., Camera, E. & Picardo, M. (2003). Chemical and instrumental approaches to treat hyperpigmentation. *Pigment Cell Melanoma Res., 16,* 101-110.

[156] Ando, H., Ichihashi, M. & Hearing, V. J. (2009). Role of the ubiquitin proteasome system in regulating skin pigmentation. *Int. J. Mol. Sci., 10,* 4428-4434.

[157] Nakayama, T., Sato, T., Fukui, Y., Yonekura-Sakakibara, K., Hayashi, H., Tanaka, Y., Kusumi, T. & Nishino, T. (2001). Specificity analysis and mechanism of aurone synthesis catalyzed by aureusidin synthase, a polyphenol oxidase homolog responsible for flower coloration. *FEBS Lett., 499,* 107-111.

[158] Jin, Y. Z., Li, G. H., Ahn, S. Y., Row, K. H. & Kim, E. K. (2006). Extraction and purification of depigmenting agents from Chinese plants. *Chem. Res. Chin. Univ., 22,* 162-167.

[159] Wang, K. H., Lin, R. D., Hsu, F. L., Huang, Y. H., Chang, H. C., Huang, C. Y. & Lee, M, H. (2006). Cosmetic applications of selected traditional Chinese herbal medicines. J. Ethnopharmacol., *106,* 353-359.

[160] Liu, S. H., Chu, I. M. & Pan, I. H. (2008). Effects of hydroxybenzyl alcohols on melanogenesis in melanocyte-keratinocyte co-culture and monolayer culture of melanocytes. *J. Enzym. Inhib. Med. Chem., 23,* 526-534.

[161] Zhong, S., Wu, Y., Soo-Mi, A., Zhao, J., Wang, K., Yang, S., Jae-Ho, Y. & Zhu, X. (2006). Depigmentation of melanocytes by the treatment of extracts from traditional Chinese herbs: a cell culture assay. *Biol. Pharm. Bull., 29,* 1947-1951.

[162] Greatens, A., Hakozaki, T., Koshoffer, A., Epstein, H., Schwemberger, S., Babcock, G., Bissett, D., Takiwaki, H., Arase, S., Wickett, R. R. & Boissy, R. E. (2005). Effective inhibition of melanosome transfer to keratinocytes by lectins and niacinamide is reversible. *Exp. Dermatol., 14,* 498-508.

[163] Yamakoshi, J., Otsuka, F., Sano, A., Tokutake, S., Saito, M., Kikuchi, M. & Kubota, Y. (2003). Lightening effect on ultraviolet-induced pigmentation of guinea pig skin by oral administration of a proanthocyanidin-rich extract from grape seeds. *Pigment Cell Melanoma Res., 16,* 629-638.

[164] Yoshimura, M., Watanabe, Y., Kasai, K., Yamakoshi, J. & Koga, T. (2005). Inhibitory effect of an ellagic acid-rich pomegranate extract on tyrosinase activity and ultraviolet-induced pigmentation. *Biosci. Biotechnol. Biochem., 69,* 2368-2373.

[165] Duval, C., Smit, N. P., Kolb, A. M., Régnier, M., Pavel, S. & Schmidt, R. (2002). Keratinocytes control the pheo/eumelanin ratio in cultured normal human melanocytes. *Pigment Cell Melanoma Res., 15,* 440-446.

[166] Choi, T. Y., Kim, J. H., Ko, D. H., Kim, C. H., Hwang, J. S., Ahn, S., Kim, S. Y., Kim, C. D., Lee, J. H. & Yoon, T. J. (2007). Zebrafish as a new model for phenotype-based screening of melanogenic regulatory compounds. *Pigment Cell Melanoma Res., 20,* 120-127.

[167] Tsujishita, Y., Asaoka, Y. & Nishizuka, Y. (1994). Regulation of phospholipase A2 in human leukemia cell lines: Its implication for intracellular signaling. *Proc. Natl. Acad. Sci. USA, 91,* 6274-6278.

[168] Chawla, A., Repa, J. J., Evans, R. M. & Mangelsdorf, D. J. (2001). Nuclear receptors and lipid physiology: Opening the X-files. *Science, 294,* 1866-1870.

[169] Clarke, S. D. (2004). The multi-dimensional regulation of gene expression by fatty acids: Polyunsaturated fats as nutrient sensors. *Curr. Opin. Lipidology, 15,* 13-18.

[170] Ando, H., Wen Z. M., Kim, H. Y., Valencia, J. C., Costin G. E., Watabe, H., Yasumoto, K., Niki, Y., Kondoh, H., Ichihashi, M. & Hearing V. J. (2006). Intracellular composition of fatty acid affects the processing and function of tyrosinase through the ubiquitin-proteasome pathway. *Biochem. J., 394,* 43-50.

[171] Ando, H., Funasaka, Y., Oka, M., Ohashi, A., Furumura, M., Matsunaga, J., Matsunaga, N., Hearing, V. J. & Ichihashi, M. (1999). Possible involvement of proteolytic degradation of tyrosinase in the regulatory effect of fatty acids on melanogenesis. *J. Lipid Res., 40,* 1312-1316.

[172] Dahlmann, B., Rutschmann, M., Kuehn, L. & Reinauer, H. (1985). Activation of the multicatalytic proteinase from rat skeletal muscle by fatty acids or sodium dodecyl sulphate. *Biochem J., 228,* 171-177.

[173] Santulli, R. J., Derian, C. K., Darrow, A. L., Tomko, K. A., Eckardt, A. J., Seiberg, M., Scarborough, R. M. & Andrade-Gordon, P. (1995). Evidence for the presence of a protease-activated receptor distinct from the thrombin receptor in human keratinocytes. *Proc. Natl. Acad. Sci. USA. 92,* 9151-9155.

[174] Sharlow, E. R., Paine, C.S., Babiarz, L., Eisinger, M., Shapiro, S. & Seiberg, M. (2000). The protease-activated receptor-2 upregulates keratinocyte phagocytosis. *J. Cell Sci., 113,* 3093-3101.

[175] Paine, C., Sharlow, E., Liebel, F., Eisinger, M., Shapiro, S. & Seiberg, M. (2001). An alternative approach to depigmentation by soybean extracts via inhibition of the PAR-2 pathway. *J. Invest. Dermatol., 116,* 587-595.

[176] Scott, G., Leopardi, S., Parker, L., Babiarz, L., Seiberg, M. & Han, R. (2003). The proteinase-activated receptor-2 mediates phagocytosis in a Rho-dependent manner in human keratinocytes. *J. Invest. Dermatol., 121,* 529-541.

[177] Saeki, Y., Kanamaru, A., Matsumoto, A. & Tada, A. (2003). The inhibitory effects of centaureidin on the outgrowth of dendrites, melanosome transfer and melanogenesis in normal human melanogenesis. Pigment Cell Melanoma Res., *16,* 593.

[178] Ito, Y., Kanamaru, A. & Tada, A. (2006). Centaureidin promotes dendrite retraction of melanocytes by activating Rho. Biochim. Biophys. Acta-Gen. Subj., *1760,* 487-494.

[179] Ito, Y., Kanamaru, A. & Tada, A. (2006). Effects of methylophiopogonanone B on melanosome transfer and dendrite retraction. *J. Dermatol. Sci., 42,* 68-70.

[180] Hakozaki, T., Minwalla, L., Zhuang, J., Chhoa, M., Matsubara, A., Miyamoto, K., Greatens, A., Hillebrand, G. G., Bissett, D. L. & Boissy, R. E. (2002). The effect of niacinamide on reducing cutaneous pigmentation and suppression of melanosome transfer. *Br. J. Dermatol., 147,* 20-31.

[181] Yoon, T. J., Lei, T. C., Yamaguchi, Y., Batzer, J., Wolber, R. & Hearing, V. J. (2003). Reconstituted 3-dimensional human skin of various ethnic origins as an in vitro model for studies of pigmentation. *Anal. Biochem., 318,* 260-269.

[182] Lei, T. C., Virador, V. M., Vieira, W. D. & Hearing, V. J. (2002). A melanocyte-keratinocyte coculture model to assess regulators of pigmentation in vitro. *Anal. Biochem., 305,* 260-268.

[183] Brenner, M. & Hearing, V. J. (2008). Modifying skin pigmentation-approaches through intrinsic biochemistry and exogenous agents. *Drug Discov. Today Dis. Mech., 5,* 189-199.

[184] Imokawa, G., Kobayashi, T., Miyagishi, M., Higashi, K. & Yada, Y. (1997). The role of endothelin-1 in epidermal hyperpigmentation and signaling mechanisms of mitogenesis and melanogenesis. *Pigment Cell Melanoma Res., 10,* 218-228.

[185] Hachiya, A., Kobayashi, A., Yoshida, Y., Kitahara, T., Takema, Y. & Imokawa, G. (2004). Biphasic expression of two paracrine melanogenic cytokines, stem cell factor and endothelin-1, in ultraviolet B-induced human melanogenesis. *Am. J. Pathol., 165,* 2099-2109.

[186] Hirobe, T. & Ootaka, H. (2007). Interleukin-1alpha stimulates the differentiation of melanocytes but inhibits the proliferation of melanoblasts from neonatal mouse epidermis. *Zool. Sci., 24,* 959-970.

[187] Hachiya, A., Kobayashi, T., Takema, Y. & Imokawa, G. (2002). Biochemical characterization of endothelin-converting enzyme-1alpha in cultured skin-derived cells and its postulated role in the stimulation of melanogenesis in human epidermis. *J. Biol. Chem., 277,* 5395-5403.

[188] Kawaguchi, Y., Mori, N. & Nakayama, A. (2001). Kit(+) melanocytes seem to contribute to melanocyte proliferation after UV exposure as precursor cells. *J. Invest. Dermatol., 116,* 920-925.

[189] Maeda, K. & Naganuma, M. (1997). Melanocyte-stimulating properties of secretory phospholipase A2, *Photochem. Photobiol., 65,* 145-149.

[190] Pentland, A. P. & Mahoney, M. G. (1990). Keratinocyte prostaglandin synthesis is enhanced by IL-1. *J. Invest. Dermatol., 94,* 43-46.

[191] Hachiya, A., Kobayashi, A., Ohuchi, A., Kitahara, T. & Takema, Y. (2001). The inhibitory effect of an extract of *Sanguisorba officinalis* L. on ultraviolet B-induced pigmentation *via* the suppression of endothelin-converting enzyme-1alpha. *Biol. Pharm. Bull., 24,* 688-692.

[192] Kobayashi, A., Hachiya, A., Ohuchi, A., Kitahara, T. & Takema, Y. (2002). Inhibitory mechanism of an extract of *Althaea officinalis* L. on endothelin-1-induced melanocyte activation. *Biol. Pharm. Bull., 25,* 229-234.

[193] Shimoda, H., Tanaka, J., Shan, S. J. & Maoka, T. (2010). Anti-pigmentary activity of fucoxanthin and its influence on skin mRNA expression of melanogenic molecules. *J. Pharm. Pharmacol., 62,* 1137-1145.

[194] Hasegawa, T., Takano, F., Takata, T., Niiyama, M. & Ohta, T. (2008). Bioactive monoterpene glycosides conjugated with gallic acid from the leaves of *Eucalyptus globulus*. *Phytochemistry, 69,* 747-753.

[195] Kawabata, T., Cui, M. Y., Hasegawa, T., Takano, F. & Ohta, T. (2011). Anti-inflammatory and anti-melanogenic steroidal saponin glycosides from Fenugreek (Trigonella foenum-graecum L.) seeds. *Planta Med., 77,* 705-710.

[196] Takashi, K. (2000). Development of new skin whitening agents. Whitening effect of Guava leaves extract. *Fragrance J, 28,* 86-90.

[197] Öhman, H. & Vahlquist, A. (1994). *In vivo* studies concerning a pH gradient in human stratum corneum and upper epidermis. *Acta Derm.-Venereol., 74,* 375-379.

[198] Sondell, B., Thornell, L.E. & Egelrud, T. (1995). Evidence that stratum corneum chymotryptic enzyme is transported to the stratum corneum extracellular space *via* lamellar bodies. *J. Invest. Dermatol., 104,* 819-823.

[199] Ekholm, I. E., Brattsand, M. & Egelrud, T. (2000). Stratum corneum tryptic enzyme in normal epidermis: a missing link in the desquamation process? *J. Invest. Dermatol., 114,* 56-63.

[200] Horikoshi, T., Arany, I., Rajaraman, S., Chen, S. H., Brysk, H., Lei, G., Tyring, S. K. & Brysk, M. M. (1998). Isoforms of cathepsin D and human epidermal differentiation. *Biochimie, 80,* 605-612.

[201] Zhu, W. & Zhang, R. (2006). Cosmetic Science and Technology Series. *In Cosmetic Formulation of Skin Care Products: Skin Lightening Agents. New York.* 205-218.

[202] Bowe, W. P. & Shalita, A. R. (2008). Effective over-the-counter acne treatments. *Semin. Cutan. Med. Surg., 27,* 170-176.

[203] Badreshia-Bansal, S. & Draelos, Z. D. (2007). Insight into skin lightening cosmeceuticals for women of color. *J. Drugs Dermatol., 6,* 32-39.

[204] Smith, W. P. (1999). The effects of topical (+) lactic Acid and ascorbic Acid on skin whitening. *Int. J. Cosmet Sci, 21,* 33-40.

[205] Yamamoto, Y., Uede, K., Yonei, N., Kishioka, A., Ohtani, T. & Furukawa, F. (2006). Effects of alpha-hydroxy acids on the human skin of Japanese subjects: the rationale for chemical peeling. *J. Dermatol., 33,* 16-22.

[206] Bellemère, G., Stamatas, G. N., Bruère, V., Bertin, C., Issachar, N. & Oddos, T. (2009). Antiaging action of retinol: from molecular to clinical. *Skin Pharmacol. Physiol., 22,* 200-209.

[207] Amer, M. & Metwalli, M. (2000). Topical liquiritin improves melasma. *Int. J. Dermatol., 39,* 299-301.

[208] Zhu, W. & Gao, J. (2008). The use of botanical extracts as topical skin-lightening agents for the improvement of skin pigmentation disorders. *J. Investig. Dermatol. Symp. Proc., 13,* 20-24.

[209] Riley, P. A. (1969). Hydroxyanisole depigmentation: *in-vitro* studies. *J. Pathol., 97,* 193-206.

[210] Naish-Byfield, S., Cooksey, C. J., Latter, A. M., Johnson, C. I. & Riley, P. A. (1991). *In vitro* assessment of the structure-activity relationship of tyrosinase-dependent cytotoxicity of a series of substitutedphenols. *Melanoma Res., 4,* 273-287.

[211] Smit, N. P., Peters, K., Menko, W., Westerhof, W., Pavel, S. & Riley, P. A. (1992). Cytotoxicity of a selected series of substituted phenols towards cultured melanoma cells. *Melanoma Res., 2,* 295-304.

[212] Sugai, T. (1992). Clinical effects of arbutin in patients with chloasma. *Skin Res. (Hifu), 34,* 522-529.

[213] Polnikorn, N. (2010). Treatment of refractory melasma with the MedLite C6 Q-switched Nd: YAG laser and alpha arbutin: a prospective study. *J Cosmet Laser Ther, 12,* 126-131.

[214] Boissy, R. E., Visscher, M. & DeLong, M. A. (2005). DeoxyArbutin: a novel reversible tyrosinase inhibitor with effective *in vivo* skin lightening potency. *Exp. Dermatol., 14,* 601-608.

[215] Chawla, S., deLong, M. A., Visscher, M. O., Wickett, R. R., Manga, P. & Boissy, R. E. (2008). Mechanism of tyrosinase inhibition by deoxyArbutin and its second-generation derivatives. *Br. J. Dermato., 159,* 1267-1274.

[216] Mishima, Y., Ohyama, Y., Shibata, T., Seto, H. & Hatae, S. (1994). Inhibitory action of kojic acid on melanogenesis and its therapeutic effect for various human hyper-pigmentation disorders. *Skin Res. (Hifu), 36,* 134-150.

[217] Takizawa, T., Mitsumori, K., Tamura, T., Nasu, M., Ueda, M., Imai, T. & Hirose, M. (2003). Hepatocellular tumor induction in heterozygous p53-deficient CBA mice by a 26-week dietary administration of kojic acid. *Toxicol. Sci., 73,* 287-293.

[218] Higa, Y., Kawabe, M., Nabae, K., Toda, Y., Kitamoto, S., Hara, T., Tanaka, N., Kariya, K. & Takahashi, M. (2007). Kojic acid -absence of tumor-initiating activity in rat liver, and of carcinogenic and photo-genotoxic potential in mouse skin. *J. Toxicol. Sci., 32,* 143-159.

[219] Kumano, Y., Sakamoto, T., Egawa, M., Iwai, I., Tanaka, M. & Yamamoto, I. (1998). *In vitro* and *in vivo* prolonged biological activities of novel vitamin C derivative, 2-O-alpha-D-glucopyranosyl-L-ascorbic acid (AA-2G), in cosmetic fields. *J. Nutr. Sci. Vitaminol., 44,* 345-359.

[220] Kameyama, K., Sakai, C., Kondoh, S., Yonemoto, K., Nishiyama, S., Tagawa, M., Murata, T., Ohnuma, T., Quigley, J., Dorsky, A., Bucks, D. & Blanock, K. (1996). Inhibitory effect of magnesium L-ascorbyl-2-phosphate (VC-PMG) on melanogenesis *in vitro* and *in vivo*. *J. Am. Acad. Dermatol, 34,* 29-33.

[221] Miyai, E., Yamamoto, I., Akiyama, J. & Yanagida, M. (1996). Inhibitory effect of ascorbic acid 2-O-α-glucoside on the pigmentation of skin by exposure to ultraviolet light. *Nishinihon J. Dermatol., 58,* 439-443.

[222] Katagiri, T., Okubo, T., Oyobikawa, M., Futaki, K., Shaku, M., Kawai, M. & Takenouchi, M. (2001). Inhibitory action of 4-n-butylresorcinol (Rucinol®) on melanogenesis and its skin whitening effects. *J. Cosmet. Chem. Jpn., 35,* 42-49.

[223] Shimogaki, H., Tanaka, Y., Tamai, H. & Masuda, M. (2000). *In vitro* and *in vivo* evaluation of ellagic acid on melanogenesis inhibition. *Int. J. Cosmet. Sci., 22,* 291-303.

[224] Kamide, R., Arase, S., Takiwaki, H., Watanabe, S., Watanabe, Y. & Kageyama, S. (1995). Clinical effects of XSC-29 formulation on UV-induced pigmentation. *Nishinihon J. Dermatol., 57,* 136-142.

[225] Ichihashi, M., Kobayashi, A., Okuda, M. & Imokawa, G. (1999). Effect of chamomilla extracts application on UV-induced pigmentation. *Skin Research (Hifu), 41,* 475-480.

[226] Kawashima, M., Okuda, M., Kobayashi, A. & Imokawa, G. (1999). Inhibitory effect of chamomilla extracts on UV-induced pigmentation. *Nishinihon J. Dermatol., 61,* 682-685.

[227] Nakamura, K., Yoshida, M., Uchiwa, H., Kawa, Y. & Mizoguchi, M. (2003). Down-regulation of melanin synthesis by a biphenyl derivative and its mechanism. *Pigment Cell Res., 16,* 494-500.

[228] Takeda, K., Yokota, T., Ikemoto, T., Kakishima, H. & Matsuo, T. (2006). Inhibitory effect of a formulation containing 0.5% Magnolignan® (5, 5'-dipropyl-biphenyl-2, 2'-diol) on UV-induced skin pigmentation. *Nishinihon J. Dermatol., 68,* 288-292.

[229] Takeda, K., Arase, S., Sagawa, Y., Shikata, Y., Okada, H., Watanabe, S., Yokota, T., Ikemoto, T., Kakishima, H. & Matsuo, T. (2006). Clinical evaluation of the topical application of Magnolignan® (5, 5'-dipropyl-biphenyl-2, 2'-diol) for hyperpigmentation on the face. *Nishinihon J. Dermatol., 68,* 293-298.

[230] Grimes, P. E. (1995). Melasma. Etiologic and therapeutic considerations. *Arch Dermatol., 131,* 1453-1457.

[231] Nguyen, Q. H. & Bui, T. P. (1995). Azelaic acid: pharmacokinetic and pharmacodynamic properties and its therapeutic role in hyperpigmentary disorders and acne. *Int. J. Dermatol., 34,* 75-84.

[232] Breathnach, A. S. (1996). Melanin hyperpigmentation of skin: melasma, topical treatment with azelaic acid, and other therapies. *Cutis, 57,* 36-45.

[233] Lowe, N. J., Rizk, D., Grimes, P., Billips, M. & Pincus, S. (1998). Azelaic acid 20% cream in the treatment of facial hyperpigmentation in darker-skinned patients. *Clin. Ther., 20,* 945-959.

[234] Verallo-Rowell, V. M., Verallo, V., Graupe, K., Lopez-Villafuerte, L. & Garcia-Lopez, M. (1989). Double-blind comparison of azelaic acid and hydroquinone in the treatment of melasma. *Acta Derm. Venereol. Suppl. (Stockh), 143,* 58-61.

[235] Chang, W. C., Shi, G. Y., Chow, Y. H., Chang, L. C., Hau, J. S., Lin, M. T., Jen, C. J., Wing, L. Y. & Wu, H. L. (1993). Human plasmin induces a receptor-mediated arachidonate release coupled with G proteins in endothelial cells. *Am. J. Physiol., 264,* C271-C281.

[236] Wang, N., Zhang, L., Miles, L. & Hoover-Plow, J. (2004). Plasminogen regulates pro-opiomelanocortin processing. *J. Thromb. Haemost., 2,* 785-796.

[237] Maeda, K. & Naganuma, M. (1998). Topical trans-4-aminomethylcyclohexane carboxylic acid prevents ultraviolet radiation-induced pigmentation. *J. Photochem. Photobiol. B-Biol., 47,* 136-141.

[238] Furukawa, F., Kanehara, S., Harano, F., Shinohara, S., Kamimura, J., Kawabata, S., Igarashi, S., Kawamura, M., Yamamoto, Y. & Miyachi, Y. (2008). Effects of adenosine 5'-monophosphate on epidermal turnover. *Arch. Dermatol. Res., 300,* 485-493.

[239] Kawashima, M., Mizuno, A. & Murata, Y. (2008). Improvement of hyperpigmentation based on accelerated epidermal turnover: Clinical effects of disodium adenosine monophosphate in patients with melasma. *Jpn. J. Clin. Dermatol., 62,* 250-257.

[240] Jimbow, K. (1991). N-acetyl-4-S-cysteaminylphenol as a new type of depigmenting agent for the melanoderma of patients with melasma. *Arch Dermatol., 127,* 1528-1534.

[241] Clinical trial group for linoleic acid-containing gel. (1998). Clinical trial for liver spots using a linoleic acid-containing gel. *Nishinihon J. Dermatol.,60,* 537-542.

[242] Ando, H., Ryu, A., Hashimoto, A., Oka, M. & Ichihashi, M. (1998). Linoleic acid and alpha-linolenic acid lightens ultraviolet-induced hyperpigmentation of the skin. *Arch. Dermatol. Res., 290,* 375-381.

[243] Shigeta, Y., Imanaka, H., Ando, H., Ryu, A., Oku, N., Baba, N. & Makino, T. (2004). Skin whitening effect of linoleic acid is enhanced by liposomal formulations. *Biol. Pharm. Bull., 27,* 591-594.

[244] Thibault, P. K., Wlodarczyk, J. & Wenck, A. (1998). A double-blind randomized clinical trial on the effectiveness of a daily glycolic acid 5% formulation in the treatment of photoaging. *Dermatol. Surg., 24,* 573-578.

[245] Javaheri, S. M., Handa, S., Kaur, I. & Kumar, B. (2001). Safety and efficacy of glycolic acid facial peel in Indian women with melasma. *Int. J. Dermatol., 40,* 354-357.

[246] Sharquie, K. E., Al-Tikreety, M. M. & Al-Mashhadani, S. A. (2005). Lactic acid as a new therapeutic peeling agent in melasma. *Dermatol. Surg., 31,* 149-154.

[247] Stiller, M. J., Bartolone, J., Stern, R., Smith, S., Kollias, N., Gillies, R. & Drake, L. A. (1996). Topical 8% glycolic acid and 8% L-lactic acid creams for the treatment of

photodamaged skin. A double-blind vehicle-controlled clinical trial. *Arch Dermatol, 132,* 631-636.

[248] Ahn, H. H. & Kim, I. H. (2006). Whitening effect of salicylic acid peels in Asian patients. *Dermatol. Surg., 32,* 372-375.

[249] Kubo, I., Kinst-Hori, I. & Yokokawa, Y. (1994). Tyrosinase inhibitors from Anacardium occidentale fruits. *J. Nat. Prod., 57,* 545-551.

[250] Chen, Y. R., Y-Y, R., Lin, T. Y., Huang, C. P., Tang, W. C., Chen, S. T. & Lin, S. B. (2009). Identification of an Alkylhydroquinone from Rhus succedanea as an Inhibitor of Tyrosinase and Melanogenesis. *J. Agric. Food Chem., 57,* 2200-2205.

[251] Kubo, I. & Kinst-Hori, I. (1999). 2-Hydroxy-4-methoxybenzaldehyde: a potent tyrosinase inhibitor from African medicinal plants. *Planta Med., 65,* 19-22.

[252] Kim, Y. J., No, J. K., Lee, J. S., Kim, M. S. & Chung, H. Y. (2006). Antimelanogenic activity of 3,4-dihydroxyacetophenone: inhibition of tyrosinase and MITF. *Biosci. Biotechnol. Biochem., 70,* 532-534.

[253] Lim, J. Y., Ishiguro, K. & Kubo, I. (1999). Tyrosinase inhibitory *p*-coumaric acid from ginseng leaves. *Phytother. Res., 13,* 371-375.

[254] An, S. M., Lee, S. I., Choi, S. W., Moon, S. W. & Boo, Y. C. (2008). *p*-Coumaric acid, a constituent of Sasa quelpaertensis Nakai, inhibits cellular melanogenesis stimulated by alpha-melanocyte stimulating hormone. *Br. J. Dermatol., 159,* 292-299.

[255] Mapunya, M. B., Hussein, A. A., Rodriguez, B. & Lall, N. (2011). Tyrosinase activity of *Greyia flanaganii* (Bolus) constituents. *Phytomedicine, 18,* 1006-1012.

[256] No, J. K., Kim, M. S., Kim, Y. J., Bae, S. J., Choi, J. S. & Chung, H. Y. (2004). Inhibition of tyrosinase by protocatechuic aldehyde. *Am. J. Chin. Med., 32,* 97-103.

[257] Kang, H. S., Choi, J. H., Cho, W. K., Park, J. C. & Choi, J. S. (2004). A sphingolipid and tyrosinase inhibitors from the fruiting body of Phellinus linteus. *Arch. Pharm. Res., 27,* 742-750.

[258] Miyazawa, M., Oshima, T., Koshio, K., Itsuzaki, Y. & Anzai, J. (2003). Tyrosinase inhibitor from black rice bran. *J. Agric Food Chem., 51,* 6953-6956.

[259] Kang, H. S., Kim, H. R., Byun, D. S., Son, B. W., Nam, T. J. & Choi, J. S. (2004). Tyrosinase inhibitors isolated from the edible brown alga *Ecklonia stolonifera. Arch. Pharm. Res., 27,* 1226-1232.

[260] Heo, S. J., Ko, S. C., Cha, S. H., Kang, D. H., Park, H. S., Choi, Y. U., Kim, D., Jung, W. K. & Jeon, Y. J. (2009). Effect of phlorotannins isolated from *Ecklonia cava* on melanogenesis and their protective effect against photo-oxidative stress induced by UV-B radiation, *Toxicol. In. Vitro., 23,* 1123-1130.

[261] Yoon, N. Y., Eom, T. K., Kim, M. M. & Kim, S. K. (2009). Inhibitory effect of phlorotannins isolated from *Ecklonia cava* on mushroom tyrosinase activity and melanin formation in mouse B16F10 melanoma cells, *J. Agric. Food Chem., 57,* 4124-4129.

[262] Ngoc, T. M., Lee, I., Ha do, T., Kim, H., Min, B. & Bae, K. (2009). Tyrosinase-inhibitory constituents from the twigs of *Cinnamomum cassia. J. Nat. Prod., 72,* 1205-1208.

[263] Lee, S. H., Choi, S. Y., Kim, H., Hwang, J. S., Lee, B. G., Gao, J. J. & Kim, S. Y. (2002). Mulberroside F isolated from the leaves of *Morus alba* inhibits melanin biosynthesis. *Biol. Pharm. Bull., 25,* 1045-1048.

[264] Shimizu, K., Kondo, R. & Sakai, K. (2000). Inhibition of tyrosinase by flavonoids, stilbenes and related 4-substituted resorcinols: structure-activity investigations. *Planta. Med., 66,* 11-15.

[265] Cho, Y., Kim, K. H., Shim, J. S. & Hwang, J. K. (2008). Inhibitory effects of macelignan isolated from *Myristica fragrans* HOUTT. on melanin biosynthesis. *Biol. Pharm. Bull., 31,* 986-989.

[266] Masuda, M., Murata, K., Fukuhama, A., Naruto, S., Fujita, T., Uwaya, A., Isami, F. & Matsuda, H. (2009). Inhibitory effects of constituents of *Morinda citrifolia* seeds on elastase and tyrosinase. *J. Nat. Med., 63,* 267-273.

[267] Iwai, K., Kishimoto, N., Kakino, Y., Mochida, K. & Fujita, T. (2004). *In vitro* antioxidative effects and tyrosinase inhibitory activities of seven hydroxycinnamoyl derivatives in green coffee beans. *J. Agric. Food Chem., 52,* 4893-4898.

[268] Lee, H. S. (2002). Tyrosinase inhibitors of *Pulsatilla cernua* root-derived materials. *J. Agric. Food Chem., 50,* 1400-1403.

[269] Wang, H., Chou, Y. T., Hong, Z. L., Chen, H. A., Chang, Y. C., Yang, W. L., Chang, H. C., Mai, C.T., & Chen, C. Y. (2011). Bioconstituents from stems of *Synsepalum dulcificum* Daniell (Sapotaceae) inhibit human melanoma proliferation, reduce mushroom tyrosinase activity and have antioxidant properties. *Journal of the Taiwan Institute of Chemical Engineers, 42,* 204-211.

[270] Cho, M., Ryu, M., Jeong, Y., Chung, Y. H., Kim, D. E., Cho, H. S., Han, J. S., Chang M. Y., Lee, C. K., Jin, M., Kim, H. J. & Oh, S. (2009). Cardamonin suppresses melanogenesis by inhibition of Wnt/beta-catenin signaling, *Biochem. Biophys. Res. Commun., 390,* 500-505.

[271] Yoon, J. H., Shim, J. S., Cho, Y., Baek, N. I., Lee, C. W., Kim, H. S., & Hwang, J. K. (2007). Depigmentation of melanocytes by isopanduratin A and 4-hydroxypanduratin A isolated from *Kaempferia pandurat*a ROXB. *Biol. Pharm. Bull., 30,* 2141-2145.

[272] Shirota, S., Miyazaki, K., Aiyama, R., Ichioka, M. & Yokokura, T. (1994). Tyrosinase inhibitors from crude drugs. *Biol. Pharm. Bull., 17,* 266-269.

[273] Kim, J. H., Sapers, G. M. & Choi, S. W. (1998). Identification of tyrosinase inhibitor from *Galla rhois*. *Food. Sci. Biotechnol, 7.* 56-59.

[274] Chen, L. G., Chang, W. L., Lee, C. J., Lee, L. T., Shih, C. M. & Wang, C. C. (2009). Melanogenesis inhibition by gallotannins from Chinese galls in B16 mouse melanoma cells. *Biol. Pharm. Bull., 32.* 1447-1452.

[275] Kubo, I., Kinst-Hori, I., Nihei, K., Soria, F., Takasaki, M., Calderon, J. S. & Cespedes, C. L. (2003). Tyrosinase inhibitors from galls of *Rhus javanica* leaves and their effects on insects. *Z. Naturforsch., 58,* 719-725.

[276] Park, J. S., Park, H. Y., Rho, H. S., Ahn, S., Kim, D. H. & Chang, I. S. (2008). Statistically designed enzymatic hydrolysis for optimized production of icariside II as a novel melanogenesis inhibitor. *J. Microbiol. Biotechnol., 18.* 110-117.

[277] Koo, J. H., Kim, H. T., Yoon, H. Y., Kwon, K. B., Choi, I. W., Jung, S. H., Kim, H. U., Park, B. H. & Park, J. W. (2008). Effect of xanthohumol on melanogenesis in B16 melanoma cells. *Exp. Mol. Med., 40,* 313-319.

[278] Okunji, C., Komarnytsky, S., Fear, G., Poulev, A., Ribnicky, D. M., Awachie, P. I., Ito, Y. & Raskin, I. (2007). Preparative isolation and identification of tyrosinase inhibitors from the seeds of *Garcinia kola* by high-speed counter-current chromatography. *J. Chromatogr. A., 1151,* 45-50.

[279] Masuda, T., Yamashita, D., Takeda, Y. & Yonemori, S. (2005). Screening for tyrosinase inhibitors among extracts of seashore plants and identification of potent inhibitors from *Garcinia subelliptica*. *Biosci. Biotechnol. Biochem., 69,* 197-201.
[280] Kubo, I., Kinst-Hori, I., Chaudhuri, S. K., Kubo, Y., Sanchez, Y. & Ogura, T. (2000). Flavonoids from *Heterotheca inuloides*: tyrosinase inhibitory activity and structural criteria. *Bioorg. Med. Chem., 8,* 1749-1755.
[281] Choi, M. Y., Song, H. S., Hur, H. S. & Sim, S. S. (2008). Whitening activity of luteolin related to the inhibition of cAMP pathway in alpha-MSH-stimulated B16 melanoma cells. *Arch. Pharm. Res., 31,* 1166-1171.
[282] Roh, J. S., Han, J. Y., Kim, J. H. & Hwang, J. K. (2004). Inhibitory effects of active compounds isolated from safflower (*Carthamus tinctorius* L.) seeds for melanogenesis. *Biol. Pharm. Bull., 27,* 1976-1978.
[283] Fujita, H., Motokawa, T., Katagiri, T., Yokota, S., Yamamoto, A., Himeno, M. & Tanaka, Y. (2009). Inulavosin, a melanogenesis inhibitor, leads to mistargeting of tyrosinase to lysosomes and accelerates its degradation. *J. Invest. Dermatol., 129,* 1489-1499.
[284] Nakashima, S., Matsuda, H., Oda, Y., Nakamura, S., Xu, F. & Yoshikawa, M. (2010). Melanogenesis inhibitors from the desert plant *Anastatica hierochuntica* in B16 melanoma cells. *Bioorg. Med. Chem., 18,* 2337-2345.
[285] Choo, S. J., Ryoo, I. J., Kim, Y. H., Xu, G. H., Kim, W. G., Kim, K. H., Moon, S. J., Son, E. D., Bae, K. & Yoo, I. D. (2009). Silymarin inhibits melanin synthesis in melanocyte cells. *J. Pharm. Pharmacol., 61,* 663-667.
[286] Chiari, M. E., Vera, D. M., Palacios, S. M. & Carpinella, M. C. (2011). Tyrosinase inhibitory activity of a 6-isoprenoid-substituted flavanone isolated from *Dalea elegans*. *Bioorg. Med. Chem., 19,* 3474-3482.
[287] Son, J. K., Park, J. S., Kim, J. A., Kim, Y., Chung, S. R. & Lee, S. H. (2003). Prenylated flavonoids from the roots of *Sophora flavescens* with tyrosinase inhibitory activity. *Planta. Med., 69,* 559-561.
[288] Ryu, Y. B., Westwood, I. M., Kang, N. S., Kim, H. Y., Kim, J. H., Moon, Y. H., & Park, K. H. (2008). Kurarinol, tyrosinase inhibitor isolated from the root of *Sophora flavescens*, *Phytomedicine, 15,* 612-618.
[289] Kim, S. J., Son, K. H., Chang, H. W., Kang, S. S. & Kim, H. P. (2003). Tyrosinase inhibitory prenylated flavonoids from *Sophora flavescens*. *Biol. Pharm. Bull., 26,* 1348-1350.
[290] Ha, T. J., Yang, M. S., Jang, D. S., Choi, S. U. & Park, K. H. (2001). Inhibitory activity of flavanone derivatives isolated from *Sophora flavescens* for melanogenesis. *Bull. Korean. Chem. Soc., 22,* 97-99.
[291] Hyun, S. K., Lee, W. H., Jeong da, M., Kim, Y. & Choi, J. S. (2008). Inhibitory effects of kurarinol, kuraridinol, and trifolirhizin from *Sophora flavescens* on tyrosinase and melanin synthesis. *Biol. Pharm. Bull., 31,* 154-158.
[292] Lo, Y. H., Lin, R. D., Lin, Y. P., Liu, Y. L. & Lee, M. H. (2009). Active constituents from *Sophora japonica* exhibiting cellular tyrosinase inhibition in human epidermal melanocytes. *J. Ethnopharmacol., 124,* 625-629.
[293] Baek, S., Kim, J., Kim, D., Lee, C. & Chung, D. K. (2008). Inhibitory effect of dalbergioidin isolated from the trunk of *Lespedeza cyrtobotrya* on melanin biosynthesis. *J. Microbiol. Biotechnol., 18,* 874-879.

[294] Kim, J. H., Baek, S. H., Kim, D. H., Choi, T. Y., Yoon, T. J., Hwang, J. S., Kim, M. R., Kwon, H. J. & Lee, C. H. (2008). Downregulation of melanin synthesis by haginin A and its application to *in vivo* lightening model. *J. Invest. Dermatol., 128,* 1227-1235.

[295] Kim, H. J., Seo, S. H., Lee, B. G. & Lee, Y. S. (2005). Identification of tyrosinase inhibitors from *Glycyrrhiza uralensis. Planta. Med., 71,* 785-787.

[296] Fu, B., Li, H., Wang, X., Lee, F. S. & Cui, S. (2005). Isolation and identification of flavonoids in licorice and a study of their inhibitory effects on tyrosinase. *J. Agric. Food Chem., 53,* 7408-7414.

[297] Kim, J. H., Kim, M. R., Lee, E. S. & Lee, C. H. (2009). Inhibitory effects of calycosin isolated from the root of *Astragalus membranaceus* on melanin biosynthesis. *Biol. Pharm. Bull., 32,* 264-268.

[298] Lee, M. H., Lin, Y. P., Hsu, F. L., Zhan, G. R. & Yen, K. Y. (2006) Bioactive constituents of *Spatholobus suberectus* in regulating tyrosinase-related proteins and mRNA in HEMn cells. *Phytochemistry, 67,* 1262-1270.

[299] Ko, R. K., Kim, G.O., Hyun, C. G., Jung, D. S. & Lee, N.H. (2011). Compounds with tyrosinase inhibition, elastase inhibition and DPPH radical scavenging activities from the branches of *Distylium racemosum* Sieb. et Zucc. *Phytother. Res.*

[300] Karioti, A., Protopappa, A., Megoulas, N. & Skaltsa, H. (2007). Identification of tyrosinase inhibitors from *Marrubium velutinum* and *Marrubium cylleneum. Bioorg. Med Chem., 15,* 2708-2714.

[301] Kubo, I. & Kinst-Hori, I. (1999). Flavonols from saffron flower: tyrosinase inhibitory activity and inhibition mechanism. *J. Agric. Food Chem., 47,* 4121-4125.

[302] Oozeki, H., Tajima, R. & Nihei, K. (2008). Molecular design of potent tyrosinase inhibitors having the bibenzyl skeleton. *Bioorg. Med. Chem. Lett., 18,* 5252-5254.

[303] Kim, D. H., Kim, J. H., Baek, S. H., Seo, J. H., Kho, Y. H., Oh, T. K. & Lee, C. H. (2004). Enhancement of tyrosinase inhibition of the extract of *Veratrum patulum* using cellulase. *Biotechnol. Bioeng., 87,* 849-854.

[304] Yagi, A., Kanbara, T. & Morinobu, N. (1987). Inhibition of mushroom-tyrosinase by *aloe* extract. *Planta Med., 53,* 515-517.

[305] Wang, Z., Li, X., Yang, Z., He, X., Tu, J. & Zhang, T. (2008). Effects of aloesin on melanogenesis in pigmented skin equivalents. *Int. J. Cosmet. Sci., 30,* 121-130.

[306] Zheng, Z. P., Cheng, K. W., To, J. T., Li, H. & Wang, M. (2008). Isolation of tyrosinase inhibitors from *Artocarpus heterophyllus* and use of its extract as antibrowning agent. *Mol. Nutr. Food Res., 52,* 1530-1538.

[307] Likhitwitayawuid, K., Sritularak, B. & De-Eknamkul, W. (2000). Tyrosinase inhibitors from *Artocarpus gomezianus. Planta Med., 66,* 275-277.

[308] Arung, E. T., Shimizu, K., Tanaka, H. & Kondo, R. (2010). 3-Prenyl luteolin, a new prenylated flavone with melanin biosynthesis inhibitory activity from wood of *Artocarpus heterophyllus. Fitoterapia, 81,* 640-643.

[309] Baek, Y. S., Ryu, Y. B., Curtis-Long, M. J., Ha, T. J., Rengasamy, R., Yang, M. S. & Park, K. H. (2009). Tyrosinase inhibitory effects of 1,3-diphenylpropanes from *Broussonetia kazinoki. Bioorg. Med. Chem., 17,* 35-41.

[310] Shimizu, K., Yasutake, S. & Kondo, R. (2003). A new stilbene with tyrosinase inhibitory activity from *Chlorophora excelsa. Chem. Pharm. Bull. (Tokyo), 51,* 318-319.

[311] Zheng, Z. P., Zhu, Q., Fan, C. L., Tan, H. Y. & Wang, M. (2011). Phenolic tyrosinase inhibitors from the stems of *Cudrania cochinchinensis*. *Food Funct., 2,* 259-264.

[312] Zhang, X., Hu, X., Hou, A. & Wang, H. (2009). Inhibitory effect of 2,4,2',4'-tetrahydroxy-3-(3-methyl-2-butenyl)-chalcone on tyrosinase activity and melanin biosynthesis. *Biol. Pharm. Bull., 32,* 86-90.

[313] Shin, N. H., Ryu, S. Y., Choi, E. J., Kang, S. H., Chang, I. M., Min, K. R. & Kim, Y. (1998). Oxyresveratrol as the potent inhibitor on dopa oxidase activity of mushroom tyrosinase. *Biochem. Biophys. Res. Commun.,243,* 801-803.

[314] Jeong, S. H., Ryu, Y. B., Curtis-Long, M. J., Ryu, H. W., Baek, Y. S., Kang, J. E., Lee, W. S. & Park, K. H. (2009). Tyrosinase inhibitory polyphenols from roots of *Morus lhou*. *J. Agric. Food Chem., 57,* 1195-1203.

[315] Nattapong, S. & Omboon, L. (2008). A new source of whitening agent from a Thai Mulberry plant and its betulinic acid quantitation. *Nat. Prod. Res., 22,* 727-734.

[316] Hanamura, T., Uchida, E. & Aoki, H. (2008). Skin-lightening effect of a polyphenol extract from Acerola (*Malpighia emarginata* DC.) fruit on UV-induced pigmentation. *Biosci. Biotechnol. Biochem., 72,* 3211-3218.

[317] Ding, H. Y., Lin, H. C. & Chang, T. S. (2009). Tyrosinase inhibitors isolated from the roots of *Paeonia suffruticosa*. *J. Cosmet. Sci., 60,* 347-352.

[318] Cheng, K. T., Hsu, F. L., Chen, S. H., Hsieh, P. K., Huang, H. S., Lee, C. K. & Lee, M. H. (2007). New constituent from *Podocarpus macrophyllus* var. *macrophyllus* shows anti-tyrosinase effect and regulates tyrosinase-related proteins and mRNA in human epidermal melanocytes. *Chem. Pharm. Bull. (Tokyo), 55,* 757-761.

[319] Leu, Y. L., Hwang, T. L., Hu, J. W. & Fang, J. Y. (2008). Anthraquinones from *Polygonum cuspidatum* as tyrosinase inhibitors for dermal use. *Phytother. Res., 22,* 552-556.

[320] Miyazawa, M. & Tamura, N. (2007). Inhibitory compound of tyrosinase activity from the sprout of *Polygonum hydropiper* L. (Benitade). *Biol. Pharm. Bull., 30,* 595-597.

[321] Fujii, T. & Saito, M. (2009). Inhibitory effect of quercetin isolated from rose hip (*Rosa canina* L.) against melanogenesis by mouse melanoma cells. *Biosci. Biotechnol. Biochem., 73,* 1989-1993.

[322] Sasaki, K. & Yoshizaki, F. (2002). Nobiletin as a tyrosinase inhibitor from the peel of *Citrus* fruit. *Biol. Pharm. Bull., 25,* 806-808.

[323] Magid, A. A., Voutquenne-Nazabadioko, L., Bontemps, G., Litaudon, M. & Lavaud, C. (2008). Tyrosinase inhibitors and sesquiterpene diglycosides from *Guioa villosa*. *Planta Med., 74,* 55-60.

[324] Momtaz, S., Mapunya, B. M., Houghton, P. J., Edgerly, C., Hussein, A., Naidoo, S. & Lall, N. (2008). Tyrosinase inhibition by extracts and constituents of *Sideroxylon inerme* L. stem bark, used in South Africa for skin lightening. *J. Ethnopharmacol., 119,* 507-512.

[325] Azhar, U. Haq., Malik, A., Khan, M. T., Anwar, U. H., Khan, S. B., Ahmad, A. & Choudhary, M. I. (2006). Tyrosinase inhibitory lignans from the methanol extract of the roots of *Vitex negundo* Linn. and their structure-activity relationship. *Phytomedicine, 13,* 255-260.

[326] Ohguchi, K., Tanaka, T., Iliya, I., Ito, T., Iinuma, M., Matsumoto, K., Akao, Y. & Nozawa, Y. (2003). Gnetol as a potent tyrosinase inhibitor from genus *Gnetum*. *Biosci. Biotechnol. Biochem., 67,* 663-665.

[327] No, J. K., Soung, D. Y., Kim, Y. J., Shim, K. H., Jun, Y. S., Rhee, S. H., Yokozawa, T. & Chung, H. Y. (1999). Inhibition of tyrosinase by green tea components. *Life Sci., 65,* PL241-246.

[328] Choi, S. W., Lee, S. K., Kim, E. O., Oh, J. H., Yoon, K. S., Parris, N., Hicks, K. B. & Moreau, R. A. (2007). Antioxidant and antimelanogenic activities of polyamine conjugates from corn bran and related hydroxycinnamic acids. *J. Agric. Food Chem., 55,* 3920-3925.

[329] Park, J. S., Kim, D. H., Lee, J. K., Lee, J. Y., Kim, D. H., Kim, H. K., Lee, H. J. & Kim, H. C. (2010). Natural ortho-dihydroxyisoflavone derivatives from aged Korean fermented soybean paste as potent tyrosinase and melanin formation inhibitors. *Bioorg. Med. Chem. Lett., 20,* 1162-1164.

[330] Kim, D. C., Rho, S. H., Shin, J. C., Park, H. H. & Kim, D. (2011). Inhibition of melanogenesis by 5,7-dihydroxyflavone (chrysin) via blocking adenylyl cyclase activity. *Biochem. Biophys. Res. Commun., 411,* 121-125.

[331] Sung, J. H., Park, S. H., Seo, D. H., Lee, J. H., Hong, S. W. & Hong, S. S. (2009). Antioxidative and skin-whitening effect of an aqueous extract of *Salicornia herbacea. Biosci. Biotechnol. Biochem., 73,* 552-556.

[332] Cho, Y. H., Kim, J. H., Park, S. M., Lee, B. C., Pyo, H. B. & Park, H. D. (2006). New cosmetic agents for skin whitening from *Angelica dahurica. J. Cosmet Sci., 57,* 11-21.

[333] Kubo, I., Yokokawa, Y. & Kinst-Hori, I. (1988). Tyrosinase inhibitors from cumin. *J. Agric. Food Chem., 46,* 5338-5341.

[334] Lee, K. K. & Choi, J. D. (1999). The effects of *Areca catechu* L extract on anti-inflammation and anti-melanogenesis. *Int. J. Cosmet. Sci., 21,* 275-284.

[335] Behera, B. C., Adawadkar, B. & Makhija, U. (2006). Tyrosinase-inhibitory activity in some species of the lichen family Graphidaceae. *J. Herb Pharmacother., 6,* 55-69.

[336] Luo, L. H., Kim, H. J., Nguyen, D. H., Lee, H. B., Lee, N. H. & Kim, E. K. (2009). Depigmentation of melanocytes by (2Z,8Z)-matricaria acid methyl ester isolated from *Erigeron breviscapus*. *Biol. Pharm Bull., 32,* 1091-1094.

[337] Chang, Y. H., Kim, C., Jung, M., Lim, Y. H., Lee, S. & Kang, S. (2007). Inhibition of melanogenesis by selina-4(14),7(11)-dien-8-one isolated from *Atractylodis Rhizoma* Alba. *Biol. Pharm. Bull., 30,* 719-723.

[338] Choi, H., Ahn, S., Lee, B. G., Chang, I. & Hwang, J. S. (2005). Inhibition of skin pigmentation by an extract of *Lepidium apetalum* and its possible implication in IL-6 mediated signaling. *Pigment Cell Res., 18,* 439-446.

[339] Wu, B., He, S., Wu, X. D. & Pan, Y. J. (2008). New tyrosinase inhibitory sesquiterpenes from *Chloranthus henryi. Chem. Biodivers., 5,* 1298-1303.

[340] Wu, B., Chen, J., Qu, H. & Cheng, Y. (2008). Complex sesquiterpenoids with tyrosinase inhibitory activity from the leaves of *Chloranthus tianmushanensis. J. Nat. Prod., 71.* 877-880.

[341] Khan, M. T., Khan, S. B. & Ather, A. (2006). Tyrosinase inhibitory cycloartane type triterpenoids from the methanol extract of the whole plant of *Amberboa ramosa* Jafri and their structure-activity relationship. *Bioorg Med. Chem., 14,* 938-943.

[342] Choi, J. Y., Choi, E. H., Jung, H. W., Oh, J. S., Lee, W. H., Lee, J. G., Son, J. K., Kim, Y. & Lee, S. H. (2008). Melanogenesis inhibitory compounds from *Saussureae Radix. Arch. Pharm. Res., 31,* 294-299.

[343] Issa, R. A., Afifi, F. U. & Amro, B. I. (2008). Studying the anti-tyrosinase effect of *Arbutus andrachne* L. extracts. *Int. J. Cosmet. Sci., 30,* 271-276.

[344] Masamoto, Y., Ando, H., Murata, Y., Shimoishi, Y., Tada, M. & Takahata, K. (2003). Mushroom tyrosinase inhibitory activity of esculetin isolated from seeds of *Euphorbia lathyris* L. *Biosci. Biotechnol. Biochem., 67,* 631-634.

[345] Sabudak, T., Tareq Hassan Khan, M., Iqbal Choudhary, M. & Oksuz, S. (2006). Potent tyrosinase inhibitors from *Trifolium balansae*. *Nat. Prod. Res., 20,* 665-670.

[346] Baurin, N., Arnoult, E., Scior, T., Do, Q. T. & Bernard, P. (2002). Preliminary screening of some tropical plants for anti-tyrosinase activity. *J. Ethnopharmacol., 82,* 155-158.

[347] Li, C. Y., Lee, E. J. & Wu, T. S. (2004). Antityrosinase principles and constituents of the petals of *Crocus sativus*. *J. Nat. Prod., 67,* 437-440.

[348] Lee, S. E., Kim, M. O., Lee, S. G., Ahn, Y. J. & Lee, H. S. (2000). Inhibitory effects of *Cinnamomum cassia* bark-derived materials on mushroom tyrosinase. *Food Sci. Biotechnol., 9,* 330-333.

[349] Wang, H. M., Chen, C. Y. & Wen, Z. H. (2011). Identifying melanogenesis inhibitors from *Cinnamomum subavenium* with *in vitro* and *in vivo* screening systems by targeting the human tyrosinase. *Exp. Dermatol., 20,* 242-248.

[350] Wang, H. M., Chen, C. Y., Chen, C. Y., Ho, M. L., Chou, Y. T., Chang, H. C., Lee, C. H., Wang, C. Z. & Chu, I. M. (2010). (-)-N-Formylanonaine from *Michelia alba* as a human tyrosinase inhibitor and antioxidant. *Bioorg. Med. Chem., 18,* 5241-5247.

[351] Jang, S. G., Jeon, K. S., Lee, E. H., Kong, W. S. & Cho, J. Y. (2009). Isolation of 1',3'-dilinolenoyl'-2'-linoleoylglycerol with tyrosinase inhibitory activity from *Flammulina velutipes*. *J. Microbiol. Biotechnol., 19,* 681-684.

[352] Chang, L. W., Juang, L. J., Wang, B. S., Wang, M. Y., Tai, H. M., Hung, W. J., Chen, Y. J. & Huang, M. H. (2011). Antioxidant and antityrosinase activity of mulberry (*Morus alba* L.) twigs and root bark. *Food Chem. Toxicol., 49,* 785-790.

[353] Kubo, I. & Kinst-Hori, I. (1999). Tyrosinase inhibitory activity of the olive oil flavor compounds. *J. Agric. Food Chem., 47,* 4574-4578.

[354] Wu, L. C., Chang L. H., Chen, S. H., Fan, N. C. & Ho, J. A. (2009). Antioxidant activity and melanogenesis inhibitory effect of the acetonic extract of *Osmanthus fragrans*: a potential natural and functional food flavor additive. LWT- *Food Sci. Technol., 42,* 1513-1519.

[355] Behera, B. C., Verma, N., Sonone, A. & Makhija, U. (2007). Tissue culture of some lichens and screening of their antioxidant, antityrosinase and antibacterial properties. *Phytother. Res., 21,* 1159-1170.

[356] Kumar, C. M., Sathisha, U. V., Dharmesh, S., Rao, A. G. & Singh, S. A. (2011). Interaction of sesamol (3,4-methylenedioxyphenol) with tyrosinase and its effect on melanin synthesis. *Biochimie., 93,* 562-569.

[357] Sharma, V. K., Choi, J., Sharma, N., Choi, M. & Seo, S. Y. (2004). *In vitro* anti-tyrosinase activity of 5-(hydroxymethyl)-2-furfural isolated from *Dictyophora indusiata*. *Phytother. Res., 18,* 841-844.

[358] Kim, K. S., Kim, J. A., Eom, S. Y., Lee, S. H., Min, K. R. & Kim, Y. (2006). Inhibitory effect of piperlonguminine on melanin production in melanoma B16 cell line by downregulation of tyrosinase expression. *Pigment Cell Res., 19,* 90-98.

[359] Masuda, T., Odaka, Y., Ogawa, N., Nakamoto, K. & Kuninaga, H. (2008). Identification of geranic acid, a tyrosinase inhibitor in lemongrass (*Cymbopogon citratus*). *J. Agric. Food Chem., 56,* 597-601.

[360] Silveira, J. E., Pereda Mdel, C., Eberlin, S., Dieamant, G. C. & Di Stasi, L. C. (2008). Effects of *Coccoloba uvifera* L. on UV-stimulated melanocytes. *Photodermatol. Photoimmunol. Photomed., 24,* 308-313.

[361] Chien, C. C., Tsai, M. L., Chen, C. C., Chang, S. J. & Tseng, C. H. (2008). Effects on tyrosinase activity by the extracts of *Ganoderma lucidum* and related mushrooms. *Mycopathologia., 166,* 117-120.

[362] Jang, J. Y., Lee, J. H., Kang, B. W., Chung, K. T., Choi, Y. H. & Choi, B. T. (2009). Dichloromethane fraction of *Cimicifuga heracleifolia* decreases the level of melanin synthesis by activating the ERK or AKT signaling pathway in B16F10 cells. *Exp. Dermatol., 18,* 232-237.

[363] Itoh, K., Hirata, N., Masuda, M., Naruto, S., Murata, K., Wakabayashi, K. & Matsuda, H. (2009). Inhibitory effects of *Citrus hassaku* extract and its flavanone glycosides on melanogenesis. *Biol. Pharm. Bull., 32,* 410-415.

[364] Rangkadilok, N., Sitthimonchai, S., Worasuttayangkurn, L., Mahidol, C., Ruchirawat, M. & Satayavivad, J. (2007). Evaluation of free radical scavenging and antityrosinase activities of standardized longan fruit extract. *Food Chem. Toxicol., 45,* 328-336.

[365] Oh, E. Y., Jang, J. Y., Choi, Y. H., Choi, Y. W. & Choi, B. T. (2010). Inhibitory effects of 1-O-methyl-fructofuranose from *Schisandra chinensis* fruit on melanogenesis in B16F0 melanoma cells. *J .Ethnopharmacol., 132,* 219-224.

[366] Husni, A., Jeon, J. S., Um, B. H., Han, N. S. & Chung, D. (2011). Tyrosinase inhibition by water and ethanol extracts of a far eastern sea cucumber, *Stichopus japonicus*. *J. Sci. Food Agric., 91,* 1541-1547.

[367] Villareal, M. O., Han, J., Yamada, P., Shigemori, H. & Isoda, H. (2010). Hirseins inhibit melanogenesis by regulating the gene expressions of Mitf and melanogenesis enzymes. *Exp. Dermatol., 19,* 450-457.

[368] Goetghebeur, M. & Kermasha, S. (1996). Inhibition of polyphenol oxidase by copper-metallothionein from *Aspergillus niger*. *Phytochemistry, 42,* 935-940.

[369] Piao, X. L., Baek, S. H., Park, M. K. & Park, J. H. (2004). Tyrosinase-inhibitory furanocoumarin from *Angelica dahurica*. *Biol. Pharm. Bull., 27,* 1144-1146.

[370] Panich, U., Kongtaphan, K., Onkoksoong, T., Jaemsak, K., Phadungrakwittaya, R., Thaworn, A., Akarasereenont, P., & Wongkajornsilp, A. (2010). Modulation of antioxidant defense by *Alpinia galanga* and *Curcuma aromatica* extracts correlates with their inhibition of UVA-induced melanogenesis. *Cell Biol. Toxicol., 26,* 103-116.

[371] Jang, J. Y., Lee, J. H., Jeong, S. Y., Chung, K. T., Choi, Y. H. & Choi, B. T. (2009). Partially purified *Curcuma longa* inhibits alpha-melanocyte-stimulating hormone-stimulated melanogenesis through extracellular signal-regulated kinase or Akt activation-mediated signalling in B16F10 cells. *Exp. Dermatol., 18,* 689-694.

[372] Jeon, H. J., Noda, M., Maruyama, M., Matoba, Y., Kumagai, T. & Sugiyama, M. (2006). Identification and kinetic study of tyrosinase inhibitors found in sake lees. *J. Agric. Food Chem., 54,* 9827-9833.

[373] Wang, B. S., Chang L.W., Wu H. C., Huang S. L., Chu H. L. & Huang M. H. (2011). Antioxidant and antityrosinase activity of aqueous extracts of green asparagus. *Food Chem., 127,* 141-146.

[374] Pinon, A., Limami, Y., Micallef, L., Cook-Moreau, J., Liagre, B., Delage, C., Duval, R. E. & Simon, A. (2011). A novel form of melanoma apoptosis resistance: melanogenesis up-regulation in apoptotic B16-F0 cells delays ursolic acid-triggered cell death. *Exp. Cell Res., 317,* 1669-1676.

[375] Ye, Y., Chu, J. H., Wang, H., Xu, H., Chou, G. X., Leung, A. K., Fong, W. F. & Yu, Z. L. (2010). Involvement of p38 MAPK signaling pathway in the anti-melanogenic effect of San-bai-tang, a Chinese herbal formula, in B16 cells. *J. Ethnopharmacol., 132,* 533-535.

[376] Minwalla, L., Zhao, Y., Cornelius, J., Babcock, G. F., Wickett, R. R., Le Poole, I. C. & Boissy, R. E. (2001). Inhibition of melanosome transfer from melanocytes to keratinocytes by lectins and neoglycoproteins in an *in vitro* model system., *Pigment Cell Res., 14,* 185-194.

[377] Brenner, M. & Hearing, V. J. (2008). Modifying skin pigmentation–approaches through intrinsic biochemistry and exogenous agents. *Drug Discov. Today Dis. Mech., 5,* 189-199.

[378] Akihisa, T., Noto, T., Takahashi, A., Fujita, Y., Banno, N., Tokuda, H., Koike, K., Suzuki, T., Yasukawa, K. & Kimura, Y. (2009). Melanogenesis inhibitory, anti-inflammatory, and chemopreventive effects of limonoids from the seeds of *Azadirachta indicia* A. Juss. (neem). *J. Oleo. Sci., 58,* 581-594.

[379] Yokota, T., Nishio, H., Kubota, Y. & Mizoguchi, M. (1998). The inhibitory effect of glabridin from licorice extracts on melanogenesis and inflammation. *Pigment Cell Res., 11,* 355-361.

[380] Kim, Y. J., Kang, K. S. & Yokozawa, T. (2008). The anti-melanogenic effect of pycnogenol by its anti-oxidative actions. *Food Chem. Toxicol., 46,* 2466-2471.

[381] Heo, S. J., Ko, S. C., Cha, S. H., Kang, D. H., Park, H. S., Choi, Y. U., Kim, D., Jung, W. K. & Jeon, Y. J. (2009). Effect of phlorotannins isolated from *Ecklonia cava* on melanogenesis and their protective effect against photo-oxidative stress induced by UV-B radiation. *Toxicol. Vitro, 23,* 1123-1130.

[382] Heo, S. J., Ko, S. C., Kang, S. M., Cha, S. H., Lee, S. H., Kang, D. H., Jung, W. K., Affan, A., Oh, C. & Jeon, Y. J. (2010). Inhibitory effect of diphlorethohydroxycarmalol on melanogenesis and its protective effect against UV-B radiation-induced cell damage. *Food Chem. Toxicol., 48,* 1355-1361.

[383] Huang, H. C., Chiu, S. H. & Chang, T. M. (2011). Inhibitory Effect of [6]-Gingerol on Melanogenesis in B16F10 Melanoma Cells and a Possible Mechanism of Action. *Biosci. Biotechnol. Biochem., 75,* 1067-1072.

[384] Hamed, S. H., Sriwiriyanont, P., de Long, M. A., Visscher, M. O., Wickett, R. R. & Boissy, R. E. (2006). Comparative efficacy and safety of deoxyarbutin, a new tyrosinase-inhibiting agent. *J. Cosmet. Sci., 57,* 291-308.

[385] Miyamoto, K., Takiwaki, H., Hillebrand, G. G. & Arase, S. (2002). Utilization of a high-resolution digital imaging system for the objective and quantitative assessment of hyperpigmented spots on the face. *Skin Res. Technol., 8,* 73-77.

[386] Kasai, K., Yoshimura, M., Koga, T., Arii, M. & Kawasaki, S. (2006). Effects of oral administration of ellagic acid-rich pomegranate extract on ultraviolet-induced pigmentation in the human skin. *J. Nutr. Sci. Vitaminol. (Tokyo), 52,* 383-388.

[387] Ertam, I., Mutlu, B., Unal, I., Alper, S., Kivcak, B. & Ozer, O. (2008). Efficiency of ellagic acid and arbutin in melasma: a randomized, prospective, open-label study. *J. Dermatol., 35,* 570-574.

[388] Mafune, E., Morimoto, Y. & Iizuka, Y. (2008). Tranexamic acid and melasma. *Farumashia., 44,* 437-442.

In: Melanin: Biosynthesis, Functions and Health Effects ISBN: 978-1-62100-991-7
Editors: Xiao-Peng Ma and Xiao-Xiao Sun

Chapter II

Fungal Melanins: Biosynthesis and Biological Functions

Rodrigo Almeida-Paes[1], Joshua Daniel Nosanchuk[2] and Rosely Maria Zancope-Oliveira[1]

[1] Laboratorio de Micologia, Instituto de Pesquisa Clínica Evandro Chagas, Fundação Oswaldo Cruz, Rio de Janeiro, Brazil

[2] Department of Medicine (Division of Infectious Diseases) and Department of Microbiology and Immunology, Albert Einstein College of Medicine, Bronx, NY, US

Abstract

Melanins are hydrophobic polymers of high molecular weight, formed by oxidative polymerization of phenolic and indolic compounds, produced by organisms in all Kingdoms. They are typically black or dark brown in color and their molecular structures are diverse. Several fungi can produce melanins and the functions of this pigment enhance microbial survival under diverse unfavorable environmental and host conditions. The major melanin type encountered among fungi is the 1,8-dihydroxynaphthalene (DHN) melanin that is synthesized from acetyl-coenzyme A via the polyketide pathway. This melanin is generated by several human pathogenic fungi, such as *Fonsecaea pedrosoi*, *Exophialla dermatitidis*, *Aspergillus fumigatus*, *Histoplasma capsulatum* and *Sporothrix schenckii*. It is also present in phytopathogenic fungi such as *Colletotrichum* spp., *Magnaporte orizae* and *Ascochyta rabiei*. In addition to DHN melanin, fungi can also produce melanin via dihydroxyphenylalanine (DOPA), in which tyrosinases or laccases hydroxylate tyrosine via DOPA to dopaquinone that then auto-oxidizes and polymerizes, resulting in a polyphenolic heteropolymer of black color known as eumelanin. *Cryptococcus neoformans* is the best known fungus to produce this type of melanin, but other fungi such as *Candida albicans*, *Paracoccidioides brasiliensis* and *S. schenckii* can also produce eumelanin. A type of soluble fungal melanin is produced from L-tyrosine through *p*-hydroxyphenylpyruvate and homogentisic acid. This pigment is called pyomelanin and it is similar to alkaptomelanin produced by humans. *A. fumigatus*, *Madurella mycetomatis* and *Yarrowia lipolytica* are examples of fungi that can produce this type of pigment. Fungal melanins play an important role in the protection of fungi from several environmental stresses, such as desiccation, UV irradiation, heavy metals, temperature fluctuation and digestion by hydrolytic enzymes. Melanins also play a role in the virulence of a broad range of pathogenic fungi. These pigments protect the fungi from host defense mechanisms and antifungal agents. Although melanins challenge the immunological strategies of host defense, they are also targets for alternative antimicrobial strategies, by the use of antibodies against melanin or inhibitors of melanin synthesis.

Introduction

Melanins are ubiquitous pigments produced by a broad range of living organisms from bacteria to humans [1, 2]. They are typically dark brown or black in color [3] and have a high molecular weight [4]. Melanins are synthesized by several pathways, all converging on the oxidative polymerization of phenolic or indolic compounds [5, 6]. Some of physical and chemical properties of melanins include a negative charge, hydrophobicity and insolubility in both aqueous and organic solvents [7].

To date, no definitive structure has been found for any type of melanin because of their insolubility, which makes studies on melanins very difficult [2, 6]. In general, fungal melanins are studied after digestion of cells with glycolitic and proteolytic enzymes followed by extraction with guanidinium isothiocyanate and hot concentrated acid (hydrochloric acid 6N). This treatment yields dark particles retaining the original cellular shape, but devoid of cytoplasm or organelles, and are referred to as melanin ghosts [8].

Structurally, melanins appear to represent a mixture of high molecular weight polymers and this structure makes them very stable and resistant to several destructive physicochemical processes such as oxidant agents, desiccation, extreme temperatures, UV light, heavy metals and other drugs [6, 9]. Electron spin resonance (ESR) characteristics have been used to define pigments with stable organic free radicals as melanins [2]. This technique generates distinctive signals (Figure 1) due to the presence of unpaired electrons in the polymer [10].

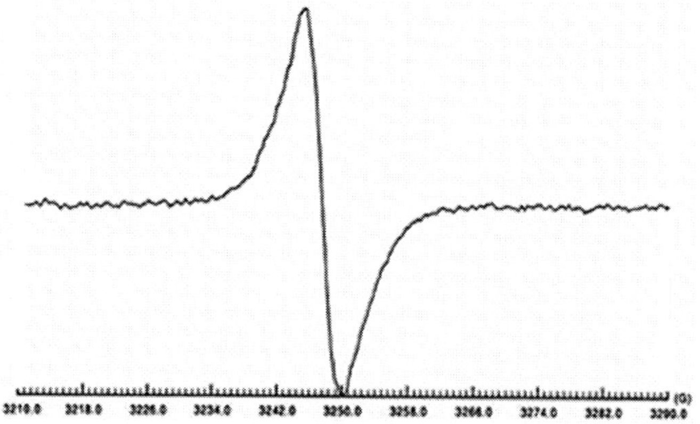

Figure 1. Electron spin resonance analysis of melanin particles generated from a representative *S. schenckii* strain IPEC 26449 on its yeast phase, cultured in minimal medium (15 mM glucose, 10 mM $MgSO_4$, 29.4 mM K_2HPO_4, 13 mM glycine, and 3.0 mM thiamine, pH 5.5) with 1 mM L-3,4-dihydroxyphenylalanine at 37°C during 10 days.

Many fungi are able to synthesize melanin through different pathways, and functions of this pigment are related to survival under diverse environmental and host conditions [1, 5]. This chapter will focus on the pathways used by different fungi to produce these dark pigments, and also on their biological function on the fungi and implications for their hosts.

Types and Biosynthesis of Fungal Melanins

Various types of melanin can be found in nature. The major type of melanin found within the Kingdom Fungi is the 1,8-dihydroxynapthalene (DHN) melanin synthesized from acetyl-coenzyme A (CoA) or malonyl-CoA via the polyketide pathway [9, 11]. Fungal polyketides are synthesized by a process similar to fatty acid biosynthesis.

The biosynthesis of this type of melanin (Figure 2) begins with the conversion of malonyl-CoA into 1,3,6,8-tetrahydroxynaphtalene (THN) by the enzyme polyketide synthase.

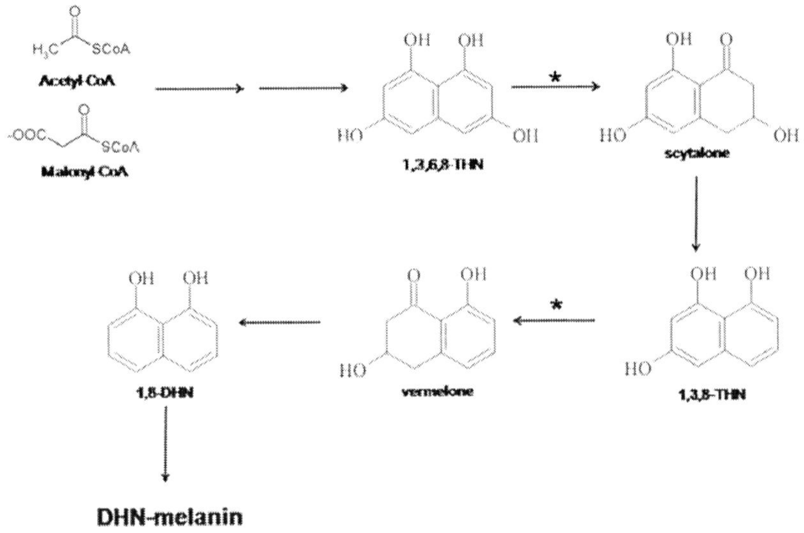

Figure 2. General biosynthetic pathway of fungal DHN melanin. Acetyl- and/or malonyl-CoA are converted by at least two enzymatic steps to 1,3,6,8-THN that after two reductions and two dehydration enzymatic reactions is converted to the 1,8-DHN precursor of melanin synthesis. The reduction steps marked with * can be blocked with tricyclazole.

Then, by successive steps of reduction and dehydration, this compound is converted to 1,8-DHN. Subsequent steps are thought to involve a dimerization of the 1,8-DHN molecules, which are finally polymerized by a fungal laccase to form the DHN melanin [11-13].

This metabolic pathway can be inhibited by the commercialized inhibitors tricyclazole (Figure 3) and fenoxanil [13, 14]. It is important to note that, since the biosynthesis of this type of melanin starts with the product of essential metabolic pathways such as glycolysis and the pentose phosphate pathway, DHN melanin can be synthesized without the presence of any precursor.

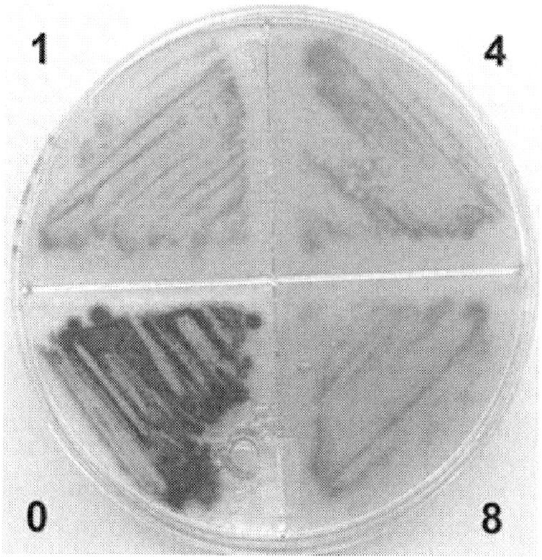

Figure 3. Influence of tricyclazole on melanization of a representative *S. schenckii* strain, IPEC 26449. Numbers indicate concentration (mg/L) of tricyclazole on cultures. Ethanol (the tricyclazole diluents) concentration was 0.6% on all media.

Other types of fungal melanins are synthesized only if a specific precursor is present during fungal growth. The most common precursor for fungal melanin synthesis is L-tyrosine. In fact, two types of melanin can be formed with this amino acid. Many fungi are able to synthesize black or dark- brown pigments from L-tyrosine via dihydroxyphenylalanine (DOPA).

The pathway for this type of melanin (Figure 4), called eumelanin, requires that tyrosinases or laccases hydroxylate tyrosine via DOPA to dopaquinone.

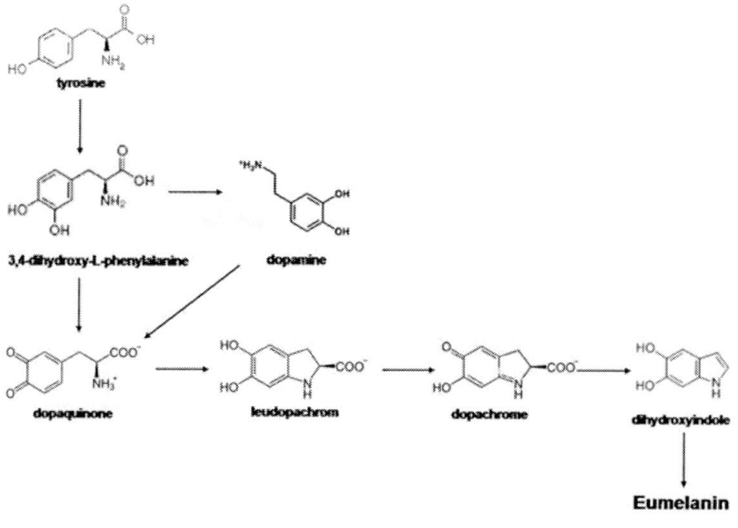

Figure 4. General biosynthetic pathway of fungal eumelanins. In this pathway, tyrosine is converted to L-DOPA and this compound to dopaquinone directly or via dopamine. Dopaquinone is converted via other intermediates to dihydroxyindole that oxidates and polymerizates to generate melanin.

Then, after a series of cyclyzation, oxidation, tautomerization and polymerization reactions, eumelanin is produced [11].

Other fungi, however, have the ability to produce brown pigments from tyrosine in a pathway leading to the accumulation and auto-oxidation of intermediates of tyrosine catabolism [15, 16]. This fungal pigment, known as pyomelanin, is similar to the human pigment alkaptomelanin.

Actually, pyomelanin and alkaptomelanin are considered different designations for the same pigment [16]. In general, homogentisic acid is the accumulated product of tyrosine catabolism (Figure 5) that, after oxidation in benzoquinoacetate and polymerization, leads to the production of pyomelanin.

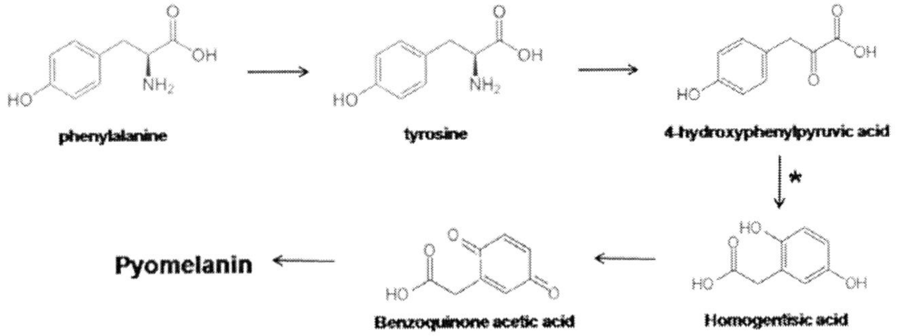

Figure 5. General biosynthetic pathway of fungal pyomelanins. Phenylalanine and tyrosine catabolisms generate homogentisic acid that can lead to the production of pyomelanin through benzoquinone acetic acid after oxidation and polymerization. The step marked with * can be blocked with sulcotrione.

It is important to note that all biosynthesis models presented are general in nature, and the pathways may vary slightly from fungus to fungus. Fungi can also produce other types of melanin, such as allomelanins, nitrogen-free macromolecular polymers of simple phenols, which have not been related to fungal virulence. The remainder of this chapter will focus on the major human fungal pathogens and also on some plant pathogens, emphasizing the importance of melanins for the fungus-host interactions and also on their implications for human health.

Melanized Fungi

Cryptococcus neoformans

Cryptococcus neoformans is a free-living ubiquitous yeast-like organism with a characteristic polysaccharide capsule that can survive in a variety of environmental niches such as soils contaminated with avian excreta and certain tree species [17-19].

This fungus and the closely related species, *Cryptococcus gattii*, cause cryptococcosis, a disease that is relatively common in individuals with suppression of the cellular immune system, but can also affect immunocompetent individuals.

The major complication of this disease is a life-threatening meningoencephalitis [20]. *C. neoformans* and *C. gattii* differ in biochemical, molecular characteristics, ecology and geographic distribution [21], though melanization properties are similar between these two species [22, 23].

C. neoformans is the most studied fungus in terms of melanization, with more than 210 published references in this field up to June 2011. Melanization was identified in this organism as early as 1962 [4]. This fungus is unable to synthesize DHN-melanin and, therefore, is incapable of *de novo* melanogenesis, relying on the presence of phenolic compounds, such as L-DOPA (Figure 6), for making eumelanin [4, 24].

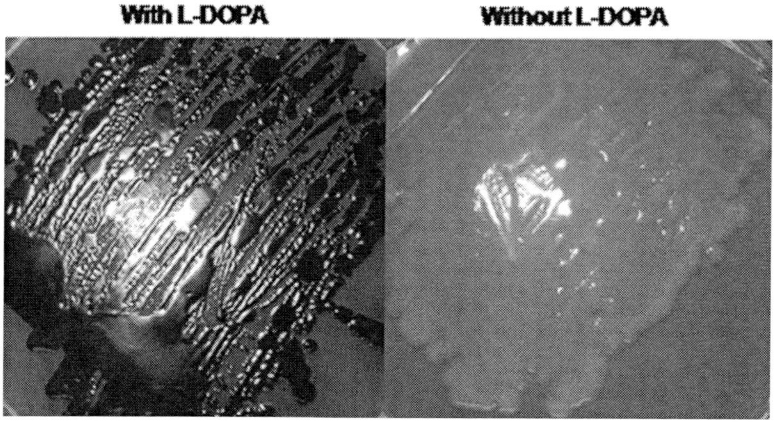

Figure 6. *Cryptococcus neoformans* [strain ATCC 24607 (serotype D)] produces a melanized phenotype when cultured in minimal medium with L-DOPA (left) and an albino phenotype when cultured in absence of L-DOPA (right). All cultures were maintained at 30°C during 14 days in the dark.

This particular feature can be utilized in the diagnosis of cryptococcosis, because when *C. neoformans* is cultured in media such as Staib Agar, rich in phenolic compounds, yeast colonies grow dark-brown whereas other pathogenic yeast produce white colonies [25, 26].

Over the past decade, researchers have advanced the concept that virulence and other aspects associated with the relationship between certain fungi and mammalian host originated from interactions between fungal cells and environmental organisms, such as bacteria, protozoan and also nematodes [27-30]. For instance, *C. neoformans* can survive and replicate within macrophages in a manner similar to that within amoebae [30]. Furthermore, the interaction between *C. neoformans* and the gram-negative bacterium *Klebsiella aerogenes* results in fungal melanization [22]. Also, *C. neoformans* is able to produce melanin using the bacterial melanin precursor homogentisic acid in a laccase dependent way [23]. The generation of pigment from bacterial products may in part explain the fact that this yeast is melanized in the environment [31, 32], since this microbe produces melanin only from exogenous substrates. As *C. neoformans* is a free-living organism that does not require mammalian parasitism in its life cycle, melanization would protect this fungus primarily from disadvantageous environmental conditions. In fact, melanization protects *C. neoformans* from enzymatic degradation by antagonist microbes in the environment [33] and by damage from UV light [34] as well as heat and cold [35].

Melanin production, as well as capsule growth (another important virulence factor of *C. neoformans*), is regulated by a G-α protein-cAMP-PKA (cAMP-dependent protein kinase A) signaling pathway [36]. Melanin is produced when a laccase of 75-kDa encoded by the *CNLAC1* gene catalyzes the oxidation of L-DOPA or dopamine to quinones, which then polymerizes to form melanin [37]. This fungus also possesses another laccase-encoding gene, *CNLAC2*, whose transcript is a 65-kDa laccase that is also associated with melanogenesis [38]. *C. neoformans* L-DOPA melanin is very similar to mammalian DOPA melanin, but the cryptococcal melanin does not contain any phaeomelanin, a thiol containing melanin type derived from tyrosine and cysteine, that is also present in mammalian melanin [11]. It is important to note that some fungi are able to synthesize eumelanin from tyrosine, but the *C. neoformans* laccase is considered a diphenol oxidase, since it produces pigment from phenolic compounds with two hydroxyl groups but not from tyrosine [39]. Some of the substrates used by *C. neoformans* laccase include L- and D-DOPA, methyl-DOPA, catechol, dopamine and norepinephrine [8, 40, 41].

In *C. neoformans*, melanin is deposited in a layer internal to the fungal cell wall, next to the plasma membrane [24, 42]. The current model for melanin synthesis is that the pigment is formed in vesicles that are secreted and retained by the chitin cell wall [43], generating a structure comprised of several layers of granular particles. Melanin porosity is a property of the assembly of these particles, with absence of specialized pore structures for nutrient acquisition. Small nutrient molecules, such as sugars and amino acids, can enter the cell by passing through the spaces between the melanin particles [42]. During asexual reproduction, melanin in the parent cell is not carried to the daughter cells, but rather is synthesized *de novo* in buds. Hence, melanin remodeling occurs during fungal cell growth in a process requiring degradation and synthesis at sites of budding [44].

Melanin is synthesized during mammalian *C. neoformans* infection [45, 46] and this black pigment is highly associated with *C. neoformans* virulence. In fact, amelanotic *C. neoformans* mutant strains are severely attenuated in animal models of infection [24, 28]. Cryptococcal melanin also impacts diverse host responses. Cryptococcal melanin is immunogenic. For instance, it activates the alternative complement pathway [47], and also elicits antibodies, some of which can inhibit fungal growth [48, 49]. It is noteworthy that monoclonal antibodies (mAbs) have been generated to cryptococcal melanin [45] that are reactive against a wide spectrum of melanin types [4]. Moreover, melanization is associated with lowered levels of pro-inflammatory cytokines in animal models of infection [50]. Melanization decreases the rate of phagocytosis and killing of *C. neoformans* by macrophages [24], probably because melanized *C. neoformans* cells are less susceptible than nonmelanized cells to the fungicidal effects of nitrogen- and oxygen-derived oxidants [51]. Melanin also down regulates immune responses early in infection [50]. Together, these studies indicate that melanin in *C. neoformans* increases virulence by reducing its susceptibility to host defense mechanisms and interfering with the development of successful immune responses [1, 4, 7, 32].

In addition to increasing resistance of *C. neoformans* to immune defenses, melanin also reduces the efficacy of certain antifungal drugs, such as amphotericin B and caspofungin [52-54].

Thus, melanization has clinical implications for *C. neoformans* infections in terms of the alteration in immunologic responses and the interference with the potency of antifungal drugs.

However, the pigment is also a potential drug target, either by antibody binding to melanin [49] or by disruption of the melanization pathway [55].

Members of the Order Chaetothyriales

The Order *Chaetothyriales* is composed by fungi with dark mycelium [56]. The dark coloration of the mycelium (Figure 7) is due to the production of melanin.

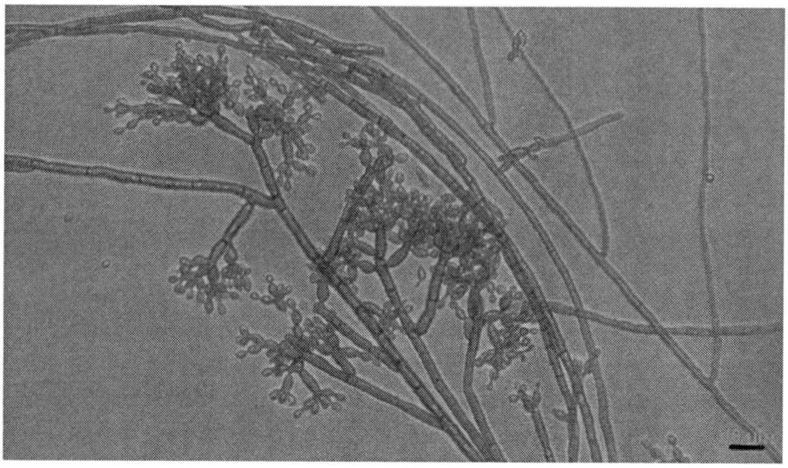

Figure 7. *Fonsecaea pedrosoi*, a member of the Order *Chaetothyriales*. Note the dark pigment (melanin) on the cell walls of hyphae, conidiophores and conidia. Bar 10μm.

These fungi generally contain DHN melanin [56], although melanin derived from L-DOPA has also been described in *Exophiala dermatitidis* [57]. Additional studies are necessary to access whether or not other members of *Chaetothyriales* produce other types of melanin. Melanin is an important factor associated with virulence of some members of this order, however the presence of melanin alone is not sufficient to explain the pathogenicity of these fungi, and additional factors, such as thermotolerance, must be involved in the pathogenesis of disease [58]. This order contains several species of medical importance, mainly *Fonsecaea pedrosoi* and *E. dermatitidis*.

Fonsecaea pedrosoi

Fonsecaea pedrosoi is the main agent of chromoblastomycosis, an important subcutaneous mycosis that is endemic worldwide although its prevalence is higher in tropical countries. The disease begins with the traumatic inoculation of pigmented moulds into the skin, and the most important species are *F. pedrosoi*, *Phialophora verrucosa* and *Cladophialophora carrionii*. Even though chromoblastomycosis is typically not fatal, it is characteristically chronic, extremely difficult to treat, and it can be complicated by lymphatic damage and neoplastic transformation [59]. This disease is characterized by the presence of muriform sclerotic bodies in tissue [60]. *F. pedrosoi* produces olivaceous to black mycelia colonies that under microscopic analysis present conidia formed from swollen denticles, giving rise to secondary and tertiary conidia; conidia may be also formed on sympodial conidiophores and occasionally from discrete phialides [56].

Inhibition of melanin synthesis with tricyclazole [61, 62] together with *de novo* melanogenesis [63, 64] confirms that *F. pedrosoi* synthesizes DHN melanin. The fungus is able to synthesize melanin on hyphae, conidia and sclerotic bodies [62, 63]. Constituents of melanin from *F. pedrosoi* comprise aromatic, aliphatic and glycosidic structures with a predominance of the latter [63]. Both extracellular and cell-wall associated melanin [62, 65, 66] are produced inside melanosome-like compartments associated with Ca^{2+} and Fe^{2+} [67]. The dispersed melanin over the fungal cell-wall is thought to have a valuable role in cross-linking distinct cell wall compounds that help maintain the normal shape of the cell [62].

Melanin from *F. pedrosoi* is immunologically active. It can elicit a humoral immune response, giving rise to human antifungal antibodies that can impair fungal growth *in vitro* and enhance the antifungal functions of phagocytes [64]. Melanin can influence the complement system activation by the alternative pathway [68]. Moreover, it has the ability to interact with immune system cells. Some studies have shown that *F. pedrosoi* melanin inhibits nitric oxide production by macrophages [69, 70] and that melanized cells are more resistant to phagocytosis [61, 65]. On the other hand, soluble melanin leads to high levels of fungal internalization by macrophages associated with an enhanced oxidative burst [64]. Thus, there are different effects of soluble and cell-wall associated melanin in *F. pedrosoi.*

Another role for the cell-wall associated melanin in *F. pedrosoi* is the reduction of specific antibody recognition. In fact, melanin masks cerebroside recognition by antibodies, conferring resistance of sclerotic cells to the antimicrobial effects of antibodies to monohexosylceramides [71]. Together, these results show a diverse role for melanin on chromoblastomycosis due to *F. pedrosoi.*

Exophiala dermatitidis

Species within the genus *Exophiala* are frequently referred to as black yeasts, due to the ability of several species to form budding yeast-like cells in addition to hyphal forms during their life cycle. *Exophiala (Wangiella) dermatitidis* is phenotypically characterized by its mucoid colonies, an ability to grow at 40°C, and a lack of nitrate assimilation as well as forming yeast cells surrounded by capsules [56]. This species causes phaeohyphomycosis and it is of particular concern as an agent of brain infections in patients from East Asia [58]. This fungus has previously been known as *Wangiella dermatitidis*, however according to a recent revision about dematiaceous fungi, this is an obsolete name [56].

The first DHN-melanin pathway in a pathogenic fungus was described for *E. dermatitidis* [72]. A polyketide synthase encoded by the gene *WdPKS1* catalyses the reactions on the first steps of the pathway [14, 73]. Detailed new molecular approaches show that *E. dermatitidis* produces DHN melanin in a pathway that requires hexaketide 2-acetyl-1,3,6,8-tetrahydroxynaphtalene as a precursor of THN [74]. These results show that, despite the high degree of similarity among fungal polyketide synthases, they have different ways to produce the necessary precursors for melanin synthesis.

In this fungus, melanin is polymerized exclusively on the fungal cell wall, and an effective chitin synthase gene is necessary for the correct deposition of the pigment [75]. Also, albino mutant strains of *E. dermatitidis* present thinner cell-walls compared to the wild type [57]. Melanin biosynthesis does not affect cell wall permeability. However, melanin affects the development of *E. dermatitidis* within the host as it is associated with invasion of the fungus *in vitro* and *in vivo* [76].

Several approaches have been used to successfully correlate melanin and virulence in *E. dermatitidis*. Initially, wild type and UV generated melanin-deficient mutant strains were used in mouse studies. These melanin deficient mutants were significantly less virulent than the wild type, with a few hyphae observed in brains of mice infected with amelanotic strains [77-79].

The molecular cloning and characterization of the *WdPKS1* gene revealed the importance of melanin synthesis during a mouse model of infection [73], probably because of its protective effects against antifungal agents [57]. Interestingly, melanin did not influence phagocytosis, but the presence of melanin protected *E. dermatitidis* from killing within the phagolysosome of neutrophils [80]. Additionally, melanin deposition on the cell wall protects this fungus from environmental stresses, such as lysing enzymes, heat and cold [57].

Treatment of phaeohyphomycosis, especially cerebral cases, is difficult, and needs early diagnosis and aggressive therapy [81]. Studies on antifungal susceptibility using UV generated melanin-deficient mutants and an agar dilution technique showed that only for itraconazole the minimum inhibitory concentration (MIC) for mutant strains was lower than for the wild type, with MICs for fluconazole, amphotericin B, amorolfine, flucytosine, terbinafine and ketoconazole being similar for melanized and non-melanized strains [82].

On the other hand, another study using a molecular approach to knock-out the *WdPKS1* gene determined by time-kill assays that melanin protects *E. dermatitidis* from amphotericin B and voriconazole [57].

Dimorphic Fungi

Dimorphic fungi comprise a special group of microbes that can reproduce in either a mycelial or a yeast-like state. Usually the mycelial saprotrophic form is present at 25°C, and the yeast-like or spherule pathogenic form is found at 37°C.

Several dimorphic fungi are also pathogenic for humans and other mammals and can cause diseases like sporotrichosis, histoplasmosis, paracoccidioidomycosis, blastomycosis, coccidioidomycosis and penicilliosis.

Sporothrix schenckii

Sporothrix schenckii in its saprophytic stage or when cultured at 25ºC is composed of hyaline, septate hyphae with conidiogenous cells arising from the undifferentiated hyphae that form conidia in groups of small, clustered denticles. Often, brown thick-walled conidia arise alongside the hyphae. Macroscopically filamentous colonies are smooth and wrinkled, white to creamy at first, but turn into brown to black after a few days, after the dematiaceous conidia are produced. This fungus is evident in both human and animal tissue as budding cigar shaped yeasts causing sporotrichosis, a subcutaneous mycosis commonly acquired by traumatic implantation of the fungus into the skin [83]. Recently, *S. schenckii* was found to be a complex of species that have morphological, physiological and molecular differences. The new described species are *Sporothrix brasiliensis*, *Sporothrix mexicana*, *Sporothrix globosa* and *Sporothrix luriei* [84, 85].

Both morphological forms of *S. schenckii* have the ability to synthesize melanin. Melanin production on *S. schenckii* dematiaceous conidia occurs through the DHN pathway [86]. Macroscopicaly, only the mycelial phase of the fungus is melanized, however melanin production on yeast cells has been demonstrated *in vitro* and during infection [87]. Recently, our group has shown that *S. schenckii* can also produce melanin, both on filamentous and yeast forms, using phenolic compounds such as L-DOPA as a precursor. Of particular interest is that on the fungal filamentous form, only conidia form melanin by the DHN pathway.

Nevertheless, if L-DOPA is accessible during fungal growth, hyphae can be melanized as well (Figure 8) [88].

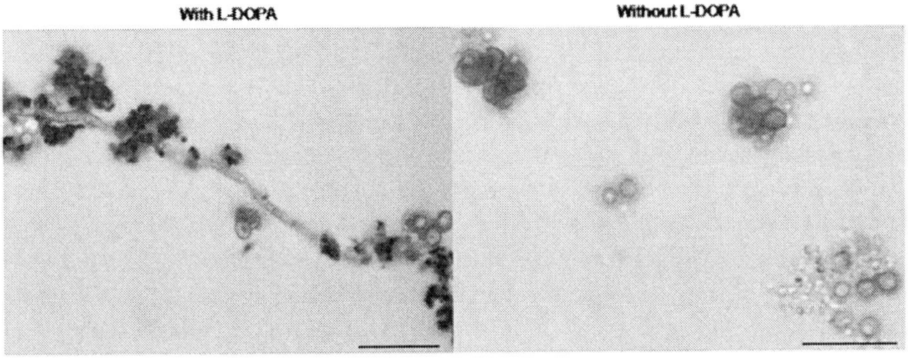

Figure 8. Melanin particles of mycelial forms of *Sporothrix schenckii* strain IPEC 18782A grown on minimal medium with (left) and without (right) L-DOPA. Bars, 10μm.

Melanization of *S. schenckii* has been proposed as a virulence characteristic originating in response to interactions with environmental predators. Yeast cells of *S. schenckii* when ingested by *Acantamoeba castellanii*, a free-living soil amoeba, are able to survive within the protozoan after ingestion, and are capable of killing the amoeba and using it as a source of nutrients. This behavior is not shared by pathogenic fungi that do not have the soil as habitat, such as *Candida albicans* or by non primary pathogenic fungi such as the yeast *Saccharomyces cerevisiae* [29].

In view of the fact that *S. schenckii* is a soil-habiting fungus that does not require host parasitism to complete its life cycle, fungal melanization must also play an important role for survival in response to unfavorable environmental conditions, since the fungus is mycelial in nature [87].

Environmental sources that enhance melanization might promote this virulence factor, contributing to the success of possible encounters between the organism and a host [89]. *In vitro* studies show that the melanization process in *S. schenckii* can be enhanced by several factors such as temperature, pH and nutrient conditions [88]. Moreover, similar culture media from different suppliers can yield differences in melanization within a single *S. schenckii* strain [90].

Conidial melanization enhances their resistance to phagocytosis by macrophages [86]. Melanization also has a role in the pathogenesis of cutaneous sporotrichosis, since pigmented wild type *S. schenckii* has a greater invasive ability than an albino mutated strain in a rat experimental model of sporotrichosis. The albino strain also was restrained in the core of granulomas, whereas the melanized strain produced multifocal granulomas [91]. Interestingly, a laboratory worker who handled large numbers of both pigmented and albino strains of *S. schenckii* developed cutaneous sporotrichosis with a dematiaceous strain [92].

Historically, *S. schenckii* melanization *in vivo* was suspected based on the identification of a brown halo on the yeast cell wall by tissue staining with Fontana-Masson, a histopathological technique originally used to demonstrate melanin on *C. neoformans* [93]. More recently, melanization has been confirmed by the findings that *Sporothrix* melanin ghosts can been isolated from tissues of infected animals and antibodies to melanin have been detected in sera from human patients with sporotrichosis [87, 88]. These sera have antibodies reacting preferentially against melanin derived from L-DOPA rather than DHN-melanin [88].

Histoplasma capsulatum

Histoplasma capsulatum is the anamorphic form of *Ajellomyces capsulatum*. *A. capsulatum* is a heterothallic fungus with two distinct mating types: (+) and (-) [94]. Although there historically have been three *H. capsulatum* varieties (*H. capsulatum* var. *capsulatum*, the etiological agent of classic histoplasmosis, a cosmopolitan fungal infection with areas of high endemicity; *H. capsultaum* var. *duboisii*, the etiological agent of African histoplasmosis; and *H. capsulatum* var. *farciminosum*, the etiological agent of epizootic lymphangitis of horses and mules [95]), recent phylogenetic work has demonstrated significant molecular interdispersion leading to the suggestion that rather than assigning strains to a variety that we recognize instead the existence of genetically distinct geographical populations or phylogenetic species [96]. In immunocompetent individuals, most primary infections result in mild or asymptomatic respiratory disease, however there is a broad spectrum of clinical manifestations of histoplasmosis, ranging from a self-limited pulmonary infection that resolves without treatment to chronic pulmonary infection to widespread disseminated lethal disease [97].

The filamentous form of *H. capsulatum* occurs at temperatures below 35°C or in the environment. This form is composed by hyaline septate hyphae that produce two different hyaline asexual reproduction structures: round to pear-shaped microconidia and large, thick-walled, round macroconidia. These macroconidia are typically tuberculate, knobby or with short cylindrical projections, though they occasionally may be smooth. In parasitism or when cultivated at 37°C in specific enriched media, *H. capsulatum* forms small hyaline ovoid yeast cells with a narrow base at the smaller end [98].

In both saprophytic and parasitic stages, *H. capsulatum* must face assorted challenging environmental conditions. In response, this dimorphic fungus produces several molecules with biological activities such as siderophores to survive iron starvation, catalase to survive oxidative stress conditions and orotidine 5-monophosphate pyrophosphorylase to endure uracil limitation [99]. Moreover, this fungus produces melanin on both conidia and yeast cells despite the production of hyaline structures on both morphological phases [100].

Melanization has been associated with the pathogenesis of histoplasmosis since 1962, when it was observed that brown phenotype filamentous *H. capsulatum* colonies were more virulent in a rabbit infection model than the albino phenotypes of *H. capsulatum* [101]. In its filamentous form, *H. capsulatum* can perform *de novo* melanogenesis, thus probably it produces DHN melanin on these structures. Since *H. capsulatum* conidia synthesize melanin in the absence of exogenous phenolic substrate, it is probable that conidia are melanized in the environment, a theory supported by the observation that melanin production genes are induced in the mycelial phase of fungal growth [102]. Thus, melanization may protect the conidia from environmental insults. Melanization of the yeast form, where a laccase-like enzymatic activity has been observed, requires compounds such as L-DOPA, (-)-epinephrine or phenolic compounds present on brain heart infusion medium [100]. Yeast melanization appears to contribute to virulence by reducing *H. capsulatum* susceptibility to host defense mechanisms and the antifungal drugs amphotericin B and capsofungin [53, 103]. Moreover, yeast L-DOPA melanin can elicit an antibody response in mice infected with *H. capsulatum* [100].

Paracoccidioides brasiliensis

Paracoccidioides brasiliensis is the dimorphic fungus agent of paracoccidioidomycosis, the main systemic mycosis on Latin America and a fungal infection that initiates with the transition of the inhaled infective *P. brasiliensis* conidia into the lungs. Upon inhalation, the conidia transform into peculiar yeast-like cells with multiple buds into the lungs. Subsequent dissemination to other organs may occur, giving rise to secondary lesions on the skin, lymph nodes and adrenal glands preferentially [104].

Melanin or melanin-like pigments can be found in conidia and yeast of *P. brasiliensis*. Treatment of conidia with proteolytic and glycolitic enzymes, denaturant and hot concentrated acid results in a the isolation of particles retaining the size and shape of the original conidia [105]. Since the conidia are obtained from a culture medium with only water and agar, conidia are thought to produce DHN-melanin.

The first analyses of *P. brasiliensis* yeast using Fontana Mason staining indicated that they were not melanized, in contrast to the positive staining for melanin in a related fungus, *Lacazzia loboi*, the etiologic agent of lobomycosis [106]. However, a more recent study has shown that, in the presence of L-DOPA, yeast cells in agar darken after 8 days, with a dark-brown pigment in the cytoplasm and in the cell wall. These cells also yield dark particles after enzymatic, denaturant and hot-acid treatments, which react with antibodies to melanin and produced the characteristic free radical signal of melanin by ESR spectroscopy [105]. *P. brasiliensis* melanin is located external to the cell wall [103]. Although a laccase-like activity has been demonstrated on cytoplasmic yeast extracts of *P. brasiliensis* by two different methods [105, 107], the enzymatic pathway to synthesize melanin has not yet been established.

Melanin is synthesized *in vivo* by *P. brasiliensis*, as demonstrated by the recognition of yeast cells by melanin-binding antibody, by the recovery of dark particles in infected tissues [105] and by the observation that melanin synthesis genes (e.g. tyrosinase gene) are up regulated during a mouse model of systemic infection [108]. Actually, this tyrosinase over expression and the aromatic L-amino acid decarboxylase expression when this fungus is in contact with human plasma [109] are strong evidences of eumelanin production by *P. brasiliensis* yeast through L-DOPA or other phenolic compounds during parasitism. The functions of these pigments have been associated with protection from the fungicidal and fungistatic effects of phagocytic cells as well as from the antifungal drugs amphotericin B, ketoconazole, fluconazole and itraconazole and also the sulfonamide antibiotic sulfamethoxazole [107]. The resistance to phagocytosis is in part due to the protective effect of melanin against nitric oxide and other reactive oxygen species, such as hypochlorite and hydrogen peroxide [110]. Finally, nonmelanized *P. brasiliensis* yeast are less pathogenic than melanized yeast cells. [110].

Other Dimorphic Fungi

Blastomyces dermatitidis is an endemic dimorphic fungal pathogen found in central USA that is the etiological agent of blastomycosis, a systemic mycosis that ranges in disease manifestations from asymptomatic cases to fatal pneumonia in immunocompetent individuals [111]. *B. dermatitidis* is mycelia in the environment and produces yeast cells of 8-10μm in diameter that display broad-based budding. *Coccidioides posadasii* and its relative species *C. immitis* are endemic to the USA, Mexico and desert and semiarid areas in Central and South America. They grow as filamentous form in soils and, after inhalation of the infective arthroconidium by a mammal host, they convert to a peculiar spherule phase in the lungs, causing coccidioidomycosis, an infection that may be asymptomatic or result in an atypical pneumonia in more than 50% of the immunocompetent infected individuals [112]. *Penicillium marneffei* is a dimorphic fungus restricted to the Southeast Asia that causes infections in both immunocompetent and immunodeficient individuals, although penicilliosis caused by *P. marneffei* in the non-HIV infected populace is extremely unusual [113].

These three fungi produce hyaline structures when observed by bright field microscopy, however their conidia, after treatment with enzymes, denaturant and hot concentrated acid result in melanin ghosts retaining the original size and shape from the intact original conidia. Also, melanin or melanin-like pigments are observed on their parasitic phases both *in vitro* and *in vivo* with the techniques developed to study melanization described earlier in this chapter for other fungi [114-116]. *P. marneffei* possesses a DHN melanin-biosynthesis gene cluster [117], but the pathways to synthesize melanin in *B. dermatitidis* and *C. posadasii* have not been elucidated, although they do not require exogenous phenolic compounds to melanize. However, *C. immitis* has a putative gene with 80% similarity to a laccase from *Botrytis cinerea* and to the enzyme Lac2 of *C. neoformans* [38]. In *B. dermatitidis*, melanin reduces susceptibility to amphotericin B, but not to voriconazole or itraconazole [114]. Melanin has been posited to play a role in the virulence of *B. dermatitidis*, *C. posadasii* and *P. marneffei*, thus affecting their pathogenesis.

Candida albicans and Other Yeasts

Several members of the genus *Candida* are commensal microorganisms in humans and other mammalians, co-existing with the host without any overt damage. This balance can be broken, however, if the defense mechanisms of the host are compromised [118]. The polymorphic fungus *Candida albicans* is the major agent of candidemia and candidiasis worldwide. This species is characterized by germ tube and chlamidospore production and has morphological, genetic and carbohydrate assimilation profiles that permits distinguishing from other species within the genus [119].

C. albicans was long believed to be a non-melanin producer, and was used as a negative control in several experiments on melanin synthesis [22, 45, 100, 105, 107]. However, it has now been shown that this yeast produces melanin *in vitro* and during infection. Melanin particles extracted from *C. albicans* yeast cells, unlike the other fungi described in this chapter up to now, does not retain the shape and size of the original cells, presenting a quarter of the size of the initial yeasts. These melanin particles were obtained from yeast cells both *in vitro* and *in vivo,* but hyphae do not yield melanin. Other peculiar aspect about *C. albicans* melanization is that the small spheres of melanin obtained do not accumulate beneath the cell wall, being more similar to melanosome structures [120]. More recently, it has been demonstrated that these melanin bodies are produced when the fungus is incubated in medium containing L-DOPA as a substrate and this melanin is externalized from the fungal cells in a chitin-dependent mechanism, where the product of the *CHS3* gene, short chitin rodlets, is required for melanin externalization and the product of the *CHS8* gene, long chitin microfibrils, impairs the process [121]. It is due to these unusual aspects of *C. albicans* melanization that led earlier studies to conclude that this species was a non-melanin producer.

Melanin production was also observed in *Candida glabrata* and *Candida famata* when cultured in the presence of L-DOPA [122]. Another yeast species, *Yarrowia lipolytica,* produces a black pigment that results from the extracellular accumulation and oxidation of an intermediate of tyrosine catabolism [15]. This pigment was shown to be pyomelanin, formed by the oxidation and polymerization of homogentisic acid accumulated on the culture medium during fungal growth [123]. *Y. lipolytica* is also able to convert L-tyrosine to L-DOPA, producing small amounts of melanin after the process [124].

However, no association between melanization and virulence has been defined for *C. albicans* [121] or other hemiascomycete yeasts. *C. albicans* yeast cells secrete complex polymers into biofilm structures that alter antifungal susceptibilities [125], and melanin may play some role in this process, since it is externalized by this yeast [120].

Aspergillus

Members of the genus *Aspergillus* are among the most abundant and widely distributed organisms in the world. Several of them produce metabolites with diverse applications. Many *Aspergillus* species have the ability of degrade agricultural products and some cause a disease known as aspergillosis in immunocompromised hosts, especially in patients receiving chemotherapy or with cystic fibrosis [126]. Melanin production by species of the genus *Aspergillus* was first reported in 1969, when melanization of *A. nidulans* was detected in batch and chemostat cultures [127, 128]. This fungus is one of the most important species for studying eukaryotic cell biology [129] and its melanin has been shown to have an antioxidant activity [130].

A. fumigatus is the major clinically relevant fungal pathogen, being the main etiological agent of human and animal aspergillosis. Although this fungus lacks some virulence traits present in other fungal species, *A. fumigatus* is able to successfully establish infection in immunosupressed patients due to its virulence factors and modulation of innate and adaptive immunological responses [131]. The putative virulence factors of *A. fumigatus* include secretion of hydrolytic enzymes and toxins, such as gliotoxin, the presence of extra-cellular matrix adhesion molecules on cell surface, and the production of pigments [132].

The DHN-melanin synthesis pathway in *A. fumigatus* is very well characterized [13, 133]. Biosynthesis of this type of melanin requires the products of six different genes, located in a cluster that is expressed during fungal conidiation. For this reason, *A. fumigatus* produce DHN melanin only in the conidia as demonstrated by the methods used to generate melanin ghosts [134]. The first characterized gene of this pathway is named *arp1* and its expression yields a scytalone dehydratase, an enzyme that converts scytalone on 1,3,8-THN [135]. Another important gene in this pathway is *alb1* whose transcript is a polyketide synthase characterized latter as a naphthopyrone synthase [136, 137]. Mutations on this gene leads to an albino conidial phenotype [136]. The *abr2* gene is also characterized and codes for a laccase that is not essential for virulence, indicating that the intermediates of the DHN pathway confer some scavenging activity to reactive oxygen species [138].

DHN-melanin plays an important role in the pathogenesis of aspergillosis. *In vitro* experiments show that melanin protects the fungus against phagocytosis and decreases its susceptibility to reactive oxygen species produced by phagocytic cells, such as alveolar and monocyte-derived macrophages and neutrophil granulocytes [136, 139, 140]. *A. fumigatus* melanin also impedes apoptosis pathways, contributing to fungal dissemination within the host [141]. The melanin interferes with cellular responses to some fungal antigenic ligands [142]. Additionally, the melanin has an indirect effect on the pathogenesis of aspergillosis, as it allows for the correct assembly of the cell wall layers of conidia, thus permitting correct expression of laminin adhesins and other virulence factors at the conidial surface [13].

Together, these results may explain the findings of a lower virulence of *alb1* mutants of *A. fumigatus* in a mouse model of disseminated aspergillosis [143]. Attachment of melanin-binding antibodies to conidia within tissue sections from patients with nasal aspergilloma also suggests that melanization occurs during infection [134]. Melanin is produced by *A. fumigatus* growing in biofilms [144, 145]. Interestingly, DHN-melanin appears to be a specific virulence factor of *A. fumigatus* in mammalian disease, since strains with mutations in the genes of the DHN-melanin synthesis cluster are more virulent than the wild type strain in an insect model of *Aspergillus* infection using *Galleria mellonella* as the host [146].

Pyomelanin has been described in *A. fumigatus*. In the presence of L-tyrosine or L-phenylalanine, this species expresses enzymes related to the degradation of these amino acids, leading to the production of pyomelanin, with homogentisic acid as the major intermediate of the pathway. This pigment probably protects the germlings and hyphae of *A. fumigatus* from the oxidative products of neutrophils [16]. This species can also utilize tyrosine and DOPA melanins as sole carbon sources, leading to the production of a third type of melanin, a fungal allomelanin, that turns typically pale mycelia dark, [147]. Whether allomelanin production occurs *in vivo* is not known and no role for this type of melanin is established in the pathogenesis of aspergillosis.

A. niger is another species that causes aspergillosis. Melanin ghosts have been extracted from its conidia and they have the ability to activate the alternative complement pathway [47]. In an elegant study, the melanin contents of *A. niger* from two environments at Mount Carmel, Israel, receiving different levels of solar radiation was measured and showed that isolates with higher levels of solar radiation have higher melanin concentration and resisted long wavelength UV radiation better than the lower radiation treatment [148]. A polyketide synthase gene, *albA*, from *A. niger* has been characterized and it is an ortholog of *alb1* gene of *A. fumigatus*, responsible for the production of melanin and other naphtho-γ-pyrone family of polyketides [149], confirming the capacity of this fungus to produce DHN melanin.

Other Human Pathogenic Fungi

Pneumocystis jirovecii is a peculiar fungus that is unable to grow *in vitro*, which grows in a yeast-like from *in vivo* and causes a life-threatening pneumonia in immunocompromised humans. *Pneumocystis carinii*, a closely related species that is able to cause infection in rats, is able to produce melanin at its cell wall, as shown by the generation of melanin ghosts from microorganisms isolated from the lungs of infected rats and by labeling of cells in tissue sections by melanin-binding antibodies [150]. Subsequent to the demonstration of melanin in *P. carinii* in rats, melanin has also be demonstrated in *Pneumocystis* isolated from mice and ferrets, as well as for *P. jiroveci* in patient biopsy specimens [151]. Additionally, melanized *Pneumocystis* are less susceptible to UV irradiation or desiccation compared to non-melanized yeasts, suggesting a role for melanin against a range of stressors [151].

Scytalidium dimidiatum is a pigmented dematiaceous coelomycete that typically causes chronic superficial skin diseases and onychomycosis, but sometimes also causes deeper infections, such as subcutaneous abscesses. This fungus produces melanin on hyphae and artroconidia. *In vivo* melanization of *S. dimidiatum* is supported due to the detection of melanin in the skin of a patient with subcutaneous disease. Interestingly, *S. hyalinum*, a species with similar morphology to *S. dimidiatum*, but does not produce pigmented mycelium, yielded no dark particles after treatment with denaturant and hot acid, supporting the theory that *S. hyalinum* is an albino mutant of *S. dimidiatum* [152].

The dermatophytes are a group of fungi classified in three anamorphic genera (*Epidermophyton, Microsporum* and *Trichophyton*) that have the ability to invade keratinized tissues to cause dermatophytosis (or ringworm). Most recently, melanin production has been demonstrated in the microconidia and macroconidia of *T. rubrum, T. mentagrophytes, E. floccosum* and *M. gypseum* [153]. Also, these species produce melanin or melanin-like pigments during infection [153]. Therefore, melanin may be a putative virulence factor for dermatophytes, as for other pathogenic fungi.

Madurella mycetomatis is the main agent of black grain eumycetoma. Melanization of *M. mycetomatis* occurs on both hyphae and grains, presumably by the DHN and pyomelanin pathways. L-DOPA has been shown to be toxic to this species. Melanization appears to be involved in fungal morphogenesis as *M. mycetomatis* cells cultured in the presence of melanin inhibitors are longer, less branched and slimmer than the melanized phenotype. Other functions of melanin in this fungal species include protection against oxidant compounds and to the antifungal agents itraconazole and ketoconazole, the main antifungal drugs used in the treatment of eumycetomas [154].

Melanization has also been described in other medically important fungi, such as the yeasts of the genus *Malassezia* [155], *Hortaea werneckii* [156], *Lacazzia loboi* [106] and the opportunistic fungal pathogens *Paecilomyces lilacinus, Scedosporium prolificans, Curvularia lunata* and *Alternaria alternata* [157-160]. In *H. werneckii* melanin appears to be responsible for the reduction in the permeability of the cell wall to glycerol, which might be one of the features that facilitates the osmotic adaptation of this halophilic fungal species [156]. Biological functions for melanin during infection caused by these species, however, are not established and more studies are necessary to determine their impact on pathogenesis.

Phytopathogenic Fungi

Given that melanin is able to protect fungi against numerous environmental stresses, it is not surprising that melanization occurs in phytopathogenic fungi.

Melanin synthesis related enzymes, especially polyketide synthase genes, are abundant in fungal genomes and are more abundant in phytopathogenic ascomycetes than in saprobic fungi [161]. DHN-melanin is required for pathogenicity of fungi that produce pigmented appressoria, such as *Colletotrichum lagenarium* and *Magnaporte oryzae*. The cell wall melanin protects and stabilizes these fungi against the enormous pressures required to build and release appressoria that enable the pathogen to penetrate plant leaves [162, 163].

Gaeumannomyces graminis var. *tritici* is hyaline in culture, however, pathogenic strains invade host roots with melanized macrohyphae, and dark infection cushions that are composed of clustered hyphopodia, which are appressorium-like structures, except that they come from the vegetative hyphae [164].

Interestingly, several phytopathogenic fungi do not require melanin as a virulence factor, as albino mutants can be as pathogenic as wild type strains. Melanization is thought to have an indirect effect on the virulence of these fungi, protecting them from environmental insults and thus positively selecting for them in nature [164].

For instance, *Ascochyta rabiei*, which causes infection of chickpeas, produces DHN-melanin in pycnidia and sexual fruting bodies, but it does not augment plant infection; however this pigment is able to protect the reproduction cells within the fruting bodies from

UV light [165]. Additionally, *Bipolaris oryzae* induces expression of the 1,3,8-THN reductase gene involved in melanin biosynthesis upon exposure to ultraviolet radiation [166]. Melanin-deficient mutants of *Monilinia fructicola* yield lesions on fruit, but their conidia are vulnerable to high temperature, desiccation, freezing, UV, mechanical pressure and hydrolytic enzymes [164].

Implications for Human Health

As described in this chapter, fungal melanins are important virulence factors for leading human fungal pathogens. Melanins contribute to fungal virulence through diverse mechanisms, both directly impacting the fungus' capacity to protect their cellular structures and functions and by modifying host effector responses. However, our understanding of the physicochemical properties and biological functions of melanins sets the stage for our being able to directly therapeutically target these amorphous polymers or interfere with their synthesis.

Since melanins are important for the pathogenesis of several fungi, disrupting their synthesis should be an interesting mechanism to combat pathogenic fungi. Glyphosate is a widely used herbicide that inhibits growth of several microbes [167] and also interferes with *C. neoformans* melanization by direct inhibition of the autoxidation of L-DOPA, oxidation of epinephrine and consequently melanin polymerization [55]. This drug has therapeutic effects in mice systemically infected with *C. neoformans*. Administration of glyphosate to infected mice prolonged animal survival and reduced lung fungal burdens [55]. Melanin affects lung inflammatory reaction during cryptococcal infection by eliciting high levels of interleukins and greater numbers of leukocytes [168] and interestingly glyphosate treatment lowered inflammation in mice lungs, where only a few defective melanin ghosts were observed [55].

Other indirect evidence that treatment with drugs that block melanin synthesis results in better outcomes for fungal infections is the fact that voriconazole, a broad-spectrum triazole that inhibits cytochrome P450 dependent 14α lanosterol demethylation and is highly active against *C. neoformans* [169, 170], inhibits melanization by a direct interaction with the fungal laccase that inhibits the enzymatic synthesis of melanin [171]. Therefore, fungal melanin-synthesis pathways appear to be promising new targets for antifungal design. Recently, a new compound ptilomycalin A, a spirocyclic guanidine alkaloid extracted from the marine sponge *Monanchora arbuscula* that acts synergistically with amphotericin B, has been shown to suppress melanogenesis in *C. neoformans* by functioning as a potent laccase inhibitor [172]. Another important observation regarding melanin-inhibiting compounds as treatments is the fact that passive immunization with melanin-binding monoclonal antibodies prolonged survival and reduced the *C. neoformans* fungal burden on infected mice [49]. Hence, targeting melanin or melanin synthesis appears to be an excellent approach to combat melanotic fungi.

Actually, the inhibitory effects of antifungal drugs on melanin synthesis can be utilized also in the treatment of non-fungal diseases. Miconazole, an imidazole antifungal drug of topic use commonly used to treat cutaneous fungal infections, inhibits tyrosinase activity and tyrosinase expression in B16 melanoma cells, slowing melanin biosynthesis and, therefore, may have beneficial effects in the treatment of hyperpigmentation disorders such as melasma and ephelis [173]. On the other hand, amphotericin B induces *de novo* synthesis of tyrosinase by neuroretinal cells, allowing these cells to produce melanin [174], suggesting that different antifungal drugs may have antagonist roles on melanin production by animal cells.

Melanized fungi inhabit some remarkably extreme environments on the planet, including Arctic and Antarctic regions and the walls of the damaged reactor at Chernobyl, where they are exposed to a high and constant radiation [175]. Melanized fungi can display increased growth relative to non-melanized cells after exposure to ionizing radiation [176], because chemical composition, free radical quenching and spherical spatial arrangement of melanins protects the fungi from the radiation and the energy absorbed through these interactions can fuel fungal growth [177]. These observations led to the creation of rationally designed melanins as novel radioprotectors, that were able to protect mammalian cells against ionizing radiation of different energies [178]. In fact, melanin-covered nanoparticles offered protection of bone marrow from ionizing radiation during external radiation or radioimmunotherapy, whereas no tumor protection by these unencapsulated melanins was observed [179]. Radiolabeled melanin-binding peptides were also successfully studied in the treatment of melanoma [180]. Another way to exploit the resistance of melanized fungi to radiation is their use in bioremediation of radioactively contaminated sites and the cleanup of industrial effluents [181].

Melanins are able to chemically bind diverse compounds especially those used in several therapies, such as antifungals, antibiotics, antipsychotic and antineoplasic drugs [53, 154, 182, 183]. In fact, the capacity of melanin to adsorb a vast variety of compounds is similar to that of medicinal activated charcoal [6].

A. fumigatus has the ability to degrade melanin [147]. Studies on cosmetic development have used melanin degrading extracts isolated from *A. fumigatus* and *S. cerevisiae*. These extracts can significantly reduce UVB induced pigmentation of human skin, suggesting the usefulness of these extracts in the development of new whitening cosmetics to modify skin color and tone [184].

Conclusion

Melanins are important virulence factors for several human and plant fungal pathogens. Virtually all fungi produce melanin under specific growth conditions and several important pathogens can synthesize melanin in the absence of phenolic or other substrates. Interestingly, some fungi accumulate melanin on their conidia, others on conidia and hyphae, some only in the yeast form, and a few secrete melanin to the external medium. In general, DHN melanin is produced during fungal growth in the environment, whereas melanins derived from L-DOPA or tyrosine appear to be preferentially (but not exclusively) expressed during pathogenic stages of fungal growth where they can interact with the immune responses of the host. Despite increasing fungal pathogenicity, melanins are interesting targets for new drug development and treatment strategies for fungal infections and their properties allow the use of melanins as adjuvants in other diseases, especially cancer.

References

[1] Nosanchuk JD, Casadevall A. The contribution of melanin to microbial pathogenesis. *Cellular microbiology*. 2003 Apr;5(4):203-23.

[2] Riley PA. Melanin. *The international journal of biochemistry and cell biology*. 1997 Nov;29(11):1235-9.

[3] Liu GY, Nizet V. Color me bad: microbial pigments as virulence factors. *Trends in microbiology*. 2009 Sep;17(9):406-13.

[4] Hamilton AJ, Gomez BL. Melanins in fungal pathogens. *Journal of medical microbiology*. 2002 Mar;51(3):189-91.

[5] Gomez BL, Nosanchuk JD. Melanin and fungi. *Current opinion in infectious diseases*. 2003 Apr;16(2):91-6.

[6] Nosanchuk JD, Casadevall A. Impact of melanin on microbial virulence and clinical resistance to antimicrobial compounds. *Antimicrobial agents and chemotherapy*. 2006 Nov;50(11):3519-28.

[7] Jacobson ES. Pathogenic roles for fungal melanins. *Clinical microbiology reviews*. 2000 Oct;13(4):708-17.

[8] Wang Y, Aisen P, Casadevall A. Melanin, melanin "ghosts," and melanin composition in *Cryptococcus neoformans*. *Infection and immunity*. 1996 Jul;64(7):2420-4.

[9] Wheeler MH, Bell AA. Melanins and their importance in pathogenic fungi. *Current topics in medical mycology*. 1988;2:338-87.

[10] Enochs WS, Nilges MJ, Swartz HM. A standardized test for the identification and characterization of melanins using electron paramagnetic resonance (EPR) spectroscopy. *Pigment cell research*. 1993 Mar;6(2):91-9.

[11] Langfelder K, Streibel M, Jahn B, Haase G, Brakhage AA. Biosynthesis of fungal melanins and their importance for human pathogenic fungi. *Fungal Genetics and Biology*. 2003 Mar;38(2):143-58.

[12] Lee JK, Jung HM, Kim SY. 1,8-dihydroxynaphthalene (DHN)-melanin biosynthesis inhibitors increase erythritol production in *Torula corallina*, and DHN-melanin inhibits erythrose reductase. *Applied and environmental microbiology*. 2003 Jun;69(6):3427-34.

[13] Pihet M, Vandeputte P, Tronchin G, Renier G, Saulnier P, Georgeault S, et al. Melanin is an essential component for the integrity of the cell wall of *Aspergillus fumigatus* conidia. *BMC microbiology*. 2009;9:177.

[14] Wheeler MH, Stipanovic RD. Melanin biosynthesis and the metabolism of flaviolin and 2-hydroxyjuglone in *Wangiella dermatitidis*. *Archives of microbiology*. 1985 Aug;142(3):234-41.

[15] Carreira A, Ferreira LM, Loureiro V. Production of brown tyrosine pigments by the yeast *Yarrowia lipolytica*. *Journal of applied microbiology*. 2001 Mar;90(3):372-9.

[16] Schmaler-Ripcke J, Sugareva V, Gebhardt P, Winkler R, Kniemeyer O, Heinekamp T, et al. Production of pyomelanin, a second type of melanin, via the tyrosine degradation pathway in *Aspergillus fumigatus*. *Applied and environmental microbiology*. 2009 Jan;75(2):493-503.

[17] Levitz SM. The ecology of *Cryptococcus neoformans* and the epidemiology of cryptococcosis. *Reviews of infectious diseases*. 1991 Nov-Dec;13(6):1163-9.

[18] Nielsen K, De Obaldia AL, Heitman J. *Cryptococcus neoformans* mates on pigeon guano: implications for the realized ecological niche and globalization. *Eukaryotic cell.* 2007 Jun;6(6):949-59.

[19] Mseddi F, Sellami A, Jarboui MA, Sellami H, Makni F, Ayadi A. First environmental isolations of *Cryptococcus neoformans* and *Cryptococcus gattii* in Tunisia and review of published studies on environmental isolations in Africa. *Mycopathologia.* 2011 May;171(5):355-60.

[20] Park BJ, Wannemuehler KA, Marston BJ, Govender N, Pappas PG, Chiller TM. Estimation of the current global burden of cryptococcal meningitis among persons living with HIV/AIDS. AIDS (London, England). 2009 Feb 20;23(4):525-30.

[21] Kwon-Chung KJ, Varma A. Do major species concepts support one, two or more species within *Cryptococcus neoformans*? FEMS yeast research. 2006 Jun;6(4):574-87.

[22] Frases S, Chaskes S, Dadachova E, Casadevall A. Induction by *Klebsiella aerogenes* of a melanin-like pigment in *Cryptococcus neoformans*. *Applied and environmental microbiology*. 2006 Feb;72(2):1542-50.

[23] Frases S, Salazar A, Dadachova E, Casadevall A. *Cryptococcus neoformans* can utilize the bacterial melanin precursor homogentisic acid for fungal melanogenesis. *Applied and environmental microbiology.* 2007 Jan;73(2):615-21.

[24] Wang Y, Aisen P, Casadevall A. *Cryptococcus neoformans* melanin and virulence: *mechanism of action. Infection and immunity.* 1995 Aug;63(8):3131-6.

[25] Severo CB, Pinto GL, Sotilli J, Garcia MR, Gazzoni AF, Oliveira FM, et al. Cryptococcuria as manifestation of disseminated cryptococcosis: Staib agar as a selective identification medium. *Mycoses*. 2011 May 30.

[26] Staib F, Seibold M, Antweiler E, Frohlich B. Staib agar supplemented with a triple antibiotic combination for the detection of *Cryptococcus neoformans* in clinical specimens. *Mycoses.* 1989 Sep;32(9):448-54.

[27] Hogan DA, Kolter R. *Pseudomonas-Candida* interactions: an ecological role for virulence factors. *Science.* 2002 Jun 21;296(5576):2229-32.

[28] Mylonakis E, Ausubel FM, Perfect JR, Heitman J, Calderwood SB. Killing of *Caenorhabditis elegans* by *Cryptococcus neoformans* as a model of yeast pathogenesis. *Proceedings of the National Academy of Sciences of the United States of America.* 2002 Nov 26;99(24):15675-80.

[29] Steenbergen JN, Nosanchuk JD, Malliaris SD, Casadevall A. Interaction of *Blastomyces dermatitidis*, *Sporothrix schenckii*, and *Histoplasma capsulatum* with *Acanthamoeba castellanii*. *Infection and immunity*. 2004 Jun;72(6):3478-88.

[30] Steenbergen JN, Shuman HA, Casadevall A. *Cryptococcus neoformans* interactions with amoebae suggest an explanation for its virulence and intracellular pathogenic strategy in macrophages. *Proceedings of the National Academy of Sciences of the United States of America*. 2001 Dec 18;98(26):15245-50.

[31] Nosanchuk JD, Rudolph J, Rosas AL, Casadevall A. Evidence that *Cryptococcus neoformans* is melanized in pigeon excreta: implications for pathogenesis. *Infection and immunity.* 1999 Oct;67(10):5477-9.

[32] Casadevall A, Rosas AL, Nosanchuk JD. Melanin and virulence in *Cryptococcus neoformans*. *Current opinion in microbiology*. 2000 Aug;3(4):354-8.

[33] Rosas AL, Casadevall A. Melanization decreases the susceptibility of *Cryptococcus neoformans* to enzymatic degradation. *Mycopathologia*. 2001;151(2):53-6.

[34] Wang Y, Casadevall A. Decreased susceptibility of melanized *Cryptococcus neoformans* to UV light. *Applied and environmental microbiology.* 1994 Oct;60(10):3864-6.

[35] Rosas AL, Casadevall A. Melanization affects susceptibility of *Cryptococcus neoformans* to heat and cold. *FEMS microbiology letters.* 1997 Aug 15;153(2):265-72.

[36] D'Souza CA, Alspaugh JA, Yue C, Harashima T, Cox GM, Perfect JR, et al. Cyclic AMP-dependent protein kinase controls virulence of the fungal pathogen *Cryptococcus neoformans. Molecular and cellular biology.* 2001 May;21(9):3179-91.

[37] Salas SD, Bennett JE, Kwon-Chung KJ, Perfect JR, Williamson PR. Effect of the laccase gene *CNLAC1*, on virulence of *Cryptococcus neoformans. The Journal of experimental medicine.* 1996 Aug 1;184(2):377-86.

[38] Missall TA, Moran JM, Corbett JA, Lodge JK. Distinct stress responses of two functional laccases in *Cryptococcus neoformans* are revealed in the absence of the thiol-specific antioxidant Tsa1. *Eukaryotic cell.* 2005 Jan;4(1):202-8.

[39] Williamson PR. Biochemical and molecular characterization of the diphenol oxidase of *Cryptococcus neoformans*: identification as a laccase. *Journal of bacteriology.* 1994 Feb;176(3):656-64.

[40] Eisenman HC, Mues M, Weber SE, Frases S, Chaskes S, Gerfen G, et al. *Cryptococcus neoformans* laccase catalyses melanin synthesis from both D- and L-DOPA. *Microbiology.* 2007 Dec;153(Pt 12):3954-62.

[41] Garcia-Rivera J, Eisenman HC, Nosanchuk JD, Aisen P, Zaragoza O, Moadel T, et al. Comparative analysis of *Cryptococcus neoformans* acid-resistant particles generated from pigmented cells grown in different laccase substrates. *Fungal Genetics and Biology.* 2005 Dec;42(12):989-98.

[42] Eisenman HC, Nosanchuk JD, Webber JB, Emerson RJ, Camesano TA, Casadevall A. Microstructure of cell wall-associated melanin in the human pathogenic fungus *Cryptococcus neoformans. Biochemistry.* 2005 Mar 15;44(10):3683-93.

[43] Eisenman HC, Frases S, Nicola AM, Rodrigues ML, Casadevall A. Vesicle-associated melanization in *Cryptococcus neoformans. Microbiology.* 2009 Dec;155(Pt 12):3860-7.

[44] Nosanchuk JD, Casadevall A. Budding of melanized *Cryptococcus neoformans* in the presence or absence of L-dopa. *Microbiology.* 2003 Jul;149(Pt 7):1945-51.

[45] Rosas AL, Nosanchuk JD, Feldmesser M, Cox GM, McDade HC, Casadevall A. Synthesis of polymerized melanin by *Cryptococcus neoformans* in infected rodents. *Infection and immunity.* 2000 May;68(5):2845-53.

[46] Nosanchuk JD, Rosas AL, Lee SC, Casadevall A. Melanisation of *Cryptococcus neoformans* in human brain tissue. *Lancet.* 2000 Jun 10;355(9220):2049-50.

[47] Rosas AL, MacGill RS, Nosanchuk JD, Kozel TR, Casadevall A. Activation of the alternative complement pathway by fungal melanins. *Clinical and diagnostic laboratory immunology.* 2002 Jan;9(1):144-8.

[48] Nosanchuk JD, Valadon P, Feldmesser M, Casadevall A. Melanization of *Cryptococcus neoformans* in murine infection. *Molecular and cellular biology.* 1999 Jan;19(1):745-50.

[49] Rosas AL, Nosanchuk JD, Casadevall A. Passive immunization with melanin-binding monoclonal antibodies prolongs survival of mice with lethal *Cryptococcus neoformans infection. Infection and immunity.* 2001 May;69(5):3410-2.

[50] Huffnagle GB, Chen GH, Curtis JL, McDonald RA, Strieter RM, Toews GB. Down-regulation of the afferent phase of T cell-mediated pulmonary inflammation and immunity by a high melanin-producing strain of *Cryptococcus neoformans*. *J. Immunol.* 1995 Oct 1;155(7):3507-16.

[51] Wang Y, Casadevall A. Susceptibility of melanized and nonmelanized *Cryptococcus neoformans* to nitrogen- and oxygen-derived oxidants. *Infection and immunity.* 1994 Jul;62(7):3004-7.

[52] Ikeda R, Sugita T, Jacobson ES, Shinoda T. Effects of melanin upon susceptibility of *Cryptococcus* to antifungals. *Microbiology and immunology.* 2003;47(4):271-7.

[53] van Duin D, Casadevall A, Nosanchuk JD. Melanization of *Cryptococcus neoformans* and *Histoplasma capsulatum* reduces their susceptibilities to amphotericin B and caspofungin. *Antimicrobial agents and chemotherapy.* 2002 Nov;46(11):3394-400.

[54] Wang Y, Casadevall A. Growth of *Cryptococcus neoformans* in presence of L-dopa decreases its susceptibility to amphotericin B. *Antimicrobial agents and chemotherapy.* 1994 Nov;38(11):2648-50.

[55] Nosanchuk JD, Ovalle R, Casadevall A. Glyphosate inhibits melanization of *Cryptococcus neoformans* and prolongs survival of mice after systemic infection. *The Journal of infectious diseases.* 2001 Apr 1;183(7):1093-9.

[56] Revankar SG, Sutton DA. Melanized fungi in human disease. *Clinical microbiology reviews.* 2010 Oct;23(4):884-928.

[57] Paolo WF, Jr., Dadachova E, Mandal P, Casadevall A, Szaniszlo PJ, Nosanchuk JD. Effects of disrupting the polyketide synthase gene *WdPKS1* in *Wangiella* [*Exophiala*] *dermatitidis* on melanin production and resistance to killing by antifungal compounds, enzymatic degradation, and extremes in temperature. *BMC microbiology.* 2006;6:55.

[58] De Hoog GS, Queiroz-Telles F, Haase G, Fernandez-Zeppenfeldt G, Attili Angelis D, Gerrits Van Den Ende AH, et al. Black fungi: clinical and pathogenic approaches. *Med. Mycol.* 2000;38 Suppl 1:243-50.

[59] Ameen M. Chromoblastomycosis: clinical presentation and management. *Clinical and experimental dermatology.* 2009 Dec;34(8):849-54.

[60] Queiroz-Telles F, Esterre P, Perez-Blanco M, Vitale RG, Salgado CG, Bonifaz A. Chromoblastomycosis: an overview of clinical manifestations, diagnosis and treatment. *Med. Mycol.* 2009 Feb;47(1):3-15.

[61] Cunha MM, Franzen AJ, Alviano DS, Zanardi E, Alviano CS, De Souza W, et al. Inhibition of melanin synthesis pathway by tricyclazole increases susceptibility of *Fonsecaea pedrosoi* against mouse macrophages. *Microscopy research and technique.* 2005 Dec 15;68(6):377-84.

[62] Franzen AJ, Cunha MM, Batista EJ, Seabra SH, De Souza W, Rozental S. Effects of tricyclazole (5-methyl-1,2,4-triazol[3,4] benzothiazole), a specific DHN-melanin inhibitor, on the morphology of *Fonsecaea pedrosoi* conidia and sclerotic cells. *Microscopy research and technique.* 2006 Sep;69(9):729-37.

[63] Alviano CS, Farbiarz SR, De Souza W, Angluster J, Travassos LR. Characterization of *Fonsecaea pedrosoi* melanin. *Journal of general microbiology.* 1991 Apr;137(4):837-44.

[64] Alviano DS, Franzen AJ, Travassos LR, Holandino C, Rozental S, Ejzemberg R, et al. Melanin from *Fonsecaea pedrosoi* induces production of human antifungal antibodies

and enhances the antimicrobial efficacy of phagocytes. *Infection and immunity*. 2004 Jan;72(1):229-37.

[65] Farbiarz SR, de Carvalho TU, Alviano C, de Souza W. Inhibitory effect of melanin on the interaction of *Fonsecaea pedrosoi* with mammalian cells in vitro. *Journal of Medical and Veterinary Mycology*. 1992;30(4):265-73.

[66] Franzen AJ, de Souza W, Farina M, Alviano CS, Rozental S. Morphometric and densitometric study of the biogenesis of electron-dense granules in *Fonsecaea pedrosoi*. *FEMS microbiology letters*. 1999 Apr 15;173(2):395-402.

[67] Franzen AJ, Cunha MM, Miranda K, Hentschel J, Plattner H, da Silva MB, et al. Ultrastructural characterization of melanosomes of the human pathogenic fungus *Fonsecaea pedrosoi*. *Journal of structural biology*. 2008 Apr;162(1):75-84.

[68] Pinto L, Granja LF, Alviano DS, da Silva MH, Alviano CS, Ejzemberg R. Activation of the human complement system by pigmented and hypopigmented mycelia of the fungus *Fonsecaea pedrosoi*. Mycoses. 2011 May 9.

[69] Bocca AL, Brito PP, Figueiredo F, Tosta CE. Inhibition of nitric oxide production by macrophages in chromoblastomycosis: a role for *Fonsecaea pedrosoi* melanin. *Mycopathologia*. 2006 Apr;161(4):195-203.

[70] Cunha MM, Franzen AJ, Seabra SH, Herbst MH, Vugman NV, Borba LP, et al. Melanin in *Fonsecaea pedrosoi*: a trap for oxidative radicals. *BMC microbiology*. 2010;10:80.

[71] Nimrichter L, Cerqueira MD, Leitao EA, Miranda K, Nakayasu ES, Almeida SR, et al. Structure, cellular distribution, antigenicity, and biological functions of *Fonsecaea pedrosoi* ceramide monohexosides. *Infection and immunity*. 2005 Dec;73(12):7860-8.

[72] Geis PA, Wheeler MH, Szaniszlo PJ. Pentaketide metabolites of melanin synthesis in the dematiaceous fungus *Wangiella dermatitidis*. *Archives of microbiology*. 1984 Apr;137(4):324-8.

[73] Feng B, Wang X, Hauser M, Kaufmann S, Jentsch S, Haase G, et al. Molecular cloning and characterization of *WdPKS1*, a gene involved in dihydroxynaphthalene melanin biosynthesis and virulence in *Wangiella* (*Exophiala*) *dermatitidis*. *Infection and immunity*. 2001 Mar;69(3):1781-94.

[74] Wheeler MH, Abramczyk D, Puckhaber LS, Naruse M, Ebizuka Y, Fujii I, et al. New biosynthetic step in the melanin pathway of *Wangiella* (*Exophiala*) *dermatitidis*: evidence for 2-acetyl-1,3,6,8-Tetrahydroxynaphthalene as a novel precursor. *Eukaryotic. cell*. 2008 Oct;7(10):1699-711.

[75] Wang Z, Zheng L, Hauser M, Becker JM, Szaniszlo PJ. WdChs4p, a homolog of chitin synthase 3 in Saccharomyces cerevisiae, alone cannot support growth of *Wangiella* (*Exophiala*) *dermatitidis* at the temperature of infection. *Infection and immunity*. 1999 Dec;67(12):6619-30.

[76] Brush L, Money NP. Invasive hyphal growth in *Wangiella dermatitidis* is induced by stab inoculation and shows dependence upon melanin biosynthesis. *Fungal Genetics and Biology*. 1999 Dec;28(3):190-200.

[77] Dixon DM, Polak A, Conner GW. Mel- mutants of *Wangiella dermatitidis* in mice: evaluation of multiple mouse and fungal strains. *Journal of Medical and Veterinary Mycology*. 1989;27(5):335-41.

[78] Dixon DM, Polak A, Szaniszlo PJ. Pathogenicity and virulence of wild-type and melanin-deficient *Wangiella dermatitidis*. *J. Med. Vet. Mycol.* 1987 Apr;25(2):97-106.

[79] Dixon DM, Migliozzi J, Cooper CR, Jr., Solis O, Breslin B, Szaniszlo PJ. Melanized and non-melanized multicellular form mutants of *Wangiella dermatitidis* in mice: mortality and histopathology studies. *Mycoses*. 1992 Jan-Feb;35(1-2):17-21.

[80] Schnitzler N, Peltroche-Llacsahuanga H, Bestier N, Zundorf J, Lutticken R, Haase G. Effect of melanin and carotenoids of *Exophiala* (*Wangiella*) *dermatitidis* on phagocytosis, oxidative burst, and killing by human neutrophils. *Infection and immunity*. 1999 Jan;67(1):94-101.

[81] Li DM, de Hoog GS. Cerebral phaeohyphomycosis--a cure at what lengths? *The Lancet infectious diseases*. 2009 Jun;9(6):376-83.

[82] Polak A, Dixon DM. Loss of melanin in *Wangiella dermatitidis* does not result in greater susceptibility to antifungal agents. *Antimicrobial agents and chemotherapy*. 1989 Sep;33(9):1639-40.

[83] Lopez-Romero E, Reyes-Montes Mdel R, Perez-Torres A, Ruiz-Baca E, Villagomez-Castro JC, Mora-Montes HM, et al. *Sporothrix schenckii* complex and sporotrichosis, an emerging health problem. *Future microbiology*. 2011 Jan;6(1):85-102.

[84] Oliveira MM, Almeida-Paes R, Muniz MM, Gutierrez-Galhardo MC, Zancope-Oliveira RM. Phenotypic and Molecular Identification of *Sporothrix* Isolates from an Epidemic Area of Sporotrichosis in Brazil. *Mycopathologia*. 2011 Oct;172(4):257-67.

[85] Marimon R, Cano J, Gene J, Sutton DA, Kawasaki M, Guarro J. *Sporothrix brasiliensis*, *S. globosa*, and *S. mexicana*, three new *Sporothrix* species of clinical interest. *Journal of clinical microbiology*. 2007 Oct;45(10):3198-206.

[86] Romero-Martinez R, Wheeler M, Guerrero-Plata A, Rico G, Torres-Guerrero H. Biosynthesis and functions of melanin in *Sporothrix schenckii*. *Infection and immunity*. 2000 Jun;68(6):3696-703.

[87] Morris-Jones R, Youngchim S, Gomez BL, Aisen P, Hay RJ, Nosanchuk JD, et al. Synthesis of melanin-like pigments by *Sporothrix schenckii* in vitro and during mammalian infection. *Infection and immunity*. 2003 Jul;71(7):4026-33.

[88] Almeida-Paes R, Frases S, Fialho Monteiro PC, Gutierrez-Galhardo MC, Zancope-Oliveira RM, Nosanchuk JD. Growth conditions influence melanization of Brazilian clinical *Sporothrix schenckii* isolates. *Microbes and infection*. 2009 Apr;11(5):554-62.

[89] Hay RJ, Morris-Jones R. Outbreaks of sporotrichosis. *Current opinion in infectious diseases*. 2008 Apr;21(2):119-21.

[90] Teixeira PA, De Castro RA, Ferreira FR, Cunha MM, Torres AP, Penha CV, et al. L-DOPA accessibility in culture medium increases melanin expression and virulence of *Sporothrix schenckii* yeast cells. *Med. Mycol*. 2010 Aug;48(5):687-95.

[91] Madrid IM, Xavier MO, Mattei AS, Fernandes CG, Guim TN, Santin R, et al. Role of melanin in the pathogenesis of cutaneous sporotrichosis. *Microbes and infection*. 2009 Feb;12(2):162-5.

[92] Cooper CR, Dixon DM, Salkin IF. Laboratory-acquired sporotrichosis. *Journal of Medical and Veterinary Mycology*. 1992;30(2):169-71.

[93] Kwon-Chung KJ, Hill WB, Bennett JE. New, special stain for histopathological diagnosis of cryptococcosis. *Journal of clinical microbiology*. 1981 Feb;13(2):383-7.

[94] Kwon-Chung KJ. Sexual stage of *Histoplasma capsulatum*. *Science*. 1972 Jan 21;175(19):326.

[95] Komori T, Sano A, Yarita K, Kitagawa T, Kamei K, Nishimura K. Phylogenetic analysis of *Histoplasma capsulatum* based on partial sequence of the D1/D2 region of the 28S rRNA gene. *Nihon Ishinkin Gakkai zasshi*. 2005;46(4):291-5.

[96] Kasuga T, White TJ, Koenig G, McEwen J, Restrepo A, Castaneda E, et al. Phylogeography of the fungal pathogen *Histoplasma capsulatum*. *Molecular ecology*. 2003 Dec;12(12):3383-401.

[97] Knox KS, Hage CA. Histoplasmosis. *Proceedings of the American Thoracic Society*. 2010 May;7(3):169-72.

[98] Maresca B, Kobayashi GS. Dimorphism in *Histoplasma capsulatum* and *Blastomyces dermatitidis*. *Contributions to microbiology*. 2000;5:201-16.

[99] Woods JP. *Histoplasma capsulatum* molecular genetics, pathogenesis, and responsiveness to its environment. *Fungal. Genet. Biol.* 2002 Mar;35(2):81-97.

[100] Nosanchuk JD, Gomez BL, Youngchim S, Diez S, Aisen P, Zancope-Oliveira RM, et al. *Histoplasma capsulatum* synthesizes melanin-like pigments *in vitro* and during mammalian infection. *Infection and immunity*. 2002 Sep;70(9):5124-31.

[101] Daniels LS, Berliner MD, Campbell CC. Varying virulence in rabbits infected with different filamentous types of *Histoplasma capsulatum*. *Journal of bacteriology*. 1968 Nov;96(5):1535-9.

[102] Hwang L, Hocking-Murray D, Bahrami AK, Andersson M, Rine J, Sil A. Identifying phase-specific genes in the fungal pathogen *Histoplasma capsulatum* using a genomic shotgun microarray. *Molecular biology of the cell*. 2003 Jun;14(6):2314-26.

[103] Taborda CP, da Silva MB, Nosanchuk JD, Travassos LR. Melanin as a virulence factor of *Paracoccidioides brasiliensis* and other dimorphic pathogenic fungi: a minireview. *Mycopathologia*. 2008 Apr-May;165(4-5):331-9.

[104] Wanke B, Aide MA. Chapter 6--paracoccidioidomycosis. *J. Bras. Pneumol.* 2009 Dec;35(12):1245-9.

[105] Gomez BL, Nosanchuk JD, Diez S, Youngchim S, Aisen P, Cano LE, et al. Detection of melanin-like pigments in the dimorphic fungal pathogen *Paracoccidioides brasiliensis in vitro* and during infection. *Infection and immunity*. 2001 Sep;69(9):5760-7.

[106] Taborda VB, Taborda PR, McGinnis MR. Constitutive melanin in the cell wall of the etiologic agent of Lobo's disease. *Revista do Instituto de Medicina Tropical de Sao Paulo*. 1999 Jan-Feb;41(1):9-12.

[107] da Silva MB, Marques AF, Nosanchuk JD, Casadevall A, Travassos LR, Taborda CP. Melanin in the dimorphic fungal pathogen *Paracoccidioides brasiliensis*: effects on phagocytosis, intracellular resistance and drug susceptibility. *Microbes and infection*. 2006 Jan;8(1):197-205.

[108] Bailao AM, Schrank A, Borges CL, Dutra V, Walquiria Ines Molinari-Madlum EE, Soares Felipe MS, et al. Differential gene expression by *Paracoccidioides brasiliensis* in host interaction conditions: representational difference analysis identifies candidate genes associated with fungal pathogenesis. *Microbes and infection*. 2006 Oct;8(12-13):2686-97.

[109] Bailao AM, Shrank A, Borges CL, Parente JA, Dutra V, Felipe MS, et al. The transcriptional profile of *Paracoccidioides brasiliensis* yeast cells is influenced by human plasma. *FEMS immunology and medical microbiology*. 2007 Oct;51(1):43-57.

[110] Silva MB, Thomaz L, Marques AF, Svidzinski AE, Nosanchuk JD, Casadevall A, et al. Resistance of melanized yeast cells of *Paracoccidioides brasiliensis* to antimicrobial oxidants and inhibition of phagocytosis using carbohydrates and monoclonal antibody to CD18. *Memorias do Instituto Oswaldo Cruz*. 2009 Jul;104(4):644-8.

[111] Bradsher RW, Chapman SW, Pappas PG. Blastomycosis. *Infectious disease clinics of North America*. 2003 Mar;17(1):21-40, vii.

[112] Deus Filho A. Chapter 2: coccidioidomycosis. *J. Bras. Pneumol.* 2009 Sep;35(9):920-30.

[113] Ustianowski AP, Sieu TP, Day JN. *Penicillium marneffei* infection in HIV. *Curr. Opin. Infect. Dis*. 2008 Feb;21(1):31-6.

[114] Nosanchuk JD, van Duin D, Mandal P, Aisen P, Legendre AM, Casadevall A. *Blastomyces dermatitidis* produces melanin *in vitro* and during infection. *FEMS microbiology letters*. 2004 Oct 1;239(1):187-93.

[115] Nosanchuk JD, Yu JJ, Hung CY, Casadevall A, Cole GT. *Coccidioides posadasii* produces melanin *in vitro* and during infection. *Fungal. Genetics and Biology*. 2007 Jun;44(6):517-20.

[116] Youngchim S, Hay RJ, Hamilton AJ. Melanization of *Penicillium marneffei in vitro* and *in vivo*. *Microbiology* (Reading, England). 2005 Jan;151(Pt 1):291-9.

[117] Woo PC, Tam EW, Chong KT, Cai JJ, Tung ET, Ngan AH, et al. High diversity of polyketide synthase genes and the melanin biosynthesis gene cluster in *Penicillium marneffei*. *The FEBS journal*. 2010 Sep;277(18):3750-8.

[118] Niewerth M, Korting HC. *Candida albicans* and the principle of opportunism. *an essay*. *Mycoses*. 2002 Oct;45(8):253-8.

[119] Ells R, Kock JL, Pohl CH. *Candida albicans* or *Candida dubliniensis*? *Mycoses*. 2011 Jan;54(1):1-16.

[120] Morris-Jones R, Gomez BL, Diez S, Uran M, Morris-Jones SD, Casadevall A, et al. Synthesis of melanin pigment by *Candida albicans* in vitro and during infection. *Infection and immunity*. 2005 Sep;73(9):6147-50.

[121] Walker CA, Gomez BL, Mora-Montes HM, Mackenzie KS, Munro CA, Brown AJ, et al. Melanin externalization in *Candida albicans* depends on cell wall chitin structures. *Eukaryotic. cell.* 2010 Sep;9(9):1329-42.

[122] Jang YH, Lee SJ, Lee JH, Chae HS, Kim SH, Choe NH. Prevalence of yeast-like fungi and evaluation of several virulence factors from feral pigeons in Seoul, Korea. *Letters in applied microbiology*. 2011 Apr;52(4):367-71.

[123] Carreira A, Ferreira LM, Loureiro V. Brown pigments produced by *Yarrowia lipolytica* result from extracellular accumulation of homogentisic acid. *Applied and environmental microbiology*. 2001 Aug;67(8):3463-8.

[124] Ali S, Shultz JL, Ikram Ul H. High performance microbiological transformation of L-tyrosine to L-dopa by *Yarrowia lipolytica* NRRL-143. *BMC biotechnology*. 2007;7:50.

[125] Kuhn DM, George T, Chandra J, Mukherjee PK, Ghannoum MA. Antifungal susceptibility of *Candida* biofilms: unique efficacy of amphotericin B lipid formulations and echinocandins. *Antimicrobial agents and chemotherapy*. 2002 Jun;46(6):1773-80.

[126] Klich MA. Identification of common *Aspergillus* species. 1 ed. Utrecht: Centraalbureau voor Schimmelcultures 2002.

[127] Pirt SJ, Rowley BI. Melanin production in *Aspergillus nidulans*. *The Biochemical journal*. 1969 Aug;114(1):9P-10P.

[128] Rowley BI, Pirt SJ. Melanin production by *Aspergillus nidulans* in batch and chemostat cultures. *Journal of general microbiology*. 1972 Oct;72(3):553-63.

[129] Osmani SA, Mirabito PM. The early impact of genetics on our understanding of cell cycle regulation in *Aspergillus nidulans*. *Fungal Genetics and Biology*. 2004 Apr;41(4):401-10.

[130] de Cassia RGR, Pombeiro-Sponchiado SR. Antioxidant activity of the melanin pigment extracted from *Aspergillus nidulans*. *Biological and pharmaceutical bulletin*. 2005 Jun;28(6):1129-31.

[131] McCormick A, Loeffler J, Ebel F. *Aspergillus fumigatus*: contours of an opportunistic human pathogen. *Cellular microbiology*. 2010 Nov;12(11):1535-43.

[132] Karkowska-Kuleta J, Rapala-Kozik M, Kozik A. Fungi pathogenic to humans: molecular bases of virulence of *Candida albicans*, *Cryptococcus neoformans* and *Aspergillus fumigatus*. *Acta biochimica Polonica*. 2009;56(2):211-24.

[133] Tsai HF, Wheeler MH, Chang YC, Kwon-Chung KJ. A developmentally regulated gene cluster involved in conidial pigment biosynthesis in *Aspergillus fumigatus*. *Journal of bacteriology*. 1999 Oct;181(20):6469-77.

[134] Youngchim S, Morris-Jones R, Hay RJ, Hamilton AJ. Production of melanin by *Aspergillus fumigatus*. *Journal of medical microbiology*. 2004 Mar;53(Pt 3):175-81.

[135] Tsai HF, Washburn RG, Chang YC, Kwon-Chung KJ. *Aspergillus fumigatus* arp1 modulates conidial pigmentation and complement deposition. *Molecular microbiology*. 1997 Oct;26(1):175-83.

[136] Tsai HF, Chang YC, Washburn RG, Wheeler MH, Kwon-Chung KJ. The developmentally regulated *alb1* gene of *Aspergillus fumigatus*: its role in modulation of conidial morphology and virulence. *Journal of bacteriology*. 1998 Jun;180(12):3031-8.

[137] Watanabe A, Fujii I, Tsai H, Chang YC, Kwon-Chung KJ, Ebizuka Y. *Aspergillus fumigatus alb1* encodes naphthopyrone synthase when expressed in *Aspergillus oryzae*. *FEMS microbiology letters*. 2000 Nov 1;192(1):39-44.

[138] Sugareva V, Hartl A, Brock M, Hubner K, Rohde M, Heinekamp T, et al. Characterisation of the laccase-encoding gene abr2 of the dihydroxynaphthalene-like melanin gene cluster of *Aspergillus fumigatus*. *Archives of microbiology*. 2006 Nov;186(5):345-55.

[139] Jahn B, Langfelder K, Schneider U, Schindel C, Brakhage AA. PKSP-dependent reduction of phagolysosome fusion and intracellular kill of *Aspergillus fumigatus* conidia by human monocyte-derived macrophages. *Cellular microbiology*. 2002 Dec;4(12):793-803.

[140] Thywissen A, Heinekamp T, Dahse HM, Schmaler-Ripcke J, Nietzsche S, Zipfel PF, et al. Conidial Dihydroxynaphthalene Melanin of the Human Pathogenic Fungus *Aspergillus fumigatus* Interferes with the Host Endocytosis Pathway. *Frontiers in microbiology*. 2011;2:96.

[141] Volling K, Thywissen A, Brakhage AA, Saluz HP. Phagocytosis of melanized *Aspergillus* conidia by macrophages exerts cytoprotective effects by sustained PI3K/Akt signalling. *Cellular microbiology*. 2011 Aug;13(8):1130-48.

[142] Chai LY, Netea MG, Sugui J, Vonk AG, van de Sande WW, Warris A, et al. *Aspergillus fumigatus* conidial melanin modulates host cytokine response. *Immunobiology*. 2010 Nov;215(11):915-20.
[143] Jahn B, Koch A, Schmidt A, Wanner G, Gehringer H, Bhakdi S, et al. Isolation and characterization of a pigmentless-conidium mutant of *Aspergillus fumigatus* with altered conidial surface and reduced virulence. *Infection and immunity*. 1997 Dec;65(12):5110-7.
[144] Muller FM, Seidler M, Beauvais A. *Aspergillus fumigatus* biofilms in the clinical setting. *Med. Mycol.* 2011 Apr;49 Suppl 1:S96-S100.
[145] Beauvais A, Schmidt C, Guadagnini S, Roux P, Perret E, Henry C, et al. An extracellular matrix glues together the aerial-grown hyphae of *Aspergillus fumigatus*. *Cellular microbiology*. 2007 Jun;9(6):1588-600.
[146] Jackson JC, Higgins LA, Lin X. Conidiation color mutants of *Aspergillus fumigatus* are highly pathogenic to the heterologous insect host *Galleria mellonella*. *PloS one*. 2009;4(1):e4224.
[147] Luther JP, Lipke H. Degradation of melanin by *Aspergillus fumigatus*. *Applied and environmental microbiology*. 1980 Jul;40(1):145-55.
[148] Singaravelan N, Grishkan I, Beharav A, Wakamatsu K, Ito S, Nevo E. Adaptive melanin response of the soil fungus *Aspergillus niger* to UV radiation stress at "Evolution Canyon", Mount Carmel, Israel. *PloS one*. 2008;3(8):e2993.
[149] Chiang YM, Meyer KM, Praseuth M, Baker SE, Bruno KS, Wang CC. Characterization of a polyketide synthase in *Aspergillus niger* whose product is a precursor for both dihydroxynaphthalene (DHN) melanin and naphtho-gamma-pyrone. *Fungal Genet Biol.* 2011 Apr;48(4):430-7.
[150] Icenhour CR, Kottom TJ, Limper AH. Evidence for a melanin cell wall component in *Pneumocystis carinii*. *Infection and immunity*. 2003 Sep;71(9):5360-3.
[151] Icenhour CR, Kottom TJ, Limper AH. *Pneumocystis* melanins confer enhanced organism viability. *Eukaryotic. cell.* 2006 Jun;5(6):916-23.
[152] Morris-Jones R, Youngchim S, Hextall JM, Gomez BL, Morris-Jones SD, Hay RJ, et al. *Scytalidium dimidiatum* causing recalcitrant subcutaneous lesions produces melanin. *Journal of clinical microbiology*. 2004 Aug;42(8):3789-94.
[153] Youngchim S, Pornsuwan S, Nosanchuk JD, Dankai W, Vanittanakom N. Melanogenesis in dermatophyte species in vitro and during infection. *Microbiology*. 2011 May 12.
[154] van de Sande WW, de Kat J, Coppens J, Ahmed AO, Fahal A, Verbrugh H, et al. Melanin biosynthesis in *Madurella mycetomatis* and its effect on susceptibility to itraconazole and ketoconazole. *Microbes and infection*. 2007 Jul;9(9):1114-23.
[155] Gaitanis G, Chasapi V, Velegraki A. Novel application of the masson-fontana stain for demonstrating *Malassezia* species melanin-like pigment production *in vitro* and in clinical specimens. *Journal of clinical microbiology*. 2005 Aug;43(8):4147-51.
[156] Kogej T, Stein M, Volkmann M, Gorbushina AA, Galinski EA, Gunde-Cimerman N. Osmotic adaptation of the halophilic fungus *Hortaea werneckii*: role of osmolytes and melanization. *Microbiology*. 2007 Dec;153(Pt 12):4261-73.
[157] Egorova AS, Gessler NN, Belozerskaya TA. Melanin pigments in the fungus *Paecilomyces lilacinus* (Thom) Samson. *Doklady*. 2011 Mar-Apr;437:84-6.

[158] Kimura N, Tsuge T. Gene cluster involved in melanin biosynthesis of the filamentous fungus *Alternaria alternata*. *Journal of bacteriology*. 1993 Jul;175(14):4427-35.

[159] Lanisnik Rizner T, Wheeler MH. Melanin biosynthesis in the fungus *Curvularia lunata* (teleomorph: *Cochliobolus lunatus*). *Canadian journal of microbiology*. 2003 Feb;49(2):110-9.

[160] Ruiz-Diez B, Martinez-Suarez JV. Isolation, characterization, and antifungal susceptibility of melanin-deficient mutants of *Scedosporium prolificans*. *Current microbiology*. 2003 Mar;46(3):228-32.

[161] Kroken S, Glass NL, Taylor JW, Yoder OC, Turgeon BG. Phylogenomic analysis of type I polyketide synthase genes in pathogenic and saprobic ascomycetes. *Proceedings of the National Academy of Sciences of the United States of America*. 2003 Dec 23;100(26):15670-5.

[162] Thines E, Weber RW, Talbot NJ. MAP kinase and protein kinase A-dependent mobilization of triacylglycerol and glycogen during appressorium turgor generation by *Magnaporthe grisea*. *The Plant cell*. 2000 Sep;12(9):1703-18.

[163] Takano Y, Kubo Y, Kawamura C, Tsuge T, Furusawa I. The *Alternaria alternata* melanin biosynthesis gene restores appressorial melanization and penetration of cellulose membranes in the melanin-deficient albino mutant of *Colletotrichum lagenarium*. *Fungal Genetics and Biology*. 1997 Feb;21(1):131-40.

[164] Henson JM, Butler MJ, Day AW. THE DARK SIDE OF THE MYCELIUM: Melanins of Phytopathogenic Fungi. *Annual review of phytopathology*. 1999;37:447-71.

[165] Akamatsu HO, Chilvers MI, Stewart JE, Peever TL. Identification and function of a polyketide synthase gene responsible for 1,8-dihydroxynaphthalene-melanin pigment biosynthesis in *Ascochyta rabiei*. *Current genetics*. 2010 Aug;56(4):349-60.

[166] Kihara J, Moriwaki A, Ito M, Arase S, Honda Y. Expression of THR1, a 1,3,8-trihydroxynaphthalene reductase gene involved in melanin biosynthesis in the phytopathogenic fungus *Bipolaris oryzae*, is enhanced by near-ultraviolet radiation. *Pigment cell research*. 2004 Feb;17(1):15-23.

[167] Bode R, Melo C, Birnbaum D. Mode of action of glyphosate in *Candida maltosa*. *Archives of microbiology*. 1984 Nov;140(1):83-5.

[168] Mednick AJ, Nosanchuk JD, Casadevall A. Melanization of *Cryptococcus neoformans* affects lung inflammatory responses during cryptococcal infection. *Infection and immunity*. 2005 Apr;73(4):2012-9.

[169] Mavrogiorgos N, Zaragoza O, Casadevall A, Nosanchuk JD. Efficacy of voriconazole in experimental *Cryptococcus neoformans* infection. *Mycopathologia*. 2006 Aug;162(2):111-4.

[170] van Duin D, Cleare W, Zaragoza O, Casadevall A, Nosanchuk JD. Effects of voriconazole on *Cryptococcus neoformans*. *Antimicrobial agents and chemotherapy*. 2004 Jun;48(6):2014-20.

[171] Martinez LR, Ntiamoah P, Gacser A, Casadevall A, Nosanchuk JD. Voriconazole inhibits melanization in *Cryptococcus neoformans*. *Antimicrobial agents and chemotherapy*. 2007 Dec;51(12):4396-400.

[172] Dalisay DS, Saludes JP, Molinski TF. Ptilomycalin A inhibits laccase and melanization in *Cryptococcus neoformans*. *Bioorganic and medicinal chemistry*. 2011 May 27.

[173] Mun YJ, Lee SW, Jeong HW, Lee KG, Kim JH, Woo WH. Inhibitory effect of miconazole on melanogenesis. *Biological and pharmaceutical bulletin.* 2004 Jun;27(6):806-9.

[174] Itoh Y, Ide H, Hama T. Induction of precocious melanogenesis of pigment cells in cultures of neuroretinal cells of chick embryo by amphotericin B. *Cell and tissue research.* 1980;209(3):353-64.

[175] Dadachova E, Casadevall A. Ionizing radiation: how fungi cope, adapt, and exploit with the help of melanin. *Current opinion in microbiology.* 2008 Dec;11(6):525-31.

[176] Dadachova E, Bryan RA, Huang X, Moadel T, Schweitzer AD, Aisen P, et al. Ionizing radiation changes the electronic properties of melanin and enhances the growth of melanized fungi. *PloS one.* 2007;2(5):e457.

[177] Dadachova E, Bryan RA, Howell RC, Schweitzer AD, Aisen P, Nosanchuk JD, et al. The radioprotective properties of fungal melanin are a function of its chemical composition, stable radical presence and spatial arrangement. *Pigment cell and melanoma research.* 2008 Apr;21(2):192-9.

[178] Schweitzer AD, Howell RC, Jiang Z, Bryan RA, Gerfen G, Chen CC, et al. Physico-chemical evaluation of rationally designed melanins as novel nature-inspired radioprotectors. *PloS one.* 2009;4(9):e7229.

[179] Schweitzer AD, Revskaya E, Chu P, Pazo V, Friedman M, Nosanchuk JD, et al. Melanin-covered nanoparticles for protection of bone marrow during radiation therapy of cancer. *International journal of radiation oncology, biology, physics.* 2010 Dec 1;78(5):1494-502.

[180] Dadachova E, Moadel T, Schweitzer AD, Bryan RA, Zhang T, Mints L, et al. Radiolabeled melanin-binding peptides are safe and effective in treatment of human pigmented melanoma in a mouse model of disease. *Cancer biotherapy and radiopharmaceuticals.* 2006 Apr;21(2):117-29.

[181] Dighton J, Tugay T, Zhdanova N. Fungi and ionizing radiation from radionuclides. *FEMS microbiology letters.* 2008 Apr;281(2):109-20.

[182] Larsson BS. Interaction between chemicals and melanin. *Pigment cell research.* 1993 Jun;6(3):127-33.

[183] Bridelli MG, Ciati A, Crippa PR. Binding of chemicals to melanins re-examined: adsorption of some drugs to the surface of melanin particles. *Biophysical chemistry.* 2006 Jan 20;119(2):137-45.

[184] Mammone T, Marenus K, Muizzuddin N, Maes D. Evidence and utility of melanin degrading enzymes. *Journal of cosmetic science.* 2004 Jan-Feb;55(1):116-7.

In: Melanin: Biosynthesis, Functions and Health Effects
Editors: Xiao-Peng Ma and Xiao-Xiao Sun
ISBN: 978-1-62100-991-7

Chapter III

The Coat Color Genes Regulate Eumelanin and Pheomelanin Synthesis in Melanocytes

Tomohisa Hirobe*
Radiation Risk Reduction Research Program,
National Institute of Radiological Sciences,
Anagawa 4-9-1, Inage-ku, Chiba 263-8555,
Chiba, Japan

Abstract

In mice, eumelanin and pheomelanin synthesis is regulated by numerous coat color genes. Eumelanin and pheomelanin contents were measured in cultured melanocytes and in the epidermis/dermis and hairs of C57BL/10JHir (B10) and its congenic mice carrying the coat color genes. Eumelanin contents in agouti and dilute melanocytes are similar to black melanocytes, whereas the contents in brown, pink-eyed dilution, slaty and ruby-eye 2^d melanocytes are reduced to one third~one thirthieth. In contrast, pheomelanin contents in agouti, dilute, slaty and ruby-eye 2^d melanocytes are similar to its content in black melanocytes, whereas the content in brown melanocytes is increased. Eumelanin and pheomelanin contents in cultured epidermal melanocytes correlate well with those in skin and hair of the congenic mice, except that agouti melanocytes do not synthesize pheomelanin in culture, the pink-eyed dilution allele does not affect pheomelanin content in hairs, and the ruby-eye 2^d allele increases pheomelanin content in hairs. These results suggest that eumelanin and pheomelanin synthesis in melanocytes is regulated by numerous coat color genes in a complicated manner.

Keywords: Melanoblast/melanocyte/coat color gene/melanocyte-stimulating hormone

* Phone: +81-43-206-3253, Fax: +81-43-206-4638, E-mail: thirobe@nirs.go.jp.

Introduction

Melanocytes are neural crest-derived cells that synthesize melanin pigments (Rawles, 1947; Mayer, 1973; Hearing, 1993, 2000; Ito, 2003). Undifferentiated precursors of melanocytes, melanoblasts, are derived from neural crest cells in embryonic skin (Rawles, 1947; Mayer, 1973; Steel et al., 1992; Aoki et al., 2009; Motohashi et al., 2011). Melanoblasts invade the epidermis (Mayer, 1973) and colonize at the same place. Mouse epidermal melanocytes are known to differentiate from melanoblasts around the time of birth (Hirobe, 1984a). Fully differentiated melanocytes are characterized by pigmentation and well-developed dendrites and can be seen mainly in hair bulbs of the skin where they secrete mature melanosomes into surrounding keratinocytes giving rise to melanized hairs (Mann, 1962; Slominski and Paus, 1993; Hirobe, 1995; Peters et al., 2002). Hair bulb melanocytes are derived from epidermal melanoblasts and melanocytes (Hirobe, 1992a). Epidermal melanocytes are found only during the early weeks after birth in the hairy skin of mice (Hirobe, 1984a). In glabrous skin, such as the ear, nose, foot sole and tail of mice, epidermal melanocytes are also found even in adult mice (Quevedo and Smith, 1963).

Melanin synthesis is mainly controlled by tyrosinase (Tyr), Tyr-related protein 1 (TRP1, Tyrp1) and TRP2 (Tyrp2, dopachrome tautomerase (Dct); Hearing, 1993, 2000; Ito, 2003; Ito and Wakamatsu, 2011). Tyr initiates melanin synthesis by catalyzing oxidation of L-tyrosine (tyr) to dopaquinone (Cooksey et al., 1997). Tyrp1 possesses 5,6-dihydroxyindole-2-carboxylic acid (DHICA) oxidase activity (Jackson et al., 1990). In contrast, TRP2 possesses dopachrome tautomerase (Dct) activity (Jackson et al., 1992; Tsukamoto et al., 1992; Kroumpouzos et al., 1994), which converts dopachrome (DC) to DHICA (Korner and Pawelek, 1980). Melanocytes produce two types of melanin: brownish-black eumelanin and yellow-reddish pheomelanin (Ito, 1993, 2003; Ito and Wakamatsu 2011). Although differences exist in molecular size and general properties, these melanins arise from a common metabolic pathway in which dopaquinone is a key intermediate (Ito and Prota, 1977; Hearing and Tsukamoto, 1991; Ito and Wakamatsu, 2008, 2011).

Melanin synthesis occurs in specialized organelles called melanosomes (Seiji et al., 1963). Melanosome maturation is categorized into four stages: stages I and II include unmelanized immature premelanosomes, while melanized melanosomes are classified into stages III and IV (Fitzpatrick et al., 1969). In mice, coat colors are regulated by melanosome transfer from melanocytes to neighboring keratinocytes in hair bulbs (Silvers, 1979; Hirobe, 1995). Melanosomes are produced in varying sizes, numbers and densities in melanocytes. Melanosomes in hair bulb melanocytes are passed on to the hair shaft where the final distribution patterns of the pigment are determined. This distribution plays an important role in determining the coat coloring of mice (Silvers, 1979). Eumelanin-containing melanosomes (eumelanosomes) are elliptical with longitudinal depositions of pigments in intraluminal fibrils (Hearing et al., 1973; Sakurai et al., 1975; Hirobe and Abe, 1999). In contrast, pheomelanin-containing melanosomes (pheomelanosomes) are spherical with granular depositions of pigments in multivesicular bodies found in yellow phase agouti melanocytes as well as in yellow (lethal yellow (A^{y}/-) and recessive yellow ($Mc1r^{e}/Mc1r^{e}$)) melanocytes (Sakurai et al., 1975; Takeuchi, 1985). Thus, the differences in melanin synthesis correspond to those in melanosome morphology.

The proliferation and differentiation of mouse melanocytes during development is regulated by numerous epigenetic and genetic factors (Hirobe, 1992a). Epigenetic factors from the surrounding tissue environment, such as keratinocytes (Imokawa, 2004; Hirobe, 2005, 2011a; Yamaguchi and Hearing, 2009; Kondo and Hearing, 2011) and fibroblasts (Imokawa, 2004; Hirobe, 2011a, Yamaguchi and Hearing, 2009; Kondo and Hearing, 2011), the blood supply of hormones and other substances from the pituitary gland and other organs (Snell and Bishitz, 1960; Hirobe, 1996, 2011a; Hirobe and Abe, 2000; Hirobe et al., 2004a), minerals, especially iron (Hirobe, 2007, 2009a, b, c, 2011b) and environmental factors such as ultraviolet (UV) radiation (Quevedo and Smith, 1963; Szabo, 1967; Gilchrest et al., 1996; Hachiya et al., 2001; Naganuma et al., 2001; Furuya et al., 2002, 2009; Imokawa, 2004;; Hirobe et al., 2002a, 2004b; Choi et al., 2010) and ionizing radiation (Chase, 1949; Quevedo and Isherwood, 1958; Hirobe and Zhou, 1990; Hirobe, 1994a; Hirobe et al., 2004c, 2011a, b; Inomata et al., 2009) are also important for the regulation of melanocyte proliferation and differentiation. Among the genetic factors, semidominant genes controlling melanocyte numbers are involved in regulating the melanocyte and melanoblast-melanocyte populations in the epidermis of newborn mouse skin (Hirobe, 1982, 1988a, b, 1995). The coat color genes are the most important (Silvers, 1979; Hirobe and Abe, 1999; Lamoreux et al., 2001, 2010; Bennett and Lamoreux, 2003; Hirobe, 2011a). In mice, more than 300 genes are involved in melanocyte proliferation and differentiation; about one half of these genes have been cloned and their functions are clarified (Mouse Genome Informatics). However, many unknown genes and their functions in melanocyte proliferation and differentiation still remain to be investigated. In this chapter, studies of the control of melanin synthesis in differentiated melanocytes by the coat color genes are reviewed and their role in melanin synthsis is discussed in detail.

Regulation by the Coat Color Genes

To clarify the mechanisms of the regulation of melanin synthesis by the coat color genes, characteristics of melanin synthesis in mouse epidermal melanocytes in serum-free primary culture of epidermal cell suspension (Hirobe, 1992b, c) were compared between two different strains of mice that possess the same genetic background except for one allele in the topical coat color locus, that is, comparison was made between C57BL/10JHir (B10) and its congenic strains. In the initial stage of this serum-free primary culture of epidermal cell suspension of B10 mice, keratinocytes proliferate well and epidermal melanoblasts and melanocytes start to proliferate around the keratinocyte colony, and after 8-9 days keratinocytes gradually die, then pure cultures of melanoblasts or melanocytes are obtained after 14 days (Hirobe, 1992b, c). Pure culture of many melanocytes is obtained by melanocyte-proliferation medium (MDMD), consisting of Ham's F10 supplemented with 10 μg/ml insulin (bovine), 0.5 mg/ml bovine serum albumin (Fraction V), 1 μM ethanolamine, 1 μM phosphoethanolamine, 10 nM sodium selenite, 0.5 mM dibutyryl adenosine 3':5'-cyclic monophosphate (DBcAMP) is used. Pure culture of numerous undifferentiated melanoblasts is obtained by melanoblast-proliferation medium (MDMDF) consisting of MDMD supplemented with 2.5 ng/ml bFGF (Hirobe, 1992b, 1994b). The differentiation and melanogenesis/dendritogenesis of mouse epidermal melanocytes are induced by cAMP-elevating agent such as α-melanocyte-stimulating hormone (α-MSH, Hirobe, 1992c), DBcAMP (0.1~1 mM, Hirobe, 1992c), 3-isobutyl-1-methylxanthine (IBMX, Hirobe, 1992c) or adrenocorticotrophic hormone (ACTH)/ACTH fragments (Hirobe and Abe, 2000). Eumelanin and pheomelanin contents in the cultured melanocytes using MDMD as well as in the epidermis, dermis and hairs derived from skins of congenic mice were measured and compared with those in B10 mice, and the role of coat color genes in the regulation of eumelanin and pheomelanin synthesis was studied.

Alleles from 7 important coat color loci, namely agouti (*A*), brown ($b/Tyrp1^b$), albino (c/Tyr^c), dilute ($d/Myo5a^d$), recessive yellow ($e/Mc1r^e$), pink-eyed dilution ($p/Oca2^p$) and slaty (slt/Dct^{slt}) were introduced to B10 background by repeated backcrosses in author's laboratory, and congenic lines of B10 mice, namely, B10-*A/A*, $-Tyrp1^b/Tyrp1^b$, $-Tyr^c/Tyr^c$, $-Myo5^d/Myo5^d$, $-Mc1r^e/Mc1r^e$, $-Oca2^p/Oca2^p$ and $-Dct^{slt}/Dct^{slt}$ were prepared (Hirobe, 1986, 2011a). The ruby-eye 2d ($ru2^d/Hps5^{ru2\text{-}d}$) allele is a spontaneous autosomal recessive mutation that occurred in B10 mice in my laboratory (Hirobe et al., 2011d). Studies using C57BL/6J (B6) congenic lines (Lamoreux et al., 2010) as well as noncongenic strains are also reviewed in this chapter.

Agouti, Mahogany, Mahoganoid and Subtle Grey

Although there are a number of loci which affect melanin synthesis in mice, two major loci is known to control the nature of the pigment formed. Namely, the numerous alleles of the agouti and extension loci are involved in regulating the relative amount and distribution of pheomelanin in hairs of the coat. In the coat color of wild type (*A/A*) mice, individual hairs possess a subterminal yellow band in otherwise black. This phenotype is called agouti pattern. The agouti pattern formation is altered by genic substitutions at the agouti locus (Sakurai et al., 1975). Animals homozygous for the *a* allele produce black eumelanin only (Silvers, 1979). The switch between eumelanin and pheomelanin synthesis is regulated by α-MSH and agouti protein or agouti signaling protein (Asip), the product of the *A* allele expressed in the hair bulb (Barsh, 1996). The Asip is produced and released from dermal papilla cells in the hair bulb. A recent study showed that loss and gain of function of β-catenin in dermal papilla cells resulted in yellow and black mice, respectively. In addition, β-catenin activity in dermal papilla cells regulates melanocyte activity (eumelanogenesis) via a mechanism that is independent of the Asip (Enshell-Seijiffers et al., 2010).

These results suggest that β-catenin plays an important role in the agouti pattern formation as well as in eumelanogenesis. Eumelanin content in agouti hairs did not differ from black mice, but pheomelanin content in agouti hairs increased dramatically (Table 1).

It appears that no influence of the genetic background in the content of eumelanin and pheomelanin in agouti hairs, since no difference in the content was observed between B10 and B6 mice (Table 1).

Table 1. Effects of the coat color genes on eumelanin and pheomelanin synthesis in cultured melanocytes and in the epidermis, dermis and hairs of mice

Gene	Strain	Eu (in)	Eu (out)	Eu (e)	Eu (d)	Eu (h)	Pheo (in)	Pheo (out)	Pheo (e)	Pheo (d)	Pheo (h)	Reference
A	B10	→	→	→		→	→	→	↑ ↑		↑ ↑	Ozeki et al., 1995; Hirobe et al., 2004d
A	B6					→					↑ ↑	Lamoreux et al., 2001
Tyrp1^{b}	B10	↓				↓	↑				↑	Ozeki et al., 1995; Hirobe et al., 1998
Tyrp1^{b}	B6					↓					↑	Lamoreux et al., 2001
Tyr^{c}	B10	0		0	0	0	0		0	0	0	Ozeki et al., 1995; Hirobe et al., 1998
Tyr$^{c\text{-}2J}$	B6					0					0	Lamoreux et al., 2001
Tyr$^{c\text{-}ch}$	B6					↓					↓	Lamoreux et al., 2001
Myo5a^{d}	B10	→				→	→				→	Ozeki et al., 1995; Hirobe et al., 1998
Mc1r^{e}	B10	↑	→	↓ ↓	↓ ↓	↓ ↓	↓	→	↑	↑ ↑ ↑	↑ ↑ ↑	Hirobe et al., 2007a, b
Mc1r^{e}	B6					↓ ↓					↑ ↑	Ozeki et al., 1995
Oca2^{p}	B10	↓ ↓	→			↓ ↓ ↓	↓	→			→	Hirobe et al., 2003, 2011c
Dct^{slt}	B10	↓	↓	↓	↓ ↓	↓	→	↑	↓	↓	→	Hirobe et al., 2006
Dct^{slt}	B6					↓					→	Ozeki et al., 1995

Table 1. (Continued)

Gene	Strain	Eu (in)	Eu (out)	Eu (e)	Eu (d)	Eu (h)	Pheo (in)	Pheo (out)	Pheo (e)	Pheo (d)	Pheo (h)	Reference
Dct$^{slt\text{-}lt}$	B6					↓					↑	Lamoreux et al., 2001
Hps5$^{ru2\text{-}d}$	B10	↓	↑	↓↓	↓↓↓	↓	→	→	↓	↓	↑	Hirobe, 2011a; ; Hirobe et al., 2011d
Pmel17^{si}	B6					→					→	Lamoreux et al., 2001
A^{y}	B6					↓↓↓					↑↑	Lamoreux et al., 2001

Effects of the coat color genes on eumelanin (Eu) and pheomelanin (Pheo) synthesis in melanocytes (B10 congenic mice) cultured in MDMD for 14 days as well as in the epidermis (e), dermis (d) and hairs (h; 5-week-old) of B10 or B6 congenic mice. PTCA and AHP (or 4-AHP) were measured in cultured melanocytes (Eu (in), Pheo (in)) and in culture supernatant (Eu (out), Phe (out)), and, in addition, in the epidermis (Eu (e), Pheo (e)), dermis (Eu (d), Pheo (d)) and hairs (Eu (h), Pheo (h)) as described in the text. →, no effects; ↑, slightly increased (~×10); ↑↑, increased (~×100); ↑↑↑, greatly increased (~×1000);↓, slightly decreased (~×1/10); ↓↓, decreased (~×1/100); ↓↓↓, greatly decreased (~×1/1000). Effects of the coat color genes were compared with control melanocytes (B10 mice) cultured in MDMD and with control epidermis (B10), dermis (B10) and hairs (B10 or B6) of mice.

The number of melanoblasts and melanocytes in the epidermis after birth does not differ between black and agouti mice (Hirobe and Abe, 1999). The proliferation of agouti melanocytes cultured in MDMD is also similar to that of black melanocytes. Agouti melanocytes exhibit normal morphology (dendritic, polygonal or epithelioid) and a similar degree of pigmentation to black melanocytes is observed. Moreover, there is no difference in Tyr, Tyrp1, Dct and Kit activity between black and agouti melanocytes (Hirobe, 2011a). Melanosomes of black and agouti melanocytes are evenly distributed within the melanocytes, and they are elliptical in morphology (Hirobe and Abe, 1999; Hirobe, 2011a).

Chemical analysis of melanin produced in cultured epidermal melanocytes revealed that the pyrrole-2,3,5-tricarboxylic acid (PTCA, a degradation product of eumelanin; Ito and Fujita, 1985; Ito and Wakamatsu, 1994) content in agouti melanocytes is similar to that in black melanocytes (Hirobe et al., 2004d). Also, the 4-aminohydroxyphenylalanine (4-AHP, a degradation product of pheomelanin; Wakamatsu and Ito, 2002; Wakamatsu et al., 2002) content in agouti melanocytes cultured in MDMD is similar to that in black melanocytes (Hirobe et al., 1998), as are the PTCA/AHP ratios. However, a 1.5-fold increase in AHP, and a 37-fold increase in 5-*S*-cysteinyldopa (5-*S*-CD, a precursor of pheomelanin), was observed in culture media derived from agouti melanocytes cultured in MDMD (Hirobe et al., 2004d). Moreover, a 11-fold increase in AHP content in the epidermis of 3.5-day-old agouti mice and a 95-fold increase in the epidermis of 5.5-day-old agouti mice were observed compared with black mice (Hirobe et al., 2004d).

Analysis of the *A* allele using reverse transcription-polymerase chain reaction (RT-PCR) revealed that cultured epidermal keratinocytes and melanocytes did not express the *A* allele. Moreover, the Asip was expressed in the dermis of 0.5-, 3.5- and 5.5-day-old agouti mice, but not in the dermis of black mice or in the epidermis of agouti or black mice (Hirobe et al., 2004d). These results suggest that epidermal melanoblasts of agouti mice can be influenced by the Asip produced in the dermis, and can continue to synthesize pheomelanin in culture conditions. Pheomelanin production in the epidermis of 3.5- and 5.5-day-old agouti mice may be derived from the influence of the Asip produced in the dermis.

The master regulator of pigment-type switching is the receptor for α-MSH, melanocortin-1 receptor (Mc1r). When α-MSH binds to Mc1r on melanocyte membrane, adenylate cyclase is activated through the stimulatory G-protein, raising levels of cAMP, thereby activating the melanogenic transcription factor, microphthalmia-associated transcription factor (Mitf; Bertolotto et al., 1998). This leads to the upregulation of many genes required for melanin synthesis such as Tyr, Tyrp1, Dct and many other genes (Levy et al., 2006). The Asip is a competitive antagonist that inhibits the eumelanogenic effect of α-MSH by competing with α-MSH for binding to the Mc1r. When viable yellow (A^{vy}/-) mice producing a mixed-type melanin were injected with α-MSH, Tyr activity increased 2-fold and more eumelanic hair was produced with a concomitant increase in total melanin (TM). When these viable yellow mice were injected with bromocriptine (inhibitor of α-MSH production in the pituitary), Tyr activity was greatly reduced and pheomelanic hair was produced along with a decrease in TM (Burchill et al., 1986). These results suggest that Tyr activity is important for controlling mixed melanogenesis; higher tyrosinase activities favor eumelanogenesis, while lower activities pheomelanogenesis.

The Asip requires two accessory proteins for pigment type switching; products of the mahogany (*mg*) and mahoganoid (*md*) loci (Walker and Gunn, 2010). The mahogany locus was identified as the mouse orthologue of the human attractin (*ATRN*) gene, and the mahoganoid locus encodes a novel RING-domain containing protein. Mice homozygous for mahogany and heterozygous for lethal yellow produce a mixed type melanin with a low level of eumelanin (ca. 15% of black) and have a reduced level of pheomelanin (ca. 60% of lethal yellow). Similarly, Gunn et al. (2001) found that three Atrn mutants, either homozygous or compound heterozygous, showed a pheomelanin content 5- to 10-fold lower than wild-type agouti C3H/ HeJ mice. Another control point in the regulation of eumelanogenesis and pheomelanogenesis is cysteine concentration in melanosomes (del Marmol et al., 1996). Chintala et al. (2005) showed that the murine subtle gray (*sut*) mutation arose because of a mutation in the *Slc7a11* gene that encodes the plasma membrane cystine/glutamate exchanger xCT. The resulting low rate of extracellular cystine transport into sut melanocytes reduces pheomelanin synthesis with minimal or no effect on eumelanin synthesis. In fact, the effect of the sut mutation on pheomelanin synthesis was greatly emphasized by the A^{y}/a background, decreasing pheomelanin levels in hairs to one-sixth of the control level.

Brown

B (*Tyrp1*), the wild type allele at the brown locus, produces black eumelanin, while *b* ($Tyrp1^{b}$), the recessive allele, produces brown eumelanin. The coat color of brown mice is lighter than that of black mice, whereas tyrosinase activity in brown mice is higher than in black mice (Foster, 1965; Hirobe, 1984b; Tamate et al., 1989). Eumelanin content in brown hairs is decreased compared with black hairs, whereas pheomelanin content is increased in both B10 (Ozeki et al., 1995) and B6 (Lamoreux et al., 2001) background (Table 1). The proliferation rate of brown (B10-$Tyrp1^{b}/Tyrp1^{b}$) melanocytes cultured in MDMD is similar to that of black (B10-*Tyrp1*/*Tyrp1*) melanocytes (Hirobe, 2011a). Brown melanocytes in culture possess normal morphology (dendritic, polygonal or epithelioid), but their pigmentation is lower than that of black melanocytes (Hirobe et al., 1998). Tyr, Dct and Kit activities in brown melanocytes in culture do not differ from that in black melanocytes in culture, but Tyrp1 activity is greatly reduced (Hirobe, 2011a). Although brown melanosomes are evenly distributed within melanocytes, their morphology is very different from that of black melanosomes. Elliptical melanosomes and mature stage IV melanosomes are rarely observed (Hirobe, 2011a). Brown melanosomes are mostly spherical stage III melanosomes with granular or lamellar depositions of pigments. In addition, eumelanin is decreased 3-fold in brown melanocytes, whereas pheomelanin is increased 3- to 4-fold (Tamate et al., 1989; Ozeki et al., 1995; Hirobe et al., 1998). The PTCA/AHP ratio in brown melanocytes is one-tenth of that in black melanocytes. The formation of elliptical eumelanosomes requires plenty of eumelanin and higher Tyrp1 activity.

Tyrp1 is believed to act as a DHICA oxidase in mice (Jimenez-Cervantes et al., 1994; Kobayashi et al., 1994a). The brown mutation encodes Tyrp1 that is not properly translocated to melanosomes, resulting in no functional Tyrp1 activity and decreased tyrosinase function (Jackson et al., 1990). Brown melanocytes seem to inhibit eumelanin synthesis (TM and PTCA values). The brown mutation does not significantly alter the proportion of DHICA in the eumelanin synthesized, but rather, brown eumelanin seems to possess a smaller molecular size compared to black eumelanin (Ozeki et al., 1997). Although the exact function of Tyrp1 is not known well, it is thought to stabilize tyrosinase and Dct (Lamoreux et al., 1995; Kobayashi et al., 1998).

Albino

The albino mice lack pigment in the coat and eyes. The inability of albino mice to produce pigment is derived not from an absence of melanoblasts, but from a deficiency of Tyr activity (Tanaka et al., 1990; Hirobe and Abe, 1999). The enzyme Tyr is encoded at the albino/tyrosinase (*C/Tyr*) locus in mice. *C* (*Tyr*), the wild-type allele of the albino locus, produces melanin, while *c* (Tyr^{c}), the recessive allele, produces no pigment in the coat and the eyes (Silvers, 1979; Yamamoto et al., 1989; Tanaka et al., 1990; Table 1). The Tyr^{c} allele is a point mutation at nucleotide residue 387 (G to C transversion) causing a Cys to Ser substitution at position 85 in one of the cysteine-rich domains of the Tyr molecule (Shibahara et al., 1990). This mutation reduces Tyr activity completely. We studied the effects of the *c* mutation on the proliferation of melanoblasts cultured in MDMD and MDMDF, and found that the proliferation rate of albino melanoblasts was about one-half that of black melanocytes (Hirobe et al., 1998), suggesting the possibility that cell proliferation is active in epidermal melanocytes with full melanogenesis such as black melanocytes, but not in epidermal melanoblasts with no melanogenesis such as albino melanoblasts. In other words, proliferation and differentiation of epidermal melanocytes in culture may be linked. Albino melanoblasts exhibit normal morphology (dendritic, polygonal or epithelioid), but no pigmentation was observed (Hirobe et al., 1998; Hirobe, 2011a). Expression of Tyr in albino melanoblasts is not observed, whereas expression of Tyrp1, Dct and Kit is similar level to that in black melanocytes (Hirobe, 2011a). Melanosomes are evenly distributed within albino melanoblasts, and morphology of stage I and II melanosomes is similar to that of black melanocytes (Hirobe, 2011a). Moreover, the number of stage I and II melanosomes is greatly increased compared with black melanocytes (Hirobe, 2011a), probably due to the inhibition of stage III and IV formation by the Tyr^{c} mutation.

The chinchilla allele ($c^{ch}/Tyr^{c\text{-}ch}$) at the albino locus encodes a partially functional Tyr whose activity is one half of that of wild type, due to a point mutation (Ala464Thr) that makes it susceptible to proteolytic cleavage (Muller et al., 1988). Therefore, this is a good model to examine the specific effects of Tyr activity on pigmentogenesis. $Tyr^{c\text{-}ch}/Tyr^{c\text{-}ch}$ hairs possessed eumelanin content about one half of that observed in *Tyr/Tyr* hairs (Lamoreux et al., 2001). Brown chinchilla ($Tyrp1^{b}/Tyrp1^{b}$; $Tyr^{c\text{-}ch}/Tyr^{c\text{-}ch}$) hairs possessed lower eumelanin content than in black chinchilla (*Tyrp1/Tyrp1*; $Tyr^{c\text{-}ch}/Tyr^{c\text{-}ch}$) hairs (Lamoreux et al., 2001). However, $Tyr^{c\text{-}ch}/Tyr^{c\text{-}ch}$ hairs possessed similar amount of pheomelanin as *Tyr/Tyr* hairs (Lamoreux et al., 2001). These results suggest that functional Tyrp1 is also necessary, in addition to high levels of Tyr, for maximal production of eumelanin. In chinchilla mice, the degree of eumelanogenesis is proportional to Tyr activity under low cysteine concentration.

Dilute, Leaden and Ashen

The recessive allele of the dilute locus, $d/Myo5a^{d}$ elicits a lighter hair pigmentation in mice. Despite the fact that the dilute mutation possesses a dilution effect when introduced into wild-type mice producing intensely pigmented eumelanic and pheomelanic hairs, this effect is not due to a decrease in eumelanin and pheomelanin content (Table 1). We investigated the effects of the dilute allele on the proliferation and differentiation of melanoblasts and melanocytes (B10-*Myo5a*^{d}/*Myo5a*^{d}) cultured in MDMD/MDMDF and found that the proliferation rate of dilute melanoblasts and melanocytes was similar to that of black melanoblasts and melanocytes (Hirobe et al., 1998). The rate of differentiation and the reactivity to dopa and dopa-premelanin reactions of dilute melanocytes cultured in MDMD was also similar to that of black melanocytes (Hirobe et al., 1998). Dilute melanocytes were dendritic, polygonal or epithelioid in morphology, but their melanosomes were distributed around the nucleus (Hirobe, 2011a). A few melanosomes were observed in the peripheral region of the cytoplasm as well as in dendrites. Expression of Tyr, Tyrp1, Dct and Kit in dilute melanocytes was similar to that in black melanocytes (Hirobe, 2011a). Dilute melanosomes were distributed around the nucleus, and the number and morphology of stage I–IV melanosomes was similar to that of black melanosomes (eumelanosome type; Hirobe, 2011a). These results suggest that the dilute allele is involved in regulating the transport of melanosomes from the perinuclear region to the dendrites, rather than in regulating dendrite formation. These findings are consistent with results of molecular analyses of the dilute allele (Mercer et al., 1991; Provance et al., 1996; Wei et al., 1997; Wu et al., 1997). The dilute gene encodes myosin Va which is a dimer of two 190 kDa heavy chains. The N-terminal head region consists of actin- and ATP-binding sites and functions as a motor domain for short range movement along actin filaments of the cytoskeleton (Westbroek et al., 2001; Wu et al., 1997).

Leaden (*ln*) is also dilute mutation when homozygous and it transforms the intensely pigmented nonagouti coat color to bluish-grey (Murray, 1931). The effects of the leaden allele on hairs are essentially the same as in dilute except that some leaden genotypes, such as chocolate leaden animals, are a little lighter in color than the corresponding dilute type (Silvers, 1979). This appears to be due to a more pronounced pigment lag in *ln/ln* hairs rather than any noticeable differences in pigment clumping (Silvers, 1979). Ashen (*ash*), recessive mutation arose in strain C3H/DiSn (Lane and Womack, 1977). The coat color of these mice mimics that of dilute and leaden. Recent molecular analysis revealed that leaden (lacking melanophilin (Mlph) protein) and ashen (lacking Rab27a protein) exhibited similar melanosome distribution and these proteins appeared to anchor to MyoVa motor on the melanosome (Wu et al., 2002; Hume et al., 2007). This mechanism allows melanosomes to be retained in dendrites and to make short myosin-driven movements along actin filaments towards the plasma membrane prior to transfer to keratinocytes.

Recessive Yellow and Lethal Yellow

The phenotype that produces mostly pheomelanin is regulated by two alleles, namely, recessive yellow (*e*/*Mc1r*^{e}) at the extension locus and lethal yellow (A^{y}) at the agouti locus. The extension (*E*/*Mc1r*) locus increases eumelanin in hair follicular melanocytes when dominant, but it blocks eumelanin synthesis, extending the range of pheomelanin when recessive (Silvers, 1979). The recessive yellow allele results from a frameshift in Mc1r that produces a prematurely terminated, nonfunctioning receptor (Robbins et al., 1993). In addition to the frameshift mutation, the *Mc1r*^{e} allele possesses a conservative point mutation,

Val101Ala (Robbins et al., 1993). Moreover, the *Mc1r*^{e} allele stimulates pheomelanin synthesis in the epidermis and dermis as well as hair follicles in B10-*Mc1r*^{e}/*Mc1r*^{e} skin (Hirobe et al., 2007a). In B6-*Mc1r*^{e}/*Mc1r*^{e} mice, epidermal and dermal melanoblasts and melanocytes are greatly reduced in number (Tamate et al., 1986).

Since we could not obtain a pure culture of yellow melanocytes producing pheomelanin only from *Mc1r*^{e}/*Mc1r*^{e} mice, we investigated the proliferation and differentiation of cultured recessive yellow melanocytes producing mainly eumelanin. The addition of DBcAMP to culture media can elicit upregulation of the PKA pathway and stimulate eumelanogenesis in melanocytes (Tamate and Takeuchi, 1984). The proliferation rate of *Mc1r*^{e}/*Mc1r*^{e} melanoblasts or melanocytes cultured in MDMDF or MDMD was decreased (by one-half) compared with that of *Mc1r/Mc1r* melanoblasts and melanocytes (Hirobe et al, 2007b). Differentiation of melanocytes cultured in MDMD was also delayed in *Mc1r*^{e}/*Mc1r*^{e} mice (Hirobe et al., 2007b). Although the expression of Tyr and Kit in *Mc1r*^{e}/*Mc1r*^{e} melanocytes was similar to that in black melanocytes, expression of Tyrp1 and Dct was decreased (Hirobe et al., 2007b). The number of stage III melanosomes did not change, while the number of stage IV melanosomes was decreased (Hirobe et al., 2007b). Excess L-tyr added to MDMD rescued the reduced proliferation rate of *Mc1r*^{e}/*Mc1r*^{e} melanocytes. L-tyr also stimulated Tyr activity and expression of Tyrp1, Dct and Kit as well as maturation of stage IV melanosomes and eumelanin synthesis (Hirobe et al., 2007b). These results suggest that the *Mc1r*^{e} mutation affects the proliferation and differentiation of melanocytes and L-tyr rescues the reduced proliferation and differentiation of *Mc1r*^{e}/*Mc1r*^{e} melanocytes by stimulating Tyr activity and expression of Tyrp1 and Dct as well as melanosome maturation and eumelanin synthesis. Even at the higher cAMP levels elicited by DBcAMP-supplemented MDMD and MDMDF, the proliferation of *Mc1r*^{e}/*Mc1r*^{e} melanoblasts and melanocytes was greatly inhibited, suggesting that the PKA pathway elicited by excess DBcAMP in *Mc1r*^{e}/*Mc1r*^{e} melanocytes is different from the PKA pathway elicited by wild-type Mc1r in *Mc1r/Mc1r* melanocytes. The altered PKA pathway in *Mc1r*^{e}/*Mc1r*^{e} melanocytes may affect crosstalk with protein kinase C (PKC) or MAP kinase (MK), and consequently the proliferation and differentiation may be inhibited. L-tyr is thought to rescue the altered PKA pathway as well as the altered crosstalk between PKA and PKC/MK.

Eumelanin content in cultured *Mc1r*^{e}/*Mc1r*^{e} melanocytes in MDMD was higher than in *Mc1r/Mc1r* melanocytes. However, eumelanin content in culture supernatant did not differ between *Mc1r*^{e}/*Mc1r*^{e} and *Mc1r/Mc1r* melanocytes (Hirobe et al., 2007b). In contrast, pheomelanin content in cultured *Mc1r*^{e}/*Mc1r*^{e} melanocytes was lower than in *Mc1r/Mc1r* melanocytes. However, pheomelanin content in culture supernatant did not differ significantly between *Mc1r*^{e}/*Mc1r*^{e} and *Mc1r/Mc1r* melanocytes (Hirobe et al., 2007b; Table 1). Eumelanin contents in the epidermis and dermis of *Mc1r*^{e}/*Mc1r*^{e} mice were much lower than those of *Mc1r/Mc1r* mice, whereas pheomelanin contents in the epidermis and dermis of *Mc1r*^{e}/*Mc1r*^{e} mice was much greater than those of *Mc1r/Mc1r* mice (Hirobe et al., 2007a). Eumelanin content in *Mc1r*^{e}/*Mc1r*^{e} hairs (5-week-old) was much lower than in *Mc1r*^{e}/*Mc1r*^{e} hairs, whereas pheomelanin content in *Mc1r*^{e}/*Mc1r*^{e} hairs was much greater than in *Mc1r/Mc1r* hairs (Hirobe et al., 2007a; Table 1).

Eumelanin and pheomelanin content in dorsal hairs of female B10-*Mc1r*^{e}/*Mc1r*^{e} mice is greater than that seen in male mice, suggesting that the expression of the recessive yellow allele is regulated in a sex-dependent manner (Hirobe et al., 2007a). We have suggested that estrogen is a main factor in determining the higher content of eumelanin and pheomelanin in the hair of female *Mc1r^e/Mc1r^e* mice (Hirobe et al., 2010).

Lethal yellow (A^y) represents the top dominant of the agouti locus. Phenotypically A^y/- mice produce mostly pheomelanic hairs. A^y/A^y embryos can be formed but display characteristic abnormalities at the morula or blastocyst stage (Kirkham, 1919) and die early on the sixth day of gestation. In the A^y mutation, there is a chromosomal rearrangement that results in the production of chimeric RNA expressed in nearly every tissue of the body. The 5' portion of this chimeric RNA contains highly expressed novel 5' sequences, but the 3' portion retains the protein-coding potential of the wild-type allele. Thus, A^y/- mice produce a plenty of the Asip and suppress the action of α-MSH toward Mc1r, consequently produce pheomelanin only during normal hair growth (Miller et al., 1993). Eumelanin and pheomelanin contents in hairs from B6-A^y/a and B6- $Mc1r^e/Mc1r^e$ are similar level (Ozeki et al., 1995; Table 1), suggesting that melanin synthesized in hair bulb melanocytes does not differ from A^y/a and $Mc1r^e/Mc1r^e$.

Pink-Eyed Dilution, Underwhite and Silver

Pink-eyed dilution mutant was discovered in the mouse fancy, and is known to reduce the pigmentation of both the coat and the eyes. The eyes of pink-eyed dilution mice resemble those of albinos, possessing a pink tent. However, in contrast to albino eyes, pink-eyed dilution genes are not entirely free of pigment (Silvers, 1979). *P* (*Oca2*), the wild-type allele at the pink-eyed dilution locus, produces an intense pigmentation of both eumelanin and pheomelanin in the skin and eyes, while *p* ($Oca2^p$), the recessive allele, greatly reduces pigmentation in both the coat and the eyes (Silvers, 1979). The pink-eyed dilution locus controls melanin synthesis, melanosome morphology and Tyr activity (Ozeki et al., 1995; Hirobe and Abe, 1999; Chen et al., 2002; Toyofuku et al., 2002). The product of the *Oca2* allele is an integral membrane protein that localizes in melanosomes (Rosemblat et al., 1994); its predicted secondary structure is a 12-transmembrane domain protein similar to a channel or transporter (Gardner et al., 1992; Rinchik et al., 1993). The *Oca2* protein seems to control processing and transport of Tyr (Toyofuku, 2002), but may not be a tyr transporter (Gahl et al., 1995). Sitaram et al. (2009) reported that the *Oca2* protein is active in melanosomes and its activity might be limited by additional sorting to lysosomes. The pH of melanosomes is abnormal in $Oca2^p$ mutant melanocytes (Puri et al., 2000).

The proliferation and differentiation of mouse melanocytes cultured in MDMD is greatly inhibited by the $Oca2^p$ mutation (Hirobe, 2011a) and L-tyr rescues both proliferation and differentiation (Hirobe et al., 2002b), though most of melanins and their precursors fail to accumulate in $Oca2^p/Oca2^p$ melanosomes (Wakamatsu et al., 2007). Moreover, in $Oca2^p/Oca2^p$ melanoblasts, only a few stage I and II melanosomes are observed (Hirobe et al., 2002b), whereas L-tyr greatly increases the number of stage II, III and IV melanosomes (Hirobe et al., 2002b). The $Oca2^p$ allele greatly inhibits eumelanin synthesis, but not pheomelanin synthesis (Hirobe et al., 2011c). Production of pheomelanin in $Oca2^p/Oca2^p$ melanocytes is not influenced by the agouti, nonagouti black and recessive yellow allele (Hirobe et al., 2011c).

Pink-eyed dilution melanoblasts possess smaller but more numerous mitochondria than black melanocytes (Hirobe et al., 2008). Treatment of $Oca2^p/Oca2^p$ melanoblasts with L-tyr decreased the number of mitochondria (Hirobe et al., 2008). Media supplemented with 2,4-dinitrophenol (DNP), an inhibitor of mitochondrial function, stimulated both proliferation and differentiation of *Oca2^p/Oca2^p* melanoblasts, and simultaneous DNP and L-tyr treatment dramatically induced the differentiation of *Oca2^p/Oca2^p* melanocytes (Hirobe et al., 2008). These results suggest that the *Oca2^p* allele is involved in regulating the function of mitochondria.

Since mitochondria are well developed in *Oca2^p/Oca2^p* melanoblasts and melanocytes, the possibility exists that apoptosis occurs in *Oca2^p/Oca2^p* melanoblasts and melanocytes. Inhibitors of apoptosis, such as caspase-9 inhibitor (C9I) and Bax-inhibiting peptide (BIP), stimulated the proliferation and differentiation of cultured *Oca2^p/Oca2^p* melanoblasts, but not of *Oca2/Oca2* melanoblasts and melanocytes. The number of apoptotic melanoblasts and keratinocytes in culture derived from *Oca2^p/Oca2^p* mice was greater than that derived from *Oca2/Oca2* mice (Hirobe, 2011a). Apoptotic melanoblasts and keratinocytes in *Oca2^p/Oca2^p* mice could be decreased by treatment with C9I and BIP. Moreover, expression of caspase-9 and Bax in *Oca2^p/Oca2^p* melanoblasts and keratinocytes was greater than in *Oca2/Oca2* melanoblasts and keratinocytes (Hirobe, 2011a). These results suggest that the increased apoptosis is related to the reduced proliferation and differentiation of *Oca2^p/Oca2^p* melanoblasts.

Eumelanin content in cultured *Oca2^p/Oca2^p* melanocytes in MDMD was much lower than in *Oca2/Oca2* melanocytes. However, eumelanin content in culture supernatant did not differ between *Oca2^p/Oca2^p* and *Oca2/Oca2* melanocytes (Hirobe et al., 2003). In contrast, pheomelanin content in cultured *Oca2^p/Oca2^p* melanocytes was lower than in *Oca2/Oca2* melanocytes. However, pheomelanin content in culture supernatant did not differ significantly between *Oca2^p/Oca2^p* and *Oca2/Oca2* melanocytes (Hirobe et al., 2003; Table 1). Eumelanin content in *Oca2^p/Oca2^p* hairs (5-week-old) was much lower than in *Oca2^p/Oca2^p* hairs, whereas pheomelanin content in *Oca2^p/Oca2^p* hairs did not differ from that in *Oca2/Oca2* hairs (Hirobe et al., 2003; Table 1).

Underwhite (*uw*) is an autosomal recessive mutation that arose spontaneously in the B6 strain (Dickie, 1964). The dorsum of *uw/uw* mice is a light buff color, whereas the ventrum is white. The eyes of *uw/uw* mice are unpigmented at birth, but darken to a dark reddish color at maturity (Green, 1966a). Molecular analysis revealed that underwhite regulates Slc45a2 protein. The Slc45a2 locus in mice encodes a membrane-associated transporter protein (Matp) that has a 12-transmembrane-spanning structure (Newton et al., 2001). All of the three mutations (*uw*, *uw^d* and *UW^dbr*) at the underwhite locus reduce the production of eumelanin more than 90% compared to wild-type mice (Lehman et al., 2000). The hypopigmentary effect of the underwhite mutation is independent of *Oca2^p*, because double mutant mice at *Slc45a2* and *Oca2^p* exhibit an albino appearance. However, Costin et al. (2003) reported that processing and trafficking of Tyr to melanosomes is disrupted and Tyr is abnormally secreted from *uw/uw* melanocytes in a similar process to that seen in *Oca2^p/Oca2^p* melanocytes.

Mutations at the silver (*si/Pmel17*) locus affect eumelanin production only slightly (20% reduction) on a nonagouti background. In contrast to nonagouti silver mice, where the animals become progressively more silvered, in agouti and yellow silver mice the silvering decreases markedly as the animals get older (Dum and Thigpen, 1930). The effects become more pronounced (40–50% reduction) when interacting with the brown locus (Lamoreux et al., 2001). Thus, the effects of the mutations at the brown and silver loci are additive. The silver protein is important for the biogenesis of early stage melanosomes (Kobayashi et al.,

1994b; Theos et al., 2005), and being the primary component of the matrix fibrils in eumelanosomes (Theos et al., 2006).

Slaty

Slaty (*slt/Dct^{slt}*) is the recessive autosomal mutation occurred in a heterogeneous stock carrying limb-deformity (*ld*) and mahogany (*mg*). On a nonagouti background, slaty homozygotes possess a slightly diluted coat pigmentation (Green, 1972). The slaty locus encodes Tyrp2/Dct and thus wild-type animals produce DHICA-rich eumelanin. The slaty mutation greatly reduce the PTCA value with a mild reduction in TM. Therefore, the PTCA/TM ratio was reduced four to six-fold, suggesting that DHICA-pour eumelanin is produced in *Dct^{slt}/Dct^{slt}* melanocytes. In addition to the original slaty mutation, slaty light (*Slt^{lt}/Dct$^{Slt\text{-}lt}$*; more severe effect) and slaty 2J (*slt^{2J}/Dct$^{slt\text{-}2J}$*; similar phenotype) have been identified (Budd and Jackson, 1995). The slaty mutation is known to change an arginine to a glutamine in the first copper-binding domain of Dct, which converts DC to DHICA in the eumelanin synthesis pathway (Korner and Pawelek, 1980; Jackson et al., 1992; Tsukamoto et al., 1992); it also yields about 10–30% of the activity of wild-type Dct in eye extracts (Jackson et al., 1992). Dct is produced by both wild-type and slaty mutant cDNA, but the protein level of Dct in the slaty mutant is greatly reduced (Kroumpouzos et al., 1994).

The slaty mutation does not affect the proliferation of cultured epidermal melanoblasts and melanocytes in MDMD (Hirobe et al, 2007c). However, the differentiation and Tyrp2 expression of cultured slaty melanocytes is greatly inhibited (Hirobe et al., 2006). The slaty mutation affects both eumelanin and pheomelanin synthesis in a developmental stage-specific and skin site-specific manner (Hirobe et al., 2007c). Eumelanin content in cultured *Dct^{slt}/Dct^{slt}* melanocytes in MDMD was lower than in *Dct/Dct* melanocytes. However, eumelanin content in culture supernatant did not differ between *Dct^{slt}/Dct^{slt}* and *Dct/Dct* melanocytes (Hirobe et al., 2006, Table 1). In contrast, pheomelanin content in cultured *Dct^{slt}/Dct^{slt}* melanocytes did not differ from that in *Dct/Dct* melanocytes. However, pheomelanin content in culture supernatant did not differ significantly between *Dct^{slt}/Dct^{slt}* and *Dct/Dct* melanocytes (Hirobe et al., 2006; Table 1). Eumelanin and pheomelanin contents in the epidermis and dermis of *Dct^{slt}/Dct^{slt}* mice were lower than those of *Dct/Dct* mice (Hirobe et al., 2006; Table 1). Eumelanin content in *Dct^{slt}/Dct^{slt}* hairs (5-week-old) was smaller than in *Dct/Dct* hairs, whereas pheomelanin content in *Dct^{slt}/Dct^{slt}* hairs did not differ from *Dct/Dct* hairs (Hirobe et al., 2006; Table 1).

In slaty melanocytes, numerous spherical melanosomes with granular depositions of pigments, black type elliptical melanosomes with longitudinal depositions of pigments in intraluminal fibrils and a mix of the two melanosome types are observed (4:1:1) (Hirobe and Abe, 2006). Moreover, in slaty melanocytes, mature stage IV melanosomes greatly decrease, while immature stage III melanosomes are more numerous than in black melanocytes (Hirobe and Abe, 2007a). In slaty melanocytes, spherical and mixed type melanosomes gradually decrease after birth, whereas elliptical melanosomes gradually increase. These results suggest that the slaty mutation blocks melanosome maturation at stage III and affects melanosome morphology (elliptical or spherical) in a developmental stage-specific manner.

Inhibition of eumelanin synthesis by the slaty mutation can be partly restored by the addition of excess L-tyr to MDMD (Hirobe et al., 2006). Eumelanin and pheomelanin may be accumulated with difficulty in slaty melanocytes and are easily released during skin development. L-tyr is thought to stimulate this release. Perhaps, L-tyr acts directly on melanoblasts and melanocytes and activates factors involved in regulating eumelanin synthesis (Coughlin et al., 1988; Imokawa, 2004; Hirobe, 2005). Another possibility is that L-tyr acts on the tissue environment, especially keratinocytes, and stimulates synthesis of melanogenic factors controlling eumelanin synthesis (Imokawa 2004; Hirobe, 2005).

When L-tyr is added to MDMD, it stimulates melanosome maturation and increases elliptical melanosomes, but decreases spherical melanosomes (Hirobe and Abe, 2007b), suggesting that L-tyr restores the reduced melanosome maturation and changes the altered morphology of melanosomes affected by the slaty mutation. L-tyr may act directly on melanocytes and activate factors involved in regulating pigmentation. Since excess L-tyr restores maturation of stage IV elliptical melanosomes, slaty melanosomes are thought to possess a normal pathway related to L-tyr transport (Hirobe and Abe, 2007b).

Thus, the possibility exists that L-tyr transport system from the cytoplasm to melanosomes is affected by the slaty mutation. If this is true, melanin synthesis would be increased by excess L-tyr, and maturation of stage IV melanosomes would be stimulated. Furthermore, L-tyr increases the total number of melanosomes, suggesting that L-tyr stimulates *de novo* melanosome formation. It has been reported that α-MSH stimulates differentiation of epidermal melanocytes of black mice *in vivo* (Hirobe and Takeuchi, 1977). Differentiation stimulated by α-MSH is associated with an increase in the total number of melanosomes. Similar mechanisms in α-MSH and L-tyr seem to be involved in the stimulation of *de novo* melanosome formation by α-MSH and L-tyr.

Ruby-Eye 2^d, Beige and Mottled

In 2006, a spontaneous autosomal recessive mutant of brown coat color with ruby eyes occurred in B10 mice in my laboratory (Hirobe et al., 2011d). The phenotype of this mutant was similar to that of ruby-eye ($ru/Hps6^{ru}$) or ruby-eye 2 ($ru2/Hps5^{ru2}$). Human Hermansky-Pudlack syndrome (HPS) is a recessively inherited disease that affects several organs such as the skin (hypopigmenation), eyes (low visual acuity), blood cells (prolonged bleeding) and lungs (interstitial pulmonary fibrosis) (Wei, 2006). Many distinct types of human HPS have been described (Wei, 2006). In mice, many naturally occurring hypopigmentation models of HPS have been characterized (Wei, 2006). Human *HPS5* corresponds to mouse $Hps5^{ru2}$ (*ru2*), and *HPS6* to $Hps6^{ru}$ (*ru*) (Zhang et al., 2003). RT-PCR analysis revealed that this novel mutation named $ru2^d/Hps5^{ru2\text{-}d}$ is a frameshift mutation by 997G deletion in *Hps5* (Hirobe et al., 2011d).

Mouse *Hps5* gene is on chromosome 7 and possesses a 3381-bp open reading frame (ORF) with 23 exons, encoding a 1126 amino acid (aa) protein (127.4 kDa), 81% homologies to the human sequence (126.3 kDa) are observed (Zhang et al., 2003). All tissues (heart, brain, spleen, lung, liver, skeletal muscle, kidney and testes) examined contained the 4.8 kb transcript. Nine murine mutations in the *Hps5* (*Ru2*) gene are known until now: the $ru2^{mr}/Hps5^{ru2\text{-}mr}$ allele is a spontaneous recessive mutation with undefined molecular characterization (Bateman, 1957); the $ru2^{hz}/Hps5^{ru2\text{-}hz}$ allele leads to a predicted loss of 118 C-terminal aa (frameshift by insertion of CCGG at E900) (Dickie, 1965; Zhang et al., 2003);

the *ru2/Hps5*^{ru2} allele contains a 1.0-kb insertion (K867) of the H2A histone sequence immediately preceding codon 868 of exon 18 (Lilly, 1966; Zhang et al., 2003); the *ru2*^{J}*/Hps5*$^{ru2\text{-}J}$ allele leads to a predicted loss of 311 aa at the C terminus (frameshift by ∆G757) (Eicher and Fox, 1977; Zhang et al., 2003); the *ru2*^{8J}*/Hps5*$^{ru2\text{-}8J}$ allele is a spontaneous recessive mutation with undefined molecular characterization (Cook, 1995); the *ru2*^{11J}*/Hps5*$^{ru2\text{-}11J}$ allele is an N-ethyl-N-nitrosourea (ENU)-induced recessive mutation with undefined molecular characterization (Gwynn et al., 2004, Mouse Genome Informatics); the *ru2*^{Btlr}*/Hps5*$^{ru2\text{-}Btlr}$ allele leads to T- to C- transition in the donor splice site of intron 9 (ENU-induced recessive mutation) (Eidendchenk et al., 2008 in Mouse Genome Informatics); and the *ru2*^{2Btlr}*/Hps5*$^{ru2\text{-}2Btlr}$ allele leads to A- to T- transversion at nucleotide position 2337 (ENU-induced recessive mutation) (Blasius et al., 2008 in Mouse Genome Informatics). We first reported the tenth allele occurred in mice, *ru2*^{d}*/Hps5*$^{ru2\text{-}d}$, caused by frameshift by deletion (∆G997). The *Hps5*$^{ru2\text{-}d}$ mutation makes large molecule protein to smaller one by a premature termination codon, and reduces mRNA expression.

Human *HPS1, 2, 3, 4, 7* and *8* correspond to mouse pale ear (*ep/Hps1*^{ep}), pearl (*pl/Ap3b1*^{pl}), cocoa (*coa/Hps3*^{coa}), light ear (*le/Hps4*^{le}), sandy (*sdy/Dtnbp1*^{sdy}) and reduced pigmentation (*rp/Bloc1S3*^{rp}), respectively (Wei, 2006). All the *HPS* mutations are characterized by hypopigmentation and several diseases, and in mice, *Hps* is a disorder of organelle biogenesis in which hypopigmentation, bleeding and pulmonary fibrosis are resulted from defects in melanosomes, platelet dense granules and lysosomes (Wei, 2006). The difference in the coat color in the *Hps* mutant seems to be due to the inhibition of melanosome formation (inner structure) and maturation. Zhang et al. (2003) reported that in the retinal pigment epithelium and choroid of B6-*Hps5*^{ru2}*/Hps5*^{ru2} mice, melanosomes were fewer and immature, and their shape were mostly spherical. Nguyen et al. (2002) reported that in the hair follicle melanocytes of the dorsal skin of 4-week-old B6-*Hps5*^{ru2}*/Hps5*^{ru2} mice, stage IV melanosomes decreased in number, and their morphology remained spherical. However, in *Hps5*$^{ru2\text{-}d}$*/Hps5*$^{ru2\text{-}d}$ melanocytes, melanosomes were elliptical, but they were fewer and immature, suggesting that the *Hps5*$^{ru2\text{-}d}$ allele controls the maturation of melanosomes, but not their internal structure. The severity of the lesion in *Hps5*$^{ru2\text{-}d}$ allele (melanosome formation and maturation) may be less than that of *Hps5*^{ru2} allele.

To clarify the mechanism of the hypopigmentation, the characteristics of the proliferation and differentiation of *Hps5*$^{ru2\text{-}d}$*/Hps5*$^{ru2\text{-}d}$ epidermal melanoblasts and melanocytes cultured in MDMD and MDMDF were investigated. The proliferation of *Hps5*$^{ru2\text{-}d}$*/Hps5*$^{ru2\text{-}d}$ melanoblasts and melanocytes did not differ from that of *Hps5/Hps5* (Hirobe et al., 2011d). However, the differentiation of *Hps5*$^{ru2\text{-}d}$*/Hps5*$^{ru2\text{-}d}$ melanocytes was greatly inhibited. Tyr activity, expression of Tyr, Tyrp1, Dct and eumelanin synthesis were markedly decreased in *Hps5*$^{ru2\text{-}d}$*/Hps5*$^{ru2\text{-}d}$ melanocytes (Hirobe et al., 2011d). However, the addition of excess L-tyr to MDMD rescued the reduced differentiation via increased Tyr activity, expression of Tyr, Tyrp1, Dct and Kit and eumelanin synthesis (Hirobe et al., 2011d). These results suggest that the *Hps5*$^{ru2\text{-}d}$ allele inhibits melanocyte differentiation, though the impaired differentiation is rescued by excess L-tyr.

In *Hps5*$^{ru2\text{-}d}$*/Hps5*$^{ru2\text{-}d}$ melanocytes, elliptical melanosomes were observed, though many immature stage III melanosomes and less stage IV melanosomes were observed (Hirobe et al., 2011d). The number of stage IV melanosomes was much smaller than in *Hps5/Hps5* melanocytes. The total number of melanosomes in *Hps5*$^{ru2\text{-}d}$*/Hps5*$^{ru2\text{-}d}$ melanocytes was also less than in *Hps5/Hps5* melanocytes. However, L-tyr markedly increased the number of stage

IV melanosomes and the total number of melanosomes in *Hps5*$^{ru2\text{-}d}$/*Hps5*$^{ru2\text{-}d}$ melanocytes (Hirobe et al., 2011d). These results suggest that the *Hps5*$^{ru2\text{-}d}$ mutation markedly inhibits melanosome formation and maturation, but its inhibition can be restored by L-tyr.

Eumelanin content in cultured *Hps5*$^{ru2\text{-}d}$/*Hps5*$^{ru2\text{-}d}$ melanocytes in MDMD was lower than in *Hps5/Hps5* melanocytes. However, eumelanin content in culture supernatant was greater than that of *Hps5/Hps5* melanocytes (Hirobe et al., 2011d, Table 1). In contrast, pheomelanin content in cultured *Hps5*$^{ru2\text{-}d}$/*Hps5*$^{ru2\text{-}d}$ melanocytes in MDMD as well as in culture supernatant did not differ from that in *Hps5/Hps5* melanocytes (Hirobe et al., 2011d, Table 1). Eumelanin contents in the epidermis, dermis and hairs (5-week-old) of *Hps5*$^{ru2\text{-}d}$/*Hps5*$^{ru2\text{-}d}$ mice were much lower than those of *Hps5/Hps5* mice (Hirobe et al., 2011d; Table 1). Pheomelanin contents in the epidermis and dermis of *Hps5*$^{ru2\text{-}d}$/*Hps5*$^{ru2\text{-}d}$ mice were lower than those of *Hps5/Hps5* mice. However, 2- to 3-fold increase in pheomelanin content in hairs of 5-week-old *Hps5*$^{ru2\text{-}d}$/*Hps5*$^{ru2\text{-}d}$ mice was observed (Hirobe, 2011a; Table 1). These results suggest that pheomelanin synthesis in *Hps5*$^{ru2\text{-}d}$/*Hps5*$^{ru2\text{-}d}$ mice is increased in hair bulbs. These results are consistent with the results that 5-*S*-CD level in plasma of *Hps5*$^{ru2\text{-}d}$/*Hps5*$^{ru2\text{-}d}$ mice was greater than that of *Hps5/Hps5* mice (Hirobe et al., unpublished). We first presented the evidence that the *Hps5*$^{ru2\text{-}d}$ allele stimulates pheomelanin synthesis in mouse hair bulb melanocytes.

Beige (*bg/bg*) is a recessive mutation affecting both coat and eye color. The eye color of *bg/bg* mice was light at birth and varied from ruby to almost black in adults. *bg/bg* mice also display reduced pigmentation in the ear and tail, and the coat color is lighter than wild-type mice, particularly at the base of the hairs (Kelly, 1957). In retinal pigment epithelia and hair bulb melanocytes of *bg/bg* mice, melanosomes decrease in number and this reduction is due both to the synthesis of fewer lysosomes and to the fusion of lysosomes into progressively larger lysosomes (Pierro, 1963). The beige gene is homozygous to Chediak-Higashi syndrome gene, and these genes are encoded by Lyst gene (Barbosa et al., 1996; Nagle et al., 1996). Lyst encodes a protein with a carboxy-terminal prenylation motif and multiple potential phosphorylation sites. The Lyst protein is predicted to form extended helical domains, and possesses a region of sequence similar to stathmin, a coiled-coil phosophoprotein that is thought to act as a relay integrating cellular signal response coupling (Barbosa et al., 1996).

The mottled (*Mo*) mutation occurred in females among the progeny of a cross-segregating for albinism, piebald (*s/Ednrb*^{s}), brown and hairlessness (*hr*) (Fraser et al., 1953). The female was *Tyrp1/-*; *Ednrb/-* and possessed many regions of light-colored hair scattered in an apparently patternless fashion over the entire body. The depth of color of the hairs in these regions varied between regions. The mottled (*Mo/Atp7a*) gene locates in X chromosome. Females which are heterozygous for the *Mo* gene possess, to varying degrees, a mottled coat with patches of white, light-colored and full-colored hairs, as well as intermingled hairs of different colors (Silvers, 1979). The activity of the copper-dependent enzyme, cyrochrome c oxidase and superoxidase dismutase are reduced in this mutant mice. The mottled gene is homologous to the gene related to human Menkes disease that is an X-linked recessive copper deficiency disorder caused by mutations in the *ATP7A (MNK)* gene. Thus, the new symbol for the mottled allele is *Atp7a*. The *MNK* gene encodes a copper-transporting P-type ATPase, MNK, which is localized predominantly in the *trans*-Golgi network (TGN). The MNK protein relocates to the plasma membrane in cells exposed to elevated copper where it functions in copper efflux (Petris et al., 2000).

Sash

Sash forms a dominant spotting pattern (*W*-locus). This mutation occurred spontaneously in a pair set up to provide a (C3H × 101) F_1 hybrid stock (Silvers, 1979). The original mutant had a broad sash of white around its body in the lumbar region and produced offspring like itself when bred with a normal animal. The semi-dominant sash mutation is characterized by a sequence inversion near the Kit gene that leads to ectopic expression of Kit (Duttlinger et al., 1993). Homozygous B10-$Kit^{W\text{-}sh}$/ $Kit^{W\text{-}sh}$ mice possess almost all-white body hair except for the ear, and in heterozygous mice, the center of the body is covered with white hair. Primary cultures of epidermal cell suspensions of sash mice have not detected any melanoblasts or melanocytes (Hirobe, 2011a). However, co-culture of black melanoblasts/melanocytes with sash keratinocytes stimulated proliferation of black melanoblasts/melanocytes in MDMDF (Hirobe, 2011a). These results suggest that the sash allele affects early melanoblast development without affecting the production of mitogens for melanoblasts in keratinocytes. Moreover, human epidermal melanocytes can be grown in hair follicles of B10-$Kit^{W\text{-}sh}$/ $Kit^{W\text{-}sh}$ mice. After plucking out all the reconstituted hairs, the secondary hairs were regrown in the same area and their colors were lighter than the first reconstituted hairs (Ideta et al., 2006). These results also support the assumption that sash keratinocytes possess a normal function in the melanocyte environment.

Conclusion

The coat color genes that were the focus of this chapter mostly act directly on melanocytes, whereas the agouti and nonagouti black alleles act on the tissue environment, especially on fibroblasts in dermal papilla.

The sash and slaty alleles affect melanoblast migration and differentiation. The albino and pink-eyed dilution alleles influence melanoblast proliferation. The brown, pink-eyed dilution and slaty alleles control formation of stage I and II melanosomes in melanoblasts.

The albino, pink-eyed dilution, recessive yellow, slaty and ruby eye 2^d alleles affect expression and activity of Tyr in melanocytes. The brown, pink-eyed dilution, slaty and ruby eye 2^d alleles affect melanosome maturation, especially stage IV melanosome maturation.

The agouti, lethal yellow, nonagouti black and recessive yellow affect the types of melanin synthesized (eumelanin or pheomelanin).

Finally, the dilute allele is involved in regulating melanosome transfer from melanocyte dendrites to keratinocytes. Eumelanin and pheomelanin synthesis are regulated by numerous coat color genes in mice. Eumelanin contents in agouti and dilute melanocytes are similar to black melanocytes, whereas the contents in brown, pink-eyed dilution, slaty and ruby-eye 2^d melanocytes are reduced to one-third~one thirthieth.

In contrast, pheomelanin contents in agouti, dilute, slaty and ruby-eye 2^d melanocytes are similar to its content in black melanocytes, whereas the content in brown melanocytes is increased.

Eumelanin and pheomelanin contents in cultured epidermal melanocytes correlate well with those in the epidermis/dermis and hairs of the mice, except that agouti melanocytes do not synthesize pheomelanin in culture, the pink-eyed dilution allele does not affect pheomelanin content in hairs, and the ruby-eye 2d allele increases pheomelanin content in hairs. Thus, eumelanin and pheomelanin synthesis in melanocytes is regulated by numerous coat color genes in a very complicated manner.

Acknowledgments

The author expresses his thanks to Prof./Drs. Takeuchi (Tohoku University, deceased in 1996), Ito/Wakamatsu (Fujita Health University), Abe (Yamagata University), Kawa/Mizoguchi/Soma (St. Marianna University), Takeuchi/Hotta/Yoshihara (Okayama University), Furuya/Akiu/Naganuma/Fukuda/Ideta/Ifuku/Hara/Horii (Shiseido), Nishikawa /Osawa (RIKEN), Eguchi-Kasai/Sugaya/Murakami (National Institute of Radiological Sciences), Ogawa/Ishizuka (Joetsu University of Education) and Ootaka/Terunuma/Kiuchi (Chiba University) for their collaboration in the original papers.

References

Aoki, H., Yamada, Y., Hara, A. and Kunisada, T. (2009). Two distinct types of mouse melanocyte: differential signaling requirement for the maintenance of non-cutaneous and dermal versus epidermal melanocytes. *Development* 136, 2511–2521.

Barbosa, M. D. F. S., Nguyen, Q.A., Tchernev, V.T., Ashley, J.A., Detter, J.C., Blaydes, S.M., Brandt, S.J., Chotai, D., Hodgman, C., Solari, R.C.E., Lovett, M. and Kingsmore, S.F. (1996). Identification of the homologous beige and Chediak–Higashi syndrome genes. *Nature* 382, 262–265.

Barsh, G.S. (1996). The genetics of pigmentation: from fancy genes to complex traits. *Trends Genet.* 12, 299–305.

Bateman, N. (1957). Maroon – allele of silver? *Mouse News Lett.* 16, 7.

Bennett, D.C. and Lamoreux, M.L. (2003). The color loci of mice – a genetic century. *Pigment Cell Res.* 16, 333–344.

Bertolotto, C., Abbe, P., Hemesath,T.J., Bille, K., Fisher, D.E., Ortonne, J.-P. and Ballotti, R. (1998). Microphthalmia gene product as a signal transducer in cAMP-induced differentiation of melanocytes. *J. Cell Biol.* 142, 827–835.

Budd, P.S. and Jackson, I.J. (1995). Structure of the mouse tyrosinase-related protein-2/Dopachrome tautomerase (*Tyrp2/Dct*) gene and sequence of two novel slaty alleles. *Genomics* 29, 35–43.

Burchill, S.A., Thody, A.J. and Ito, S. (1986). Melanocyte-stimulating hormone, tyrosinase activity and regulation of eumelanogenesis and pheomelanogenesis in the hair follicular melanocytes of the mouse. *J. Endocrinol.* 109, 15–21.

Chase, H.B. (1949). Greying of hair. I. Effects produced by single doses of X-rays on mice. *J. Morphol.* 84, 57–80.

Chen, K., Manga, P. and Orlow, S.J. (2002). Pink-eyed dilution protein controls the processing of tyrosinase. *Mol. Biol. Cell* 13, 1953–1964.

Chintala, S., Li, W., Lamoreux, M.L., Ito, S., Wakamatsu, K., Sviderskaya, E.V., Bennett, D.C,, Park, Y.M., Gahl, W.A., Huizing, M., Spritz, R.A., Ben, S., Novak, E.K., Tan, J.

and Swank, R.T. (2005). Slc7a11 gene controls production of pheomelanin pigment and proliferation of cultured cell. *Proc. Natl Acad. Sci. USA* 102, 10964–10969.

Choi, W., Miyamura, Y., Wolber, R., Smuda, C., Reinhold, W., Liu, H., Kolbe, L. and Hearing, V.J. (2010). Regulation of human skin pigmentation *in situ* by repetitive UV exposure: molecular characterization of responses to UVA and/or UVB. *J. Invest. Dermatol.* 130, 1685–1696.

Cook, S. (1995). Spontaneous remutation (*ru2*^{8J}). *Mouse Genome* 93, 862.

Cooksey, C.J., Garratt, P.J., Land, E.J., Pavel, S., Ramsden, C.A., Riley, P.A. and Smit, N.P.M. (1997). Evidence of the indirect formation of the catecholic intermediate substrate responsible for the autoactivation kinetics of tyrosinase. *J. Biol. Chem.* 272, 26226–26235.

Costin, G.E., Valencia, J.C., Vieira, W.D., Lamoreux, M.L. and Hearing, V.J. (2003). Tyrosinase processing and intracellular trafficking is disrupted in mouse primary melanocytes carrying the underwhite (*uw*) mutation. A model for oculocutaneous albinism (OCA) type 4. *J. Cell Sci.* 116, 3203–3212.

Coughlin, S.R., Barr, P.J., Cousens, L.S., Fretto, L.J. and Williams, L.T. (1988). Acidic and basic fibroblast growth factors stimulate tyrosine kinase activity in vivo. *J. Biol. Chem.* 263, 988–993.

del Marmol, V., Ito, S., Bouchard, B., Libert, A., Wakamatsu, K., Ghanem, G. and Solano, F. (1996). Cysteine deprivation promotes eumelanogenesis in human melanoma cells. *J. Invest. Dermatol.* 107, 698–702.

Dickie, M.M. (1964). Private communication. *Mouse News Lett.* 30, 30.

Dickie, M.M. (1965). Haze. *Mouse News Lett.* 32, 44.

Dunn, L.C. and Thigpen, L.W. (1930). The silver mouse, a recessive color variation. *J. Hered.* 21, 495–498.

Duttlinger, R., Manova, K., Chu, T.Y., Gyssler, C., Zelenetz, A.D., Bachvarova, R.F. and Besmer, P. (1993). *W-sash* affects positive and negative elements controlling c-kit expression: ectopic c-*kit* expression at sites of kit-ligand expression affects melanogenesis. *Development* 118, 705–717.

Eicher, E.M. and Fox, S. (1977). *hz* and *mr* alleles of *ru-2*. *Mouse News Lett.* 56, 42.

Enshell-Seijffers, D., Lindon, C., Wu, E., Taketo, M.M. and Morgan, B.A. (2010). β-catenin activity in the dermal papilla of the hair follicle regulates pigment-type switching. *Proc. Natl. Acad. Sci., USA.* 107, 21564–21569.

Fitzpatrick, T. B., Hori, Y., Toda, K. and Seiji, M. (1969). Melanin 1969: some definitions and problems. *Jpn. J. Dermatol.* (Ser. B), 79, 278–282.

Foster, M. (1965). Mammalian pigment genetics. *Adv. Genet.* 13, 311–339.

Fraser, A.S., Sobey, S. and Spicer, C.C. (1953). Mottled, a sex-modified lethal in the house mouse. *J. Genet.* 51, 217–221.

Furuya, R., Akiu, S., Ideta, R., Naganuma, M., Fukuda, M. and Hirobe, T. (2002). Chages in the proliferative activity of epidermal melanocytes in serum-free primary culture during the development of ultraviolet radiation B-induced pigmented spots in hairless mice. *Pigment Cell Res.* 15, 348–356.

Furuya, R., Yoshida, Y., Moro, O., Tsunenaga, M., Aoki, H., Kishimoto, J., Ifuku, O. and Hirobe, T. (2009). Immunohistochemical survey of the distribution of epidermal melanoblasts and melanocytes during the development of UVB-induced pigmented spots. *J. Dermatol. Sci.* 55, 99–107.

Gahl, W. A., Potterf, B., Durham-Pierre, D., Brilliant, M.H. and Hearing, V.J. (1995). Melanosomal tyrosine transport in normal and pink-eyed dilution murine melanocytes. *Pigment Cell Res.* 8, 229–233.
Gardner, J.M., Nakatsu, Y., Gondo, Y., Lee, S., Lyon, M.F., King, R.A. and Brilliant, M.H. (1992). The mouse pink-eyed dilution gene: association with human Prader-Willi and Angelman syndromes. *Science* 257, 1121–1124.
Gilchrest, B.A., Park, H.Y., Eller, M.S. and Yaar, M. (1996). Mechanisms of ultraviolet light induced pigmentation. *Photochem. Photobiol.* 63, 1–10.
Green, M.C. (1966) Mutant genes and linkages. In Biology of the Laboratory Mouse, 2nd ed. E. L. Green (ed.), pp87–150. McGraw-Hill, New York.
Green, M.C. (1972). Private communication. *Mouse News Lett.* 47, 36.
Gunn, T.M., Inui, T., Kitada, K., Ito, S., Wakamatsu, K., He, L., Bouley, D.M., Serikawa, T. and Barsh, G.S. (2001). Molecular and phenotypic analysis of attractin mutant mice. *Genetics* 158, 1683–1695.
Gwynn, B., Martina, J.A., Bonifacino, J.S., Sviderskaya, E.V., Lamoreux, M.L., Bennett, D.C., Moriyama, K., Huizing, M., Helip-Wooley, A., Gahl, W.A., Webb, L.S., Lambert, A.J. and Peters, L.L. (2004). Reduced pigmentation (*rp*), a mouse model of Hermansky-Pudlak syndrome, encodes a novel component of the BLOC-1 complex. *Blood* 15, 3181–3189.
Hachiya, A., Kobayashi, A., Ohuchi, A., Takema, Y. and Imokawa, G. (2001). The paracrine role of stem cell factor/c-kit signaling in the activation of human melanocytes in ultraviolet-B-induced pigmentation. *J. Invest. Dermatol.* 116, 578–586.
Hearing, V.J. (1993). Unraveling the melanocyte. Am. *J. Hum. Genet.* 52, 1–7.
Hearing, V.J. (2000). The melanosome: the perfect model for cellular response to the environment. *Pigment Cell Res.* 13 (Suppl. 8), 23–34.
Hearing, V.J. and Tsukamoto, K. (1991). Enzymatic control of pigmentation in mammals. *FASEB J.* 5, 2902–2909.
Hearing, V.J., Phillips, P. and Lutzner, M.A. (1973). The fine structure of melanogenesis in coat color mutants of the mouse. *J. Ultrast. Res.* 43, 88–106.
Hirobe, T. (1982). Genes involved in regulating the melanocyte and melanoblast-melanocyte populations in the epidermis of newborn mouse skin. *J. Exp. Zool.* 223, 257–264.
Hirobe, T. (1984a). Histochemical survey of the distribution of the epidermal melanoblasts and melanocytes in the mouse during fetal and postnatal periods. *Anat. Rec.,* 208, 589–594.
Hirobe, T. (1984b). Effects of genic substitution at the brown locus on the differentiation of epidermal melanocytes in newborn mouse skin. *Anat. Rec.,* 209, 425–432.
Hirobe, T. (1986). Mouse stock. *Mouse News Lett.* 76, 28–29.
Hirobe, T. (1988a). Developmental changes of the proliferative response of mouse epidermal melanocytes to skin wounding. *Development* 102, 567–574.
Hirobe, T. (1988b). Genetic factors controlling the proliferative activity of mouse epidermal melanocytes during the healing of skin wounds. *Genetics* 120, 551–558.
Hirobe, T. (1992a). Control of melanocyte proliferation and differentiation in the mouse epidermis. *Pigment Cell Res.* 5, 1–11.
Hirobe, T. (1992b). Basic fibroblast growth factor stimulates the sustained proliferation of mouse epidermal melanoblasts in serum-free medium in the presence of dibutyryl cyclic AMP and keratinocytes. *Development* 114, 435–445.

Hirobe, T. (1992c). Melanocyte stimulating hormone induces the differentiation of mouse epidermal melanocytes in serum-free culture. *J. Cell. Physiol.* 152, 337–345.

Hirobe, T. (1994a). Effects of γ-irradiation on the yield of mid-ventral white spots in mice in different genetic backgrounds and at different times during development. *Mutation Res.* 322, 213–220.

Hirobe, T. (1994b). Keratiocytes are involved in regulating the developmental changes in the proliferative activity of mouse epidermal melanoblasts in serum-free culture. *Dev. Biol.* 161, 59–69.

Hirobe, T. (1995). Structure and function of melanocytes: microscopic morphology and cell biology of mouse melanocytes in the epidermis and hair follicle. *Histol. Histopathol.* 10, 223–237.

Hirobe, T. (1996). Hydrocortisone is involved in regulating the proliferation and differentiation of mouse epidermal melanoblasts in serum-free culture in the presence of keratiocytes. *Eur. J. Cell Biol.* 71, 387–394.

Hirobe, T. (2005). Role of keratinocyte-derived factors involved in regulating the proliferation and differentiation of mammalian epidermal melanocytes. *Pigment Cell Res.* 18, 2–12.

Hirobe, T. (2007). Ferrous ferric chloride stimulates the proliferation and differentiation of cultured keratinocytes and melanocytes in the epidermis of neonatal mouse skin. *J. Health Sci.* 53, 576–584.

Hirobe, T. (2009a). Ferrous ferric chloride induces the differentiation of cultured mouse epidermal melanocytes additionally with herbal medicines. *J. Health Sci.* 55, 86–94.

Hirobe, T. (2009b). Ferrous ferric chloride stimulates the proliferation of human skin keratinocytes, melanocytes, and fibroblasts in culture. *J. Health Sci.* 55, 447–455.

Hirobe, T. (2009c). Ferrous ferric chloride stimulates the skin cell function and hair growth in mice. *Biol. Pharm. Bull.* 32, 1347–1453.

Hirobe, T. (2011a). How are proliferation and differentiation of melanocytes regulated? *Pigment Cell Melanoma Res.*, 24, 462–478.

Hirobe, T. (2011b). Stimulation of the proliferation and differentiation of skin cells by ferrous ferric chloride from a distance. *Biol. Pharm. Bull.* 34, 987–995.

Hirobe, T. and Takeuchi, T. (1977). Induction of melanogenesis in the epidermal melanoblasts of newborn mouse skin by MSH. *J. Embryol. Exp. Morphol.* 37, 79–90.

Hirobe, T. and Zhou, X. (1990). Effects of gamma-radiation on the differentiation of mouse melanocytes in the hair follicles. *Mutation Res.* 234, 91–96.

Hirobe, T. and Abe, H. (1999). Genetic and epigenetic control of the proliferation and differentiation of mouse epidermal melanocytes in culture. *Pigment Cell Res.* 12, 147–163.

Hirobe, T. and Abe, H. (2000). $ACTH_{4\text{-}12}$ is the minimal message sequence required to induce the differentiation of mouse epidermal melanocytes in serum-free primary culture. *J. Exp. Zool.* 286, 632–640.

Hirobe, T and Abe, H. (2006). The slaty mutation affects the morphology and maturation of melanosomes in the mouse melanocytes. *Pigment Cell Res.* 19, 454–459.

Hirobe, T. and Abe, H. (2007a). Changes of melanosome morphology associated with the differentiation of epidermal melanocytes in slaty mice. *Anat. Rec.* 290, 981–993.

Hirobe, T and Abe, H. (2007b). Excess tyrosine restores the morphology and maturation of melanosomes affected by the murine slaty mutation. *Zool. Sci.* 24, 338–345.

Hirobe, T., Wakamatsu, K. and Ito, S. (1998). Effects of genic substitution at the agouti, brown, albino, dilute, and pink-eyed dilution loci on the proliferation and differentiation of mouse epidermal melanocytes in serum-free culture. *Eur. J. Cell Biol.* 75, 184–191.

Hirobe, T., Furuya R., Akiu, S., Ifuku, O. and Fukuda, M. (2002a). Keratinocytes control the proliferation and differentiation of cultured epidermal melanocytes from ultraviolet radiation B-induced pigmented spots in the dorsal skin of hairless mice. *Pigment Cell Res.* 15, 391–399.

Hirobe, T., Wakamatsu, K., Ito, S., Abe, H., Kawa, Y. and Mizoguchi, M. (2002b). Stimulation of the proliferation and differentiation of mouse pink-eyed dilution epidermal melanocytes by excess tyrosine in serum-free primary culture. *J. Cell. Physiol.* 191, 162–172.

Hirobe T., Wakamatsu, K. and Ito, S. (2003). Changes in the proliferation and differentiation of neonatal mouse pink-eyed dilution melanocytes in the presence of excess tyrosine. *Pigment Cell Res.* 16, 619–628.

Hirobe, T., Takeuchi, S. and Hotta, E. (2004a). The melanocortin receptor-1 gene but not the proopiomelanocortin gene is expressed in melanoblasts and contributes their differentiation in the mouse skin. *Pigment Cell Res.* 17, 627–635.

Hirobe, T., Furuya, R., Hara, E., Horii, I., Tsunenaga, M. and Ifuku, O. (2004b). Granulocyte-macrophage colony-stimulating factor controls the proliferation and differentiation of mouse epidermal melanocytes from pigmented spots induced by ultraviolet radiation B. *Pigment Cell Res.* 17, 230–240.

Hirobe, T., Eguchi-Kasai, K. and Murakami, M. (2004c). Effects of carbon ion-radiations on the postnatal development of mice as well as on the yield of white spots in the mid-ventrum and the tail-tips. *Radiat. Res.* 162, 580–584.

Hirobe, T., Takeuchi, S., Hotta, E., Wakamatsu, K. and Ito, S. (2004d). Pheomelanin production in the epidermis from newborn agouti mice is induced by the expression of the agouti gene in the dermis. *Pigment Cell Research* 17, 506–514.

Hirobe, T., Wakamatsu, K., Ito, S., Kawa, Y., Soma, Y. and Mizoguchi, M. (2006). The slaty mutation affects eumelanin and pheomelanin synthesis in mouse melanocytes. *Eur. J. Cell Biol.* 85, 537–549.

Hirobe, T., Wakamatsu, K. and Ito, S. (2007a). The eumelanin and pheomelanin contents in dorsal hairs of female recessive yellow mice are greater than in male. *J. Dermatol. Sci.* 45, 55–62.

Hirobe, T., Abe, H., Wakamatsu, K., Ito, S., Kawa, Y., Soma, Y. and Mizoguchi, M. (2007b). Excess tyrosine rescues the reduced activity of proliferation and differentiation of cultured recessive yellow melanocytes derived from neonatal mouse epidermis. *Eur. J. Cell Biol.* 86, 315–330.

Hirobe, T., Wakamatsu, K. and Ito, S. (2007c). Excess tyrosine stimulates eumelanin and pheomelanin synthesis in cultured slaty melanocytes from neonatal mouse epidermis. *Zool. Sci.* 24, 209–217.

Hirobe, T., Ishizuka, K., Ogawa, S. and Abe, H. (2008). Mitochondria are more numerous and smaller in pink-eyed dilution melanoblasts and melanocytes than in wild-type melanocytes in the neonatal mouse epidermis. *Zool. Sci.* 25, 1057–1065.

Hirobe, T., Kiuchi, M., Wakamatsu, K. and Ito, S. (2010). Estrogen increases hair pigmentation in female recessive yellow mice. *Zool. Sci.* 27, 470–476.

Hirobe, T., Eguchi-Kasai, K., Sugaya, K. and Murakami, M. (2011a). Effects of low-dose heavy ions on the postnatal development of mice and the yield of white spots in the mid-ventrum and tail-tips. *J. Radiat. Res.* 52, 278–286.

Hirobe, T., Eguchi-Kasai, K., Sugaya, K. and Murakami, M. (2011b). Effects of low-dose γ-rays on the embryonic development of mouse melanoblasts and melanocytes in the epidermis and hair bulbs. *Zool. Sci.* 28, 389–396.

Hirobe, T., Ito, S. and Wakamatsu, K. (2011c). The mouse pink-eyed dilution allele of the P-gene greatly inhibits eumelanin, but not pheomelanin synthesis as studied by chemical analysis. *Pigment Cell Melanoma Res.* 24, 241–246.

Hirobe, T., Yoshihara, C., Takeuchi, S., Wakamatsu, K., Ito, S., Abe, H., Kawa, Y. and Soma, Y. (2011d). A novel deletion mutation of mouse ruby-eye 2 named $ru2^d/Hps5^{ru2-d}$ inhibits melanocyte differentiation and its impaired differentiation is rescued by L-tyrosine. *Zool. Sci.* 28, 790–801.

Hume, A.N., Ushakov, D.S., Tarafder, A.K., Ferenczi, M.A. and Seabra, M.C. (2007). Rab27a and MyoVa are the primary Mlph interactions regulating melanosome transport in melanocytes. *J. Cell Sci.* 120, 3111–3122.

Ideta, R., Hirobe, T. and Tsunenaga, M. (2006). Expression of human cultured epidermal melanocytes in the reconstituted mice hair. *Pigment Cell Res.* 19, 653.

Imokawa, G. (2004). Autocrine and paracrine regulation of melanocytes in human skin and in pigmentary disorders. *Pigment Cell Res.* 17, 96–110.

Inomata, K., Aoto, T., Binh, N.T., Okamoto, N., Tanimura, S., Wakayama, T., Iseki, S., Hara, E., Masunaga, T., Shimizu, H. and Nishimura, E.K. (2009). Genotoxic stress abrogates renewal of melanocyte stem cells by triggering their differentiation. *Cell* 131, 1088–1099.

Ito, S. (1993). High-performance liquid chromatography (HPLC) analysis of eu- and pheomelanin in melanogenesis control. *J. Invest. Dermatol.* 100, 166s–171s.

Ito, S. (2003). A chemist's view of melanogenesis. *Pigment Cell Res.* 16, 230–236.

Ito, S. and Prota, G. (1977). A facile one-step synthesis of cysteinyldopas using mushroom tyrosinase. *Experientia* 33, 1118–1119.

Ito, S. and Fujita, K. (1985). Microanalysis of eumelanin and pheomelanin in hair and melanomas by chemical degradation and liquid chromatography. *Anal. Biochem.* 144, 527–536.

Ito S, and Wakamatsu, K. (1994). An improved modification of permanganate oxidation of eumelanin that gives a constant yield of pyrrole-2,3,5-tricarboxylic acid. *Pigment Cell Res.* 7, 141–144.

Ito, S. and Wakamatsu, K. (2008). Chemistry of mixed melanogenesis–pivotal roles of dopaquinone. *Photochem. Photobiol.* 84, 582–592.

Ito, S. and Wakamatsu, K. (2011). Human hair melanins: what we have learned and have not learned from mouse coat color pigmentation. *Pigment Cell Melanoma Res* 24, 63–74.

Jackson, I.J., Chambers, D., Rinchik, E.M. and Bennett, D.C. (1990). Characterization of TRP-1 mRNA levels in dominant and recessive mutations at the mouse brown (*b*) locus. *Genetics* 126, 451–459.

Jackson, I.J., Chambers, D.M., Tsukamoto, K., Copeland, N.G., Gilbert, D.M., Jenkins, N.A. and Hearing, V.J. (1992). A second tyrosinase-related protein, TRP-2 maps to and is mutated at the mouse slaty locus. *EMBO J.* 11, 527–535.

Jimenez-Cervantes, C., Solano, F., Kobayashi, T., Urabe, K., Hearing, V.J., Lozano, J.A. and Garcıa-Borron, J.C. (1994). A new enzymatic function in the melanogenic pathway. The

5,6-dihydroxyindole-2-carboxylic acid oxidase activity of tyrosinase related protein-1 (TRP1). *J. Biol. Chem.* 269, 17993–18000.

Kelly, E.M. (1957). Private communication. *Mouse News Lett.* 16, 36.

Kirkham, W.B. (1919). The fate of homozygous yellow mice. *J. Exp. Zool.* 28, 125-135.

Kobayashi, T., Urabe, K., Winder, A.J., Jimenez-Cervantes, C., Imokawa, G., Brewington, T., Solano, F., Garcia-Borron, J.C. and Hearing, V.J. (1994a). Tyrosinase related protein 1 (TRP1) functions as a DHICA oxidase in melanin biosynthesis. *EMBO J.* 13, 5818–5825.

Kobayashi, T., Urabe, K., Orlow, S.J., Higashi, K., Imokawa, G., Kwon, B.S., Potterf, S.B. and Hearing, V.J. (1994b). The Pmel17/silver locus protein. Characterization and investigation of its melanogenic function. *J. Biol. Chem.* 269, 29198–29205.

Kobayashi, T., Imokawa, G., Bennett, D.C. and Hearing, V.J. (1998). Tyrosinase stabilization of Tyrp1 (the brown locus protein). *J. Biol. Chem.* 273, 31801–31805.

Kondo, T. and Hearing, V.J. (2011). Update on the regulation of mammalian melanocyte function and skin pigmentation. *Expert Rev. Dermatol.* 6, 97–108.

Korner, A.M. and Pawelek, J. (1980). DOPAchrome conversion: a possible control point in melanin biosynthesis. *J. Invest. Dermatol.* 75, 192–195.

Kroumpouzos, G., Urabe, K., Kobayashi, T., Sakai, C. and Hearing, V.J. (1994). Functional analysis of the slaty gene product (TRP2) as dopachrome tautomerase and the effect of a point mutation on its catalytic fuction. *Biochem. Biophys. Res. Comm.* 202, 1060–1068.

Lamoreux, M.L., Zhou, B.-K., Rosemblat, S. and Orlow, S.J. (1995). The pink eyed-dilution protein and the eumelanin/pheomelani switch: in support of a unifying hypothesis. *Pigment Cell Res.* 8, 263–270.

Lamoreux, M.L., Wakamatsu, K. and Ito, S. (2001). Interaction of major coat color gene functions in mice as studied by chemical analysis of eumelanin and pheomelanin. *Pigment Cell Res.* 14, 23–31.

Lamoreux, M.L., Delmas, V., Larue, L. and Bennett, D.C. (2010). The Colors of Mice. A Model Genetic Network. Oxford, Wiley-Blackwell.

Lane, P.W. and Womack, J.E. (1977). Private communication. *Mouse News Lett.* 57, 18.

Lehman, A.L., Silvers, W.K., Puri, N., Wakamatsu, K., Ito, S. and Brilliant, M.H. (2000). The underwhite (uw) locus acts autonomously and reduces the production of melanin. *J. Invest. Dermatol.* 115, 601–606.

Levy, C., Khaled, M. and Fisher, D.E. (2006). MITF: master regulator of melanocyte development and melanoma oncogene. *Trends Mol. Med.* 12, 406–414.

Lilly, F. (1966). The genetic basis of susceptibility and resistance of mice to the Gross and Friend leukemia viruses. *Mouse News Lett.* 34, 14.

Mann, S.J. (1962). Prenatal formation of hair types. Anat. Rec. 144, 135–141.

Mayer, T.C. (1973). The migratory pathway of neural crest cells into the skin of mouse embryos. *Dev. Biol.,* 34, 39–46.

Mercer, J.A., Seperack, P.K., Strobel, M.C., Copeland, N.G. and Jenkins, N.A. (1991). Novel myosin heavy chain encoded by murine dilute coat colour locus. *Nature* 349, 709–713.

Miller, M.W., Duhl, D.M., Vrieling, H., Cordes, S.P., Ollmann, M.M., Winkes, B.M. and Barsh, G.S. (1993). Cloning of the mouse agouti gene predicts a secreted protein ubiquitously expressed in mice carrying the lethal yellow mutation. *Genes Dev.* 7, 454–467.

Motohashi, T., Yamanaka, K., Chiba, K., Miyajima, K., Aoki, H., Hirobe, T. and Kunisada, T. (2011). Neural crest cells retain their capability for multipotential differentiation even after lineage-restricted stages. *Dev. Dynam.* 240, 1681–1693.

Muller, G., Ruppert, S., Schmid, E. and Schutz, G. (1988). Functional analysis of alternatively spliced tyrosinase gene transcripts. *EMBO J.* 7, 2723–2730.

Murray, J.M. (1931). A preliminary note on the occurrence of a color mutation in the mouse (Mus musculus). *Science* 73, 482.

Naganuma, M., Yagi, E. and Fukuda, M. (2001). Delayed induction of pigmented spots on UVB-irradiated hairless mice. *J. Dermatol. Sci.* 25, 29–35.

Nagle, D.L., Karim, M.A., Woolf, E.A., Holmgren, L., Bork, P., Misumi, D.J., McGrail, S.H., Dussault, B.J., Jr., Perou, C.M., Boissy, R.E., Duyk, G.M., Spritz, R.A. and Moore, K.J. (1996). Identification and mutation analysis of the complete gene for Chediak-Higashi syndrome. *Nat. Genet.* 14, 307–311.

Newton, J.M., Cohen-Barak, O., Hagiwara, N., Gardner, J.M., Davisson, M.T., King, R.A. and Brilliant, M.H. (2001). Mutations in the human orthologue of the mouse underwhite gene (uw) underlie a new form of oculocutaneous albinism, OCA4. *Am. J. Hum. Genet.* 69, 981–988.

Nguyen, T., Novak, E.K., Kermani, M., Fluhr, J., Peters, L.L., Swank, R.T. and Wei, M. (2002). Melanosome morphologies in murine models of Hermansky-Pudlak syndrome reflect blocks in organelle development. *J. Invest. Dermatol.* 119, 1156–1164.

Ozeki, H., Ito, S., Wakamatsu, K. and Hirobe, T. (1995). Chemical characterization of hair melanins in various coat-color mutants of mice. *J. Invest. Dermatol.* 105, 361–364.

Ozeki, H., Wakamatsu, K., Ito, S. and Ishiguro, I. (1997). Chemical characterization of eumelanins with special emphasis on 5,6-dihydroxyindole-2-carboxylic acid content and molecular size. *Anal. Biochem.* 248, 149–157.

Peters, E.M.J., Tobin, D.J., Botchkareva, N., Maurer, M. and Paus, R. (2002). Migration of melanoblasts into the developing murine hair follicle is accompanied by transient c-kit expression. *J. Histochem. Cytochem.* 50, 751–766.

Petris, M.J., Strausak, D. and Mercer, J.F. (2000). The Menkes copper transporter is required for the activation of tyrosinase. *Hum. Mol. Genet.* 9, 2845–2851.

Pierro, L.J. (1963). Pigment granule formation in slate, a coat color mutant in the mouse. *Anat. Rec.* 146, 365–371.

Provance, D.W., Jr., Wei, M., Ipe, V. and Mercer, J.A. (1996). Cultured melanocytes from dilute mutant mice exhibit dendritic morphology and altered melanosome distribution. *Proc. Natl. Acad. Sci. USA* 93, 14554–4558.

Puri, N., Gardner, J.M. and Brilliant, M.H. (2000). Aberrant pH of melanosomes in pink-eyed dilution (p) mutant melanocytes. *J. Invest. Dermatol.* 115, 607–613.

Quevedo, W. C., Jr. and Isherwood, J.E. (1958). "Dopa oxidase" in melanocytes of X-irradiated quiescent (telogen) hair follicles. *Proc. Soc. Exp. Biol. Med.* 99, 748–750.

Quevedo, W. C., Jr. and Smith, J.A. (1963). Studies on radiation-induced tanning of skin. *Ann. N. Y. Acad. Sci.* 100, 364–388.

Rawles, M.E. (1947). Origin of pigment cells from the neural crest in the mouse embryo. *Physiol. Zool.* 20, 248–266.

Rinchik, E.M., Bultman, S.J., Horsthemke, B., Lee, S.-T., Strunk, K.M., Spritz, R.A., Avidano, K.M., Jong, M.T.C. and Nicholls, R.D. (1993). A gene for the mouse pink-eyed dilution locus and for human type II oculocutaneous albinism. *Nature* 361, 72–76.

Robbins, L.S., Nadeau, J.H., Johnson, K.R., Kelly, M.A., Roselli-Rehfuss, L., Baack, E., Mountjoy, K.G. and Cone, R.D. (1993). Pigmentation phenotypes of variant extension locus alleles result from point mutations that alter MSH receptor function. *Cell* 72, 827–834.

Rosemblat, S., Durham-Pierre, D., Gardner, J.M., Nakatsu, Y., Brilliant, M.H. and Orlow, S.J. (1994). Identification of a melanosomal membrane protein encoded by the pink-eyed dilution (type II oculocutaneous albinism) gene. *Proc. Natl. Acad. Sci. USA* 91, 12071–12075.

Sakurai, T., Ochiai, H and Takeuchi, T. (1975). Ultrastructural change of melanosomes associated with agouti pattern formation in mouse hair. *Dev. Biol.* 47, 466–471.

Seiji, M., Shimao, K., Birbeck, M.S.C. and Fitzpatrick, T.B. (1963). Subcellular localization of melanin biosynthesis. *Ann. N. Y. Acad. Sci.* 100, 497–533.

Shibahara, S., Okinaga, S., Tomita, Y., Takeda, A., Yamamoto, H., Sato, M. and Takeuchi, T. (1990). A point mutation in the tyrosinase gene of BALB/c albino mouse causing the cysteine → serine substitution at position 85. *Eur. J. Biochem.* 189, 455–461.

Silvers, W.K. (1979). The Coat Colors of Mice. Springer-Verlag, Berlin.

Sitaram, A., Piccirillo, R., Palmisano, I., Harper, D.C., Dell'Angelica, E.C., Schiaffino, M.V. and Marks, M.S. (2009). Localization to mature melanosomes by virtue of cytoplasmic dileucine motifs is required for human OCA2 function. *Mol. Biol. Cell* 20, 1464–1477.

Slominski, A. and Paus, R. (1993). Melanogenesis is coupled to murine anagen: toward new concepts for the role of melanocytes and the regulation of melanogenesis in hair growth. *J. Invest. Dermatol.* 101, 90S–97S.

Snell, R.S. and Bischitz, P.G. (1960). The effect of large doses of estrogen and estrogen and progesterone on melanin pigmentation. *J. Invest. Dermatol.* 35, 73–82.

Steel, K.P., Davidson, D.R. and Jackson, I.J. (1992). TRP-2/DT, a new early melanoblast marker, shows that steel growth factor (c-kit ligand) is a survival factor. *Development,* 115, 1111–1119.

Szabo, G. (1967). The regional anatomy of the human integument with special reference to the distribution of hair follicles, sweat glands and melanocytes. *Phil. Trans. R. Soc. London (Biol.)* 252, 447-485.

Takeuchi, T. (1985). Genes controlling intercellular communication during melanocyte differentiation in the mouse. *Zool. Sci.* 2, 823–831.

Tamate, H.B. and Takeuchi, T. (1984). Action of the e locus of mice in the response of phaeomelanic hair follicles to α-melanocyte-stimulating hormone in vitro. *Science* 224, 1241–1242.

Tamate, H.B., Hirobe, T. and Takeuchi, T. (1986) Effects of the lethal yellow (A^y) and recessive yellow (e) genes on the population of epidermal melanocytes in newborn mice. *J. Exp. Zool.* 238, 235–240.

Tamate, H.B., Hirobe, T., Wakamatsu, K., Ito, S., Shibahara, S. and Ishikawa, K. (1989). Levels of tyrosinase and its mRNA in coat-color mutants of C57BL/10J congenic mice: effects of genic substitution at the agouti, brown, albino, dilute, and pink-eyed dilution loci. *J. Exp. Zool.* 250, 304–311.

Tanaka, S., Yamamoto, H., Takeuchi, S. and Takeuchi, T. (1990). Melanization in albino mice transformed by introducing cloned mouse tyrosinase gene. *Development* 108, 223–227.

Theos, A.C., Truschel, S.T., Raposo, G. and Marks, M.S. (2005). The silver locus product Pmel17 / gp100 / Silv / ME20: controversial in name and in function. *Pigment Cell Res.* 18, 322–336.

Theos, A.C., Berson, J.F., Theos, S.C., Herman, K.E., Harper, D.C., Tenza, D., Sviderskaya, E.V., Lamoreux, M.L., Bennett, D.C., Raposo, G. and Marks, M.S. (2006). Dual loss of ER export and endocytic signals with altered melanosome morphology in the silver mutation of Pmel17. *Mol. Biol. Cell* 17, 3598–3612.

Toyofuku, K., Valencia, J.C., Kushimoto, T., Costin, G-E., Virador, V.M., Viera, W.D., Ferrans, V.J. and Hearing, V.J. (2002). The etiology of oculocutaneous albinism (OCA) type II: the pink protein modulates the processing and transport of tyrosinase. *Pigment Cell Res.* 15, 217–224.

Tsukamoto, K., Jackson, I.J., Urabe, K., Montague, P. and Hearing, V.J. (1992). A melanogenic enzyme termed DOPAchrome tautomerase is a novel tyrosinase-related protein, TRP-2. *EMBO J.* 11, 527–535.

Wakamatsu, K. and Ito, S. (2002). Advanced chemical methods in melanin determination. *Pigment Cell Res.* 15, 174–183.

Wakamatsu, K., Ito, S. and Rees, J.L. (2002). The usefulness of 4-amino-3-hydroxyphenylalanine as a specific marker of pheomelanin. *Pigment Cell Res.* 15, 225–232.

Wakamatsu, K., Hirobe, T. and Ito, S. (2007). High levels of melanin-related metabolites in plasma from pink-eyed dilution mice. *Pigment Cell Res.* 20, 222–224.

Walker, W.P. and Gunn, T.M. (2010). Shades of meaning: the pigment-type switching system as a tool for discovery. *Pigment Cell Melanoma Res.* 23, 485–495.

Wei, Q., Wu, X. and Hammer, J.A., III. (1997). The predominant defect in dilute melanocytes is in melanosome distribution and not cell shape, supporting a role for myosin V in melanosome transport. *J. Muscle Res. Cell Mot.* 18, 517–527.

Wei, M. L. (2006). Hermansky–Pudlak syndrome: a disease of protein trafficking and organelle function. *Pigment Cell Res.* 19, 19–42.

Westbroek, W., Lambert, J. and Naeyaert, J.M. (2001). The dilute locus and Griscelli syndrome: gateway towards a better understanding of melanosome transport. *Pigment Cell Res.* 14, 320–327.

Wu, X., Bowers, B., Wei, Q., Kocher, B. and Hammer, J.A., III. (1997). Myosin V associates with melanosomes in mouse melanocytes: evidence that myosin V is an organelle motor. *J. Cell Sci.* 110, 847–859.

Wu, X.S., Rao, K., Zhang, H., Wang, F., Sellers, J.R., Matesic, L.E., Copeland, N.G., Jenkins, N.A. and Hammer, J.A., III. (2002). Identification of an organelle receptor for myosin-Va. *Nat. Cell Biol.* 4, 271–278.

Yamaguchi, Y. and Hearing, V.J. (2009). Physiological factors that regulate skin pigmentation. *Biofactors* 35, 193–199.

Yamamoto, H., Takeuchi, S., Kudo, T., Sato, C. and Takeuchi, T. (1989). Melanin production in cultured albino melanocytes transfected with mouse tyrosinase cDNA. *Jpn. J. Genet.* 64, 121–135.

Zhang, Q., Zhao, B., Li, W., Oiso, N., Novak, E. K., Rusiniak, M. E., Gautam, R., Chintala, S., O'Brien, E. P., Zhang Y., Roe, B.A., Elliott, R.W., Eicher, E.M., Liang, P., Kratz, C., Legius, E., Spritz, R.A., O'Sullivan, T.N., Copeland, N.G., Jenkins, N.A. and Swank,

R.T. (2003). Ru2 and Ru encode mouse orthologs of the genes mutated in human Hermansky-Pudlak syndrome types 5 and 6. *Nat. Genet.* 33, 145–153.

In: Melanin: Biosynthesis, Functions and Health Effects
Editors: Xiao-Peng Ma and Xiao-Xiao Sun
ISBN: 978-1-62100-991-7

Chapter IV

The Role of Melanin Production in *Gaeumannomyces Graminis* Infection of Cereal Plants

***Hanafy Fouly*[1], *Shelby Henning*[2], *Osman Radwan*[2], *Henry Wilkinson*[3] *and Bruce Martin*[1]**
[1]Department of Entomology, Soil and Plant Sciences, Clemson University, SC, US
[2]Department of Crop Sciences, University of Illinois, Urbana, IL, US
[3]Department of Natural Resources and Environmental Sciences, US

Abstract

Gaeumannomyces graminis var. *graminis* (*Ggg*) is an ascomycete that causes black sheath rot disease of rice (*Oryza sativa* L.) and take-all root rot of several turfgrass species. *G. g.* var. *graminis* synthesizes melanin and deposits it in hyphal cell walls. Our research indicates that the nature of the association between *Ggg* and plant root is parasitic, but can change to pathogenic and ultimately terminate as saprophytic. Melanin plays several roles during fungal growth and throughout infection and colonization of plant roots. First, hyphal morphology (diameter, shape and melanin concentration) appears to change as the fungus invades and colonizes the tissues of the root. Second, melanin appears to be a determinant of fungal pathogenicity. Wild-type isolates of *Ggg* were pathogenic, and colonized plants showed more severe symptoms of infection while isolates lacking melanin were able to ectotrophically colonize and penetrate roots as a parasite, but no macroscopic symptoms of take-all were observed to indicate pathogenicity.

Introduction

Gaeumannomyces graminis (Sacc.) Arx & D.L. Olivier var. *graminis* (*Ggg*) is an ascomycete that infects roots of rice (*Oryza sativa* L.) and several turfgrasses (Hawksworth, 1995; Walker, 1981). It is an aggressive pathogen of rice causing black sheath rot disease.

Gaeumannomyces graminis var. *graminis* is an aggressive colonist but a somewhat weak pathogen of turfgrasses including centipedegrass (*Eremochloa ophiuroides* (Munro) Hack.) (Wilkinson, 1994), bermudagrass (*Cynodon dactylon* L.) (Elliot, 1991), zoysiagrass (*Zoysia japonica* Steudel) (Wilkinson, 1993), and St. Augustinegrass (*Stenotaphrum secundatum* (Walt.) Kuntze) (Elliot, et al. 1993). It is a primary colonist, forming a perennial association with vegetatively cloned grasses and an annual association with rice. In general, the pathogen acts as a primary colonist of newly formed roots and crowns. As an aggressive colonist, it mantles the root surface with highly melanized, ectotrophic hypha. Ectotrophic colonization is supported by endotrophic root colonization of the epidermal and cortical tissues. Subsequent invasion and colonization of the endodermis and stele tissues results in vascular occlusion which compromises the host's capacity to conduct water and store, transport, or utilize available photosynthates (Jones & Clifford, 1978). Foliage discoloration and root rotting are followed by plant death only when drought and/or heat stress occur over time.. Finally, seed formation is severely limited, or inhibited if root colonization is extensive.

Melanins are dark colored pigments produced by various organisms of all biological kingdoms (Hill, 1992). Chemically, there are three different kinds of melanins that are produced by living organisms (Bell and Wheeler, 1986). Brown and black pigments manufactured from dihydroxyphenylalanine (DOPA) are termed eumelanins. Red and yellow pigments derived from DOPA and cysteine are known as phaeomelanins. Melanins derived from phenols and catechols which lack nitrogen are known generically as melanin (Bell and Wheeler, 1986). In addition to cellulolytic and pectinolytic enzymes that aid in the infection of host cells, it is important to acknowledge the presence of melanin in the hyphae of *Gaeumannomyces*. Cellular synthesis of the biopolymer melanin has been linked to the pathogenicity of fungi (Brush and Money, 1999; Henson et al., 1999; Hill, 1992; and Hornby, 1998). For example, melanin deficient mutants of the rice-blast fungus, *Magnaporthe grisea*, have been demonstrated to be avirulent (Henson et al., 1999). Due to the fact that *Gaeumannomyces* species are characteristically melanizied, the presence of melanin in hyphae may play a role in the pathogenicity of *Gaeumannomyces graminis* (Henson et. al., 1999).

Gaeumannomyces graminis melanin is formed by the 1, 8 DHN pathway (Henson et al., 1999). Using wild-type and melanin deficient mutant isolates of *Ggg*, Frederick, et al. (1999) showed melanin was deposited on *Ggg* hyphal cell walls while Bell and Wheeler (1986) reported melanin was deposited as a layer at the exterior surface of the fungal cell wall and/or as electron dense granules distributed within the cell wall of the melanized yeast *Phaeococcomyces*. The potential benefits that DHN melanins could confer to hypha that synthesize them are considerable. Melanin protects fungal hypha from the negative effects of UV irradiation (Bell and Wheeler, 1986), temperature extremes (Hill, 1992), over-and under-abundance of moisture (Hill, 1992), toxic concentrations of metal ions (Caesar-Tonthat et. al., 1998), attack from antagonistic microbes (Henson et al., 1999), and extreme pH conditions (Frederick et al., 1999).

While melanin has been implicated in the fungal colonization and infection of plants, it has also been shown in work using melanin deficient mutatnts, that that the presence of melanin in hyphae may not be required for infection (Frederick et al., 1999; Henson et al., 1999). However, restoring melanin production restored pathogenicity in some non-melanized, non-pathogenic mutants that evidently depend on the presence of melanin to penetrate host tissues. In one study, a melanin-deficient mutant of the human pathogen, *Wangiella dermatitidis* was non-pathogenic (Brush and Money, 1999). However, when melanin production was restored, it was able to penetrate and colonize animal tissues.

This research was divided into two phases. The objectives of the first phase were to determine the role of melanin on linear growth, hyphal width and branch formation, and to quantify melanin in wild-type isolates and melanin-minus mutants of *Ggg*. The objectives of second phase were: to observe and measure changes in the melanin content of *Gaeumannomyces graminis var. graminis* (*Ggg*) during pathogenesis (inoculation through colonization of the stele) to determine if melanin content had an effect on the ability of *Ggg* to infect and colonize host roots and to;. A third objective of the second phase determine the nature of the host and parasite association as it is affected by the ability of *Ggg* to produce melanin.

Materials and Methods

Fungal Isolates and Culturing

The fungal isolates of *Gaeumannomyces graminis* var. *graminis* used in this research were designated WT1+, M1-, WT2+, and M2- (Table 1). Isolates WT1+ and M1- were obtained from Joan M. Henson, Department of Microbiology, Lewis Hall 109 Bozeman, MT 59717. Isolate WT1+ was originally isolated from soybean (*Glycine max* L.). Isolate WT1+ is a wild-type fungus that was used to produce the hyaline, melanin deficient mutant M1- using nitroquinolene oxide (NQO) as the mutagenic agent (Epstein, *et.al.*, 1994). Isolate WT2+ is a wild-type of *Ggg* obtained from Monica Elliot, University of Florida, Fort Lauderdale REC 3205 College Avenue, Ft. Lauderdale FL 33314. Isolate M2- is a hyaline, melanin deficient mutant produced from WT2+ by the method of Frederick, et.al. (1999). All isolates were maintained on potato dextrose agar (PDA) (Sigma-Aldrich, St. Louis, MO, USA) and transferred every 7 days to fresh media.

Hyphal Morphology and Vegetative Growth Rate

To determine the effect of melanin on hyphal morphology, measurements of hyphal width (W) and distance between hyphal branches (DBB) were recorded where isolates grew in culture. Each isolate was cultured and evaluated on three different media: Luria-Bertani agar (LBA, 5g tryptone, 10g NaCl, 5g yeast extract, 15g agar/1L water), vegetable juice agar (V8, 200ml V8 juice, 1.8g CaCO3, 15g agar/1L water) and Czapek-Dox agar (CDA, 3g NaNO3, 0.5g KCl, 0.5g MgSO4, 0.01g $FeSO_4$, 1g K_2HPO_4, 30g sucrose, 15g agar/1L water) using 3 repetitions (1 petri-plate = 1 repetition). When the leading edge of a colony had extended to the perimeter of the petri plate, or 7 days had elapsed, measurements of hyphal width and distance between branching were recorded. Distance between branching was defined by two consecutive points of intersection formed between the main hypha and the hyphal branch. Within these randomly selected areas of a culture, 10 measurements per area were recorded. Each experiment was replicated 3 times and repeated 3 times. Measurements were made using an ocular micrometer and an Olympus BH-2 light microscope (40 x).

Table 1. Gaeumannomyces graminis var. graminis isolates

Desig-nation*	Plant Source	Descri-ption	Coloration of Adult Thallus	Hypho-podia	Reference/Source
WT1+	Soybean	wild type	black	lobed, melanized	Frederick, 1999
M1-	Soybean	NQO mutant of WT1+	hyaline	lobed, melanized	Frederick, 1999
WT2+	Bermu-dagrass	wild type	black	lobed, melanized	M. Elliot, FL.
M2-	Bermu-dagrass	NQO mutant of WT2+	hyaline	simple, hyaline	S. Henning

* WT= wild-type; reference number; + = pigmented; and - = non-pigmentation, NQO = 4-Nitroquinoline-1-oxide.

To determine the effect of melanin on the vegetative growth of isolates in culture, studies comparing radial growth on agar media were conducted. Each isolate was cultured on LBA, CDA, and V8A media. The diameter (mm) of each colony was recorded using digital calipers. Measurements were recorded every 24h from the time of seeding and until the leading edge of a colony had reached the edge of the petri plate or 7 days had elapsed. Growth experiments were repeated 3 times, with 3 replications per experiment. The data were used to calculate mean daily growth rate (mm).

Melanin Quantification

Purification of Melanin from Wild-type Hyphae

Melanin concentration was estimated using Azure A as a melanin binding agent. Melanin was produced by culturing WT1+ in LB broth (LBB, 5g tryptone, 10g NaCl, 5g yeast extract/1L water). The LBB was seeded with 10 culture plugs (1.0 mm diameter) of WT1+ taken from leading edge of a colony growing on LBA. The LBB cultures were incubated at room temperature (20-23 ^{0}C) on an orbital shaker (150 rpm) for 7 days. The LBB medium was then separated from the hyphae by gentle vacuum filtration and discarded. The fungal mat was cut into 5 mm pieces, submersed in acetone and heated to 50 ^{0}C for 30 minutes. The acetone was then separated from the hyphae by vacuum filtration and discarded. The fungal mass was then washed three times by pouring 100 ml distilled water (20 ^{0}C) over the fungal tissue. The fungal tissue was then immersed in 200 ml absolute ethanol and heated to 85 ^{0}C for 3 hours in a hot water-bath. The fungal tissue was separated and washed as described previously. The fungal tissue was then placed into a 500 ml single neck boiling flask equipped with a dry reflux condenser. To the fungal mass, 200 ml 38% HCl were added via the reflux condenser and heated to 85 ^{0}C for 18 hours in a fume hood. The resulting melanin granules were collected from the resulting black suspension by ultra-centrifugation (13,200 rpm, 60 sec.), washed 3 times with 38 ml distilled water, dried over anhydrous $CaCl_2$ under vacuum and stored at -80 ^{0}C. The resulting material was considered concentrated melanin.

Absorption of Azure A by Melanin

The melanin-Azure A binding coefficient was determined from a reaction of concentrated melanin and a stock solution of Azure A (4.75 mg Azure A/1L 0.1M HCl). The Azure A solution (4.75 μg Azure A/1ml 0.1M HCl) had an absorbance of 0.6 O.D. at 610 nm. Serial dilutions of the reaction solution resulted in a proportional decrease in absorbance with a lower limit of detection estimated at 10 μg/ml. Triplicate samples of melanin (250, 500, 1000 μg) were each placed into 15 ml Corex tubes and 3 mls of Azure A stock solution was added. The reactions were incubated for 60 minutes at 20 °C with slight shaking (50 rpm). The melanin-Azure complex was then separated from the Azure A solution using an ultra-centrifuge (13,200 rpm, 60 sec.). The optical density of the Azure A remaining in solution was measured at 610 nm and recorded. It was calculated that a 1 milligram of concentrated melanin absorbed 873 μg of Azure A in solution and that 1 milligram of melanin would decrease the optical density (610 nm) of the Azure A stock solution by 0.13 units.

Quantification of Melanin in Mycelia

Measurement of mycelial melanin was made using a modification of melanin quantification reported by Butler and LaChance (1986). Fungal tissue used for melanin quantification was cultured in Erlenmeyer flasks (125 ml) containing 60 ml LBB. Cultures were started with 3 plugs of an isolate taken from the leading edge of a colony on LBA using a Pasteur pipette and sterile technique as previously described. Cultures were shaken at 150 rpm and maintained at laboratory temperature (20-22 °C) for 7, 14, 21, or 28 days. At the end of each growth period, fungal material was collected by removing the LBB using vacuum filtration, washed as previously described and then lyophilized for 24 hours. Hyphal melanin was assayed by reacting triplicate samples of lyophilized hyphae (2000 μg) and Azure A stock solution as described above. The reactions were incubated at 20 °C for 60 minutes with orbital shaking (50 rpm). The hyphae were then separated from the Azure A solution using an ultra-centrifuge (13200 rpm, 60 sec.). The optical density of the Azure A solution was measured (610 nm) and recorded. The loss in optical density of the Azure A solution was compared with losses in optical density resulting from concentrated melanin to determine the melanin concentration (μg melanin/mg hyphae).

Morphological experiments were complete randomized designs with sub-sampling and three replicates. Isolate and media type were the fixed factors for both experiments with treatment comparisons performed using contrast statements. Growth rate and melanin content were analyzed over time for isolate and media combinations using linear regression. All statistics were performed using general linear model or regression procedures of SAS statistical software (SAS Institute Inc., Cary, NC, USA). Every experiment was repeated at least once.

Pathogenicity Tests

Inoculation of Rice Using Conetainer Assay

The fungal isolates of *Gaeumannomyces graminis* var. *graminis* WT2+ and its melanin deficient counterpart isolate WT2- were used in this study. Inoculum was produced in Erlenmeyer flasks containing millet (*Panicum miliaceum* L.) seed (50 ml) and deionized water (50 ml), autoclave-sterilized (32 psi, 161^{0}C) for 1 hour. The moist grain was allowed to cool for 24 hours and then was autoclaved a second time. Upon cooling, the grain was seeded with culture plugs of WT2= or WT2- (5 plugs ca. 5 mm square) excised from the leading edge of a young fungal colony. The flasks were vigorously shaken every 24 hours for the first 2 days to uniformly distribute inoculum with the millet. After the millet appeared covered with fungal mycelium, it was removed from the container and dried under a laminar flow hood for 48 hours. The dried inoculum was stored at room temperature in the dark and periodically evaluated for contamination and viability by plating 1-20 millet kernels on the surface of PDA.

The procedure used for host inoculation was a modification of a conetainer assay previously reported by Wilkinson et al. (1985). A cotton ball was placed at the bottom of a small conetainer (16 x 4 cm) (Ray Leach, Inc. Canby, OR). The conetainer was then filled to within 4 cm of the top with double-autoclaved vermiculite. Five colonized millet seeds were placed on top of the vermiculite layer. Upon this layer of inoculum, a 0.5 cm thick layer of double-autoclaved vermiculite was added. Three surface-sterilized rice (*Oryza sativa* 'Cypress') seeds (1 minute soaking in 2.5% sodium hypochlorite, rinsed with sterile water until no smell of bleach remained) of a host species are placed on top of the vermiculite and covered with an additional 0.5 cm thick layer of double-autoclaved vermiculite. The filled conetainer was then placed into a holding rack. A total of 16 conetainers were prepared for each treatment. Eight additional conetainers were prepared lacking the pathogen and these served as control treatments. The conetainers were placed on a mist bench (10 seconds misted water/15 minutes) until the vegetative growth of each species was approximately 2.54 cm tall. Then, the conetainers were placed in a growth chamber (15 or 30C, 18 hours of light/6 hours of darkness cycle). Each conetainer was kept moist by topical applications of distilled water.

Inoculated rice plants were rated for disease severity using a modified version of a previously reported assay (Wilkinson et al., 1985) using a randomized block design. Each week, for a total of 4 weeks after being placed in the growth chamber, 4 conetainers per treatment as well as 2 non-inoculated control treatments were randomly removed from incubation, the roots washed free of vermiculite, and the roots rated for disease severity as follows: (no disease present, DS=0); (1-25% of roots with necrotic tissue, DS=1); (26 –50% necrotic, DS=2); (51-75% necrotic, DS=3); (76-100% necrotic, DS=4). All treatments were replicated 3 times as 3 independent biological replicates. Statistical analysis of the data was performed by SAS statistical analysis software (SAS Institute Inc., Cary, NC, USA) using analysis over time and standard deviations are given.

Inoculation of Rice Using a Petri-plate Assay

Rice was also inoculated using a Petri plate assay. Isolates used for the plate assay were wild-type WT2+ and WT1+, and their respective melanin-deficient counterparts M2- and M1-. Rice seeds were prepared by removing the outer husk and surface disinfesting them in 3 percent aqueous solution of hydrogen peroxide containing 100 ul of polyoxyethylenesorbitan (Sigma# P139). The disinfesting solution was decanted and the seeds allowed to dry on sterile paper towels. Three surface disinfested seeds were then placed at the outer edges of 90 mm Petri plates containing 10 ml potato dextrose agar. Plates were then placed under constant fluorescent lighting until germinated roots were approximately 6 cm long. Using sterile technique, seedling roots were inoculated with one 2-mm^2 plug cut from the leading edge of an actively growing colony cultured on PDA. The inoculum plug was placed in the center of the Petri pate containing germinated seeds. Inoculated plates were then placed under fluorescent lighting and monitored to determine when the fungus intersected a root. Plants were harvested 28 days following the initial contact between the fungus and the root. Samples were then embedded and sectioned for microscopicobservation.

Wax Embedment and Sectioning of Rice Roots Harvested from Conetainer Assay

Roots harvested from the conetainer assay were submerged in formalin-acetic acid-alcohol (FAA) solution for 48 hours to fix both host and fungus tissues. The fixed samples were dissected. Pieces (2 cm in length) of the main root from the area closest to the inoculum were excised, initially dehydrated in a graded water/ethanol series, and finally dehydrated a graded ethanol/xylene series. Dehydrated samples were prepared for sectioning by infiltrating them with molten Paraplast (Sigma# P3558) at 60 °C over a 24-hour time period. The infiltrated samples were placed into hand folded cube-shaped tin-foil molds, and embedded in molten paraplast. Thin section (10 µm) were then cut with a hand-operated rotary microtome, floated on 7% formaldehyde solution on gelatin (Sigma# G6144) coated slides, and incubated at 30 °C for 24 h. Paraplast was removed from sections on slides by immersing them in several changes of xylene until no paraplast was observed when viewed at 400 X. Sections were stained by immersing slides in hematoxylin solution (0.2% aqueous hematoxylin (Sigma# H3136), and 0.2% potassium iodide) for 2 hours, followed by rinsing briefly under gently flowing tap-water. Sections were further stained by placing them in 1% aqueous Fast Green (Sigma# F758) for 30 seconds, and rinsing briefly. Hematoxylin-Fast Green stained slides were quickly dehydrated in an ethanol/water series (70:30, 95:5, 100:0; 20-30 seconds in each solution), dipped in xylene, and allowed to air dry. Slides were then mounted in 3 drops of permount (Electron Microscopy Sciences, 1560 Industry Rd., Box 550 Hatfield, PA 19440), covered with 80-mm cover slips and allowed to dry overnight previous to examination with an Olympus BH-2 compound microscope (40-100X).

Agarose Embedment and Sectioning of Rice Roots Harvested from Petri-plate Assay

Roots from plants harvested from the Petri plate assay were excised and embedded in molten 3% agarose contained in 2.5 ml cryovials (Sigma# V9380). Following agarose solidification (about 15 minutes), the embedded roots were removed from cryovial containers and hand-sectioned underwater using a half of a double-edged razor blade under magnification (dissecting microscope at 40x). Sections were placed on microscope slides, observed at 100-1000X, and digital images photographically captured. Samples were observed either stained or not. Samples were stained by placing one drop of Azure A stain (Sigma# A918, 1g Azure A/L in 95% ethanol) on them prior to application of a cover slip.

Results

The Effect of Melanin Hyphal Width

There was no significant difference in hyphal width between *Ggg* wild-type isolates when cultured on LBA or V8A media (Table 2). There were significant differences in hyphal width between the two wild-type *Ggg*'s cultured on CDA where WT1+ was wider (27%) than WT2+. Wild-type WT1+ and its corresponding melanin-deficient mutant (M1-) displayed significant differences in hyphal width on all tested media. Wild-type WT1+ hyphae were wider than M1- on CDA (19%) and V8A (28%) media. Melanin-deficient mutant M1- was wider (26%) compared to WT1+ on LBA media. Wild-type WT2+ and its' corresponding melanin-deficient mutant M2- showed differences in hyphal width. When cultured on CDA, M2- hyphae were wider (24%) compared to wild-type WT2+. When grown on V8A, WT2+ had wider (19%) hyphae than M2-. There were no differences in hyphal width between WT2+ and M2- cultured on LBA medium.

Table 2. Mean Hyphal width of wild-type and melanin deficient *Gaeumannomyces graminis* var. *graminis* isolates

Isolate Contrasts	CDA	LBA	V8A
WT1+	3.90	2.89	3.63
WT2+	2.85	3.12	3.86
	**	NS	NS
WT1+	3.90	2.89	3.63
M1-	3.16	3.90	2.61
	**	**	**
WT2+	2.85	3.12	3.86
M2-	3.78	3.28	3.12
	**	NS	**

Mean hyphal widths (um) were calculated using the datda from three separate experiments. Each experiment was replicated 3x and repeated 3x (n=90). * and ** represent an alpha level of 0.05 and <0.001, respectively. NS = not significant. Ten measurements of hyphal diameter were recorded by randomly selecting 10 different hyphae from within each of those randomly selected areas of a culture. WT = wild type and M = mutant ;CDA= Czapek-Dox Agar, LBA= Luria-Bertani agar, and V8A= vegetable juice agar.

The Effect of Melanin on Hyphal Distance between Branches

In general, the distance between hyphal branches was longer for wild-type isolates than their respective mutants. Distances between hyphal branches (DBB) were significantly different between the two wild-type isolates cultured on each of the three media tested (Table 3). On CDA, WT1+ had an 18% longer DBB than WT2+. On LBA and V8A, respectively, WT2+ exhibited 12% and 27% longer DBB, respectively, compared to WT1+. In comparing the wild-type with their respective mutants, WT1+ displayed longer DBB on both CDA (22%) and LBA (26%) media compared to M1-. On V8A medium, WT1+ and M1- showed no differences in DBB. Isolate WT2+ exhibited a significantly longer DBB on CDA (41%), LBA (50%), and V8A (67%) compared to M2-.

Fungal Vegetative Growth in Different Cultures

All fungal isolates were grown on LBA medium displayed differences in hyphal growth rates (Table 4). WT2+ (15.3 mm/day) grew faster than WT1+ (12.2 mm/day) on LBA. Isolate WT2+ grew faster (15.3 mm/day) than M2- (0.5 mm/day) on LBA medium. M1- grew faster (14.6 mm/day) than WT1+ (12.2 mm/day).

Table 3. Mean Distance between branches of wild-type and melanin deficient *Gaeumannomyces graminis* var. *graminis*

Isolate Contrasts	CDA	LBA	V8A
WT1+	64.88	67.72	59.32
WT2+	53.29	77.11	82.08
	**	*	**
WT1+	64.88	67.72	59.32
M1_	50.38	49.96	57.54
	**	**	NS
WT2+	53.29	77.11	82.08
M2-	31.45	38.86	27.14
	**	**	**

Mean hyphal widths (um) were calculated using the data from three separate experiments. Each experiment was replicated 3x and repeated 3x (n=90). * and ** represent an alpha level of 0.05 and <0.001, respectively. NS = not significant. Ten measurements of hyphal diameter were recorded by randomly selecting 10 different hyphae from within each of those randomly selected areas of a culture. WT = wild type and M = mutant ;CDA= Czapek-Dox Agar, LBA= Luria-Bertani agar, and V8A= vegetable juice agar.

When fungal isolates were cultured on CDA medium, there were significant differences in growth rate between the wild-type isolates and between each wild-type isolate and their corresponding melanin deficient mutant (Table 5). WT1+ grew significantly faster (10.8 mm/day) compared to WT2+ (3.6 mm/day). Wild-type isolates grew significantly slower than their corresponding melanin deficient mutants. Isolate WT1+ grew at a slower (10.8 mm/day) than M1- (15.2 mm/day) when cultured on CDA. Wild-type WT2+ grew slower (3.6 mm/day) compared to M2- (5.3 mm/day) on CDA.

Table 4. Regression equations and contrasts of analysis of growth rate of *Geaumannomyces graminis var. graminis* isolates cultured on Luria-Bertani agar

Isolate	Regression equation
WT1+	y = 12.168x -3.968
M1-	y = 14.562x -1.696
WT2+	y = 15.326x -11.88
M2-	y = 0.502x -8.26
Contrasts of Growth Rates	p-value
WT1+ vs. WT2+	< .0001
WT1+ vs. M1-	0.0025
WT2+ vs. M2-	< .0001

Regression equations were generated from regression lines fitted to growth rate (mm/day) of wild-type (WT1+ &WT2+) and melanin deficient mutant (M1- & M2-) *Gaeumannomyces graminis* var. *graminis*. Experiments were repeated 3 times, with 3 repetitions per experiment. Alpha level = 0.05.

Table 5. Regression equations and contrasts of analysis of growth rate of *Geaumannomyces graminis var. graminis* isolates cultured on Czapek-Dox agar

Isolate	Regression equation
WT1+	y = 10.774x -3.447
M1-	y = 15.169x -7.016
WT2+	y = 3.61x + 0.103
M2-	y = 5.292x +3.192
Contrasts of growth rate	p-value
WT1+ vs. WT2+	< .0001
WT1+ vs. M1-	0.0333
WT2+ vs. M2-	< .0001

Regression equations were generated from regression lines fitted to growth rate (mm/day) of wild-type (WT1+ &WT2+) and melanin deficient mutant (M1- & M2-) *Gaeumannomyces graminis* var. *graminis*. Experiments were repeated 3 times, with 3 repetitions per experiment. Alpha level = 0.05.

Quantification of Melanin in *Gaeumannomyces Graminis* var. *graminis* Hypha

Melanin concentration was calculated using changes in the optical density at 610 nm of Azure A in solution. Extracted, purified, and concentrated *Ggg* melanin had a binding coefficient of 873 μg Azure A/mg melanin. Both wild-type isolates of *Ggg* showed no significant difference in melanin concentration throughout the experiment (Figure 1). Wild type isolates and their corresponding melanin deficient mutants were not significantly different in melanin production at the first sampling(7days of growth). Melanin concentration appeared to reach a maximum by day 14 for the wild-type isolates (Figures 2 & 3). After 14 days of fungal growth, each wild-type had a mean of 233 μg melanin/mg hyphae. Melanin deficient mutants M1- and M2- displayed means of 65 and 33 μg melanin/mg hyphae, respectively (Figures 2 & 3).

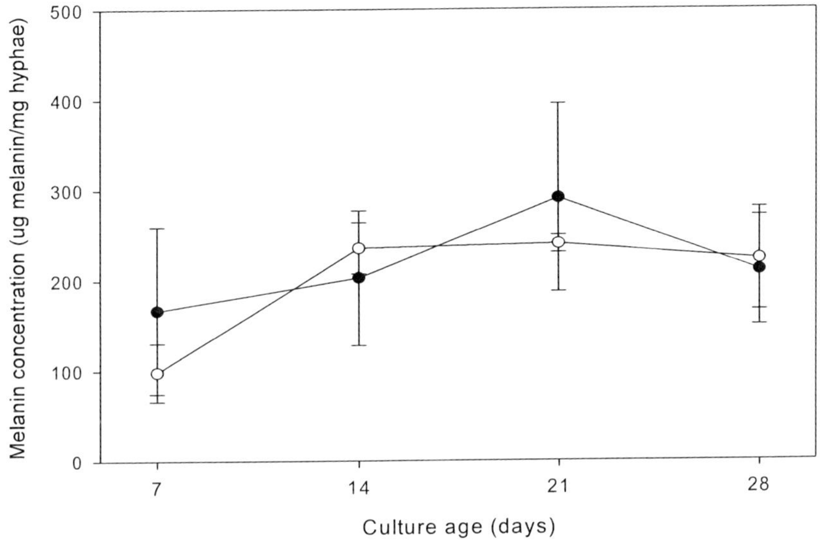

Figure 1. Melanin concentration (ug melanin/mg hyphae) of wild-type WT1+ (●) and WT2+ (○) *Gaeumannomyces graminis* var. *graminis* cultured in Luria-Bertani broth. Each point represents the mean of 3 repeated trials with 3 replications per treatment. Where standard error bars cross, there is no statistically significant difference in the data.

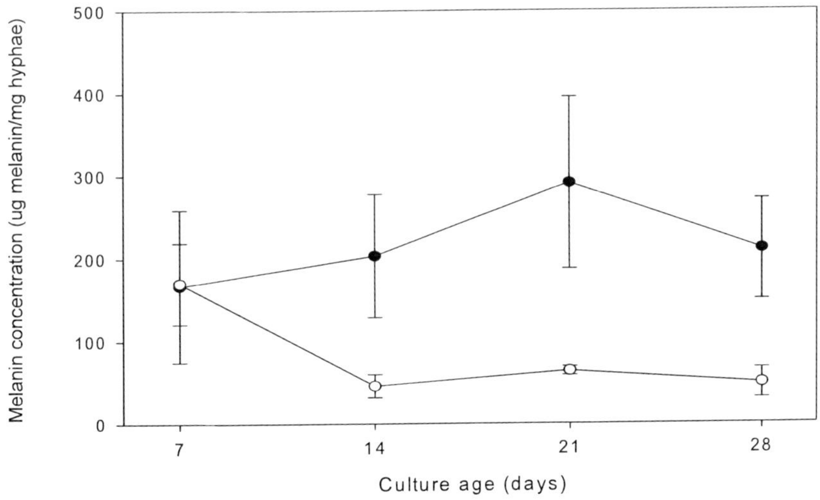

Figure 2. Melanin concentration (ug melanin/mg hyphae) of wild-type WT1+ (●) and melanin-deficient M1- (○) *Gaeumannomyces graminis* var. *graminis* cultured in Luria-Bertani broth. Each point represents the mean of 3 repeated trials with 3 replications per treatment. Where standard error bars cross, there is no statistically significant difference in the data.

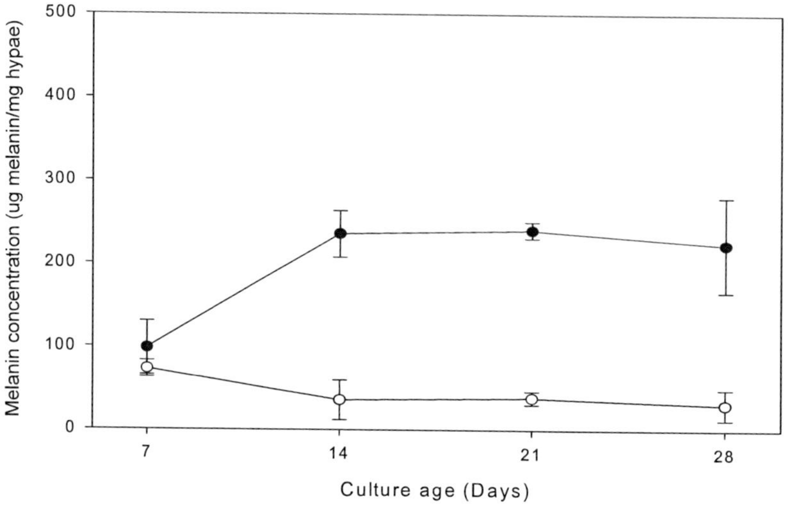

Figure 3. Melanin concentration (ug melanin/mg hyphae) of wild-type WT1+ (•) and melanin-deficient M2- (○) *Gaeumannomyces graminis* var. *graminis* cultured in Luria-Bertani broth. Each point represents the mean of 3 repeated trials with 3 replications per treatment. Where standard error bars cross, there is no statistically significant difference in the data.

Disease Severity and Ectotrophic Colonization of Rice in Conetainer Assay

Rice plants generated by conetainer assay were examined macroscopically after 28 days of incubation (n=24). Plants inoculated with wild-type WT2+ were all severely diseased, with all rated a 4 for mean disease severity (MDS), ..., and those inoculated with melanin-deficient M2- were free of disease, with all rated a 0 (MDS) for each experiment (n=24). Using the conetainer assay, wild-type WT2+ displayed extensive ectotrophic colonization (Figure 4) of the root epidermis at the time the roots were prepared for histopathological observation (ca 28 days incubation)(Figure 4). The roots of plants inoculated with the wild-type isolate were a uniform black color. Ectotrophic large diameter runner hyphae (5um) were darkly pigmented, and branched extensively forming a mantle of mycelia on the root epidermis. Plants inoculated with *Ggg* isolate M2- (melanin-deficient) displayed no evidence of lesions, or other symptoms commonly observed for root ectotrophic colonization after 28 days of incubation (Figure 4). Plants inoculated with M2- were indistinguishable from controls at 28 days of age. At the time they were prepared for sectioning, roots of M2- inoculated rice plants exhibited no observed mycelium on the outer surface of the roots, and the roots displayed no symptoms. Uninoculated rice plants displayed no symptoms of disease or discoloration (Figure 4). Roots were uniform in their appearance among treatments.

Histopathological Observations of Rice Inoculated in Conetainer Assay

Unstained roots inoculated with the wild-type WT2+ isolate exhibited darkly pigmented runner hyphae on their epidermal surfaces. Darkly pigmented hyphopodia were also detected on roots inoculated with WT2+. Unstained root sections inoculated with WT2+ did not show infection hyphae in the epidermis, cortex, or stele. Mycelia of the melanin-deficient isolate

M2- were not detected in any tissues of inoculated, unstained, sectioned, root material (n=24). Unstained sections of controls did not show the presence of fungi on or in any root tissues. Colonizing mycelium in inoculated root samples were elucidated by staining with Hematoxylin/Fast Green. Stained hypha were readily identified both ecto- and endotrophically. Dark runner hyphae were easily detected without staining, and their appearance was enhanced by staining with hematoxylin (Figure 5). Hematoxylin stained runner hyphae were a rich, dark brown color. Runner hyphae were also observed to develop infection pegs on the host surface, and these exhibited the same staining reaction (dark brown) as runner hyphae (Figure 5). Infection hyphae of the wild-type fungus did not appear melanized, and were visible in the epidermal, cortical, and vascular tissue of infected plants only after treatment with fast green (Figure 5; n=24). Infection hyphae stained by fast green were green/blue in color, and colonized root tissues in an intracellular manner (Figure 5).

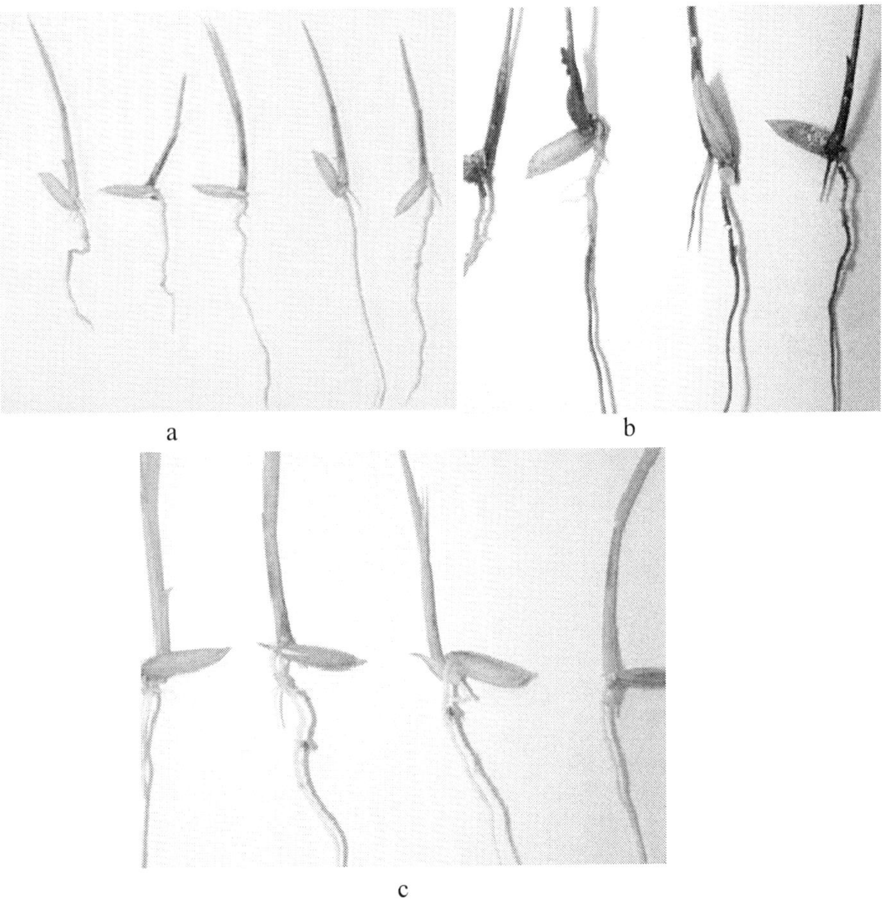

Figure 4. Rice inoculated with *Gaeumannomyces graminis* var. *graminis* using a container system and incubated at 15C. Uninoculated controls (A.); wild-type inoculated WT2+ (B.); melanin-deficient M2-inoculated rice (C.).

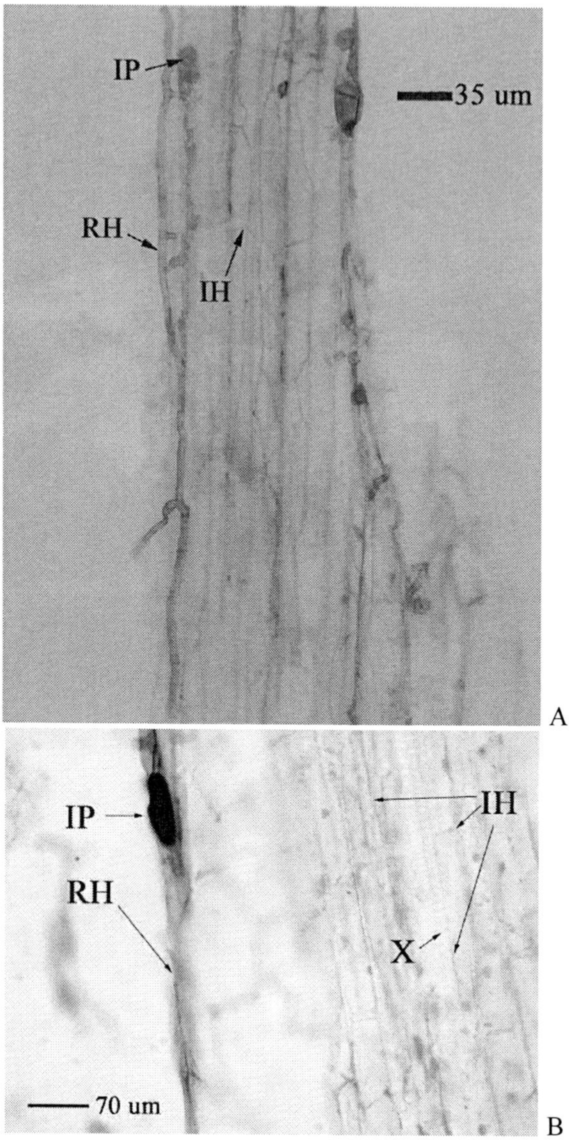

Figure 5. Rice roots after inoculation with *Gaeumannomyces graminis* var. *graminis* wild-type isolate WT2+. Longitudinal section stained with hematoxylin and fast green (A.) shows infection pegs (IP); runner hyphae (RH); and infection hyphae (IH). Longitudinal section stained with hematoxylin and fast green (B.) shows infection pegs (IP); runner hyphae (RH); infection hyphae (IH), and xylem (X).

The fungus appeared hyaline as it traversed the endodermis and entered the stele. A color change indicating re-melanization of hyphae at the endodermal tissue layer was not detected in roots inoculated with the wild-type fungus after 28 days of incubation. Hematoxylin did not appear to cause a staining reaction in infection hyphae as they traversed the endodermis and entered the stele. Identification of infection hyphae was easiest in longitudinally sectioned samples. After treatment with fast green, sectioned samples of rice roots inoculated with M2- did not exhibit stained hyphae inter- or intracellularly colonizing the epidermis, epidermal, cortical, or vascular tissues. Sections produced from M2- inoculated roots (n=24) and un-inoculated controls (n=4) were microscopically indistinguishable from each other.

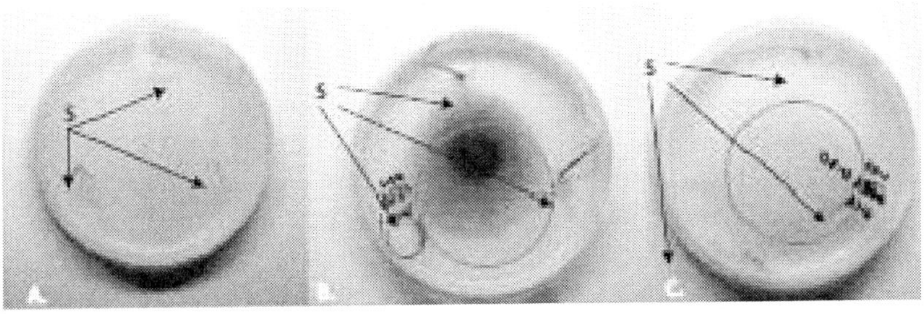

Figure 6. Rice inoculated with *Gaeumannomyces graminis* var. *graminis*: un-inoculated (A); wild-type WT2+ (B); melanin-deficient M2- (C). Red circle denotes border of fungal colony. Germinated seeds are labeled as "S".

Disease Severity and Ectotrophic Colonization of Rice in Petri-plate Assay

Rice plants inoculated with *Ggg* and incubated in the Petri plate assay were extensively colonized by ectotrophic hyphae after 28 days (Figure 6). As cultures grew across the Petri-plate, they grew over and obscured the rice roots on the plate with a mycelial mat. Inoculated plants removed from the plates were entirely mantled by the fungi and their roots were often embedded in the agar. The hyphae formed a much denser mantle around the roots compared to the colonization observed on roots cultured in the conetainer assay. Wild-type isolates WT1+ and WT2+ produced ectotrophic mycelium that was melanized and mantled the roots. Wild-type isolates (WT1+ & WT2+) caused macroscopic lesions on black roots in inoculated plants that coalesced (n=18 each). Melanin-deficient mutant isolates M1- and M2- were also observed colonizing the exterior root surface and forming a mantle. These hyphae were hyaline. The densities of the mycelial mantle of wild-type and melanin-deficient isolates were judged to be equivalent. Melanin-deficient isolate M1- inoculated roots showed reddish colored lesions While M2- displayed no color change or other symptoms (n=18).

Histopathological Observation of Rice Inoculated in Petri-plate Assay

Unstained rice roots inoculated with *Ggg* isolate WT1+ showed uniformly light brown hyphae in the epidermal, cortical, and vascular tissues by 28 days of incubation. Melanized runner hyphae were not observed to be produced by WT1+ on the surface of inoculated roots cultured in the Petri plate assay. Hyphae inside of plant roots appeared the same diameter (6 μm) in each tissue. A change in hyphal coloration (darkening) indicating re-melanization of WT1+ hypha when entering the stele was not detected in any unstained sections (n=18). Unstained sections of WT2+ infected plant material inoculated with wild-type isolate WT2+ showed that it had colonized all tissues of the root at the time of sectioning (Figure 7; n=18). Melanized runner hyphae were not observed to be produced by WT2+ on the surface of inoculated roots cultured in the Petri plate assay. In unstained sections, WT2+ hypha were a uniform brown color in each tissue (epidermis, cortex and stele) of an infected root (n=18).

These hyphae appeared to be the same diameter (6 μm) in each tissue. Sections of rice roots indicated that WT2+ hyphae did not change hyphal coloration throughout the process of pathogenesis. In addition, a change in hyphal coloration (darkening) indicating re-melanization of WT2+ hypha when entering the stele was not detected in sections of unstained inoculated roots (n=18). Unstained root sections of melanin-deficient mutant M1-inoculated plants did not indicate the presence of hyphae in any of the roots tissues. Unstained root sections of melanin-deficient mutant M1- inoculated plants showed lignitubers being produced by the host in epidermal and cortical tissues at 28D of inoculation. Unstained root sections of melanin-deficient mutant M2- inoculated plants did not indicate the presence of hyphae in any of the roots tissues.

Staining with Azure A allowed the fungus to be readily observed in sections produced from plants in Petri-plate assay. Azure A stained the anticlinal plant cell walls dark purple while fungal hyphae were stained with light purple color (Figure 8). Stained roots inoculated with *Ggg* isolate WT1+ showed light purple hyphae in the epidermal, cortical, and vascular tissues by 28 days of incubation (Figure 8). Hyphae inside plant roots appeared the same diameter (6 μm) in each tissue. A change in hyphal coloration (darkening) indicating re-melanization of WT1+ hypha when entering the stele was not detected in any stained sections. Azure A stained sections of WT 1+ inoculated plants showed colonizing mycelia infecting the root in an intracellular manner. Stained roots inoculated with *Ggg* isolate WT2+ showed light purple hyphae in the epidermal, cortical, and vascular tissues by 28 days of incubation. Hyphae inside of plant roots appeared the same diameter (6 μm) in each tissue. A change in hyphal coloration (darkening) indicating re-melanization of WT2+ hypha when entering the stele was not detected in any stained sections.

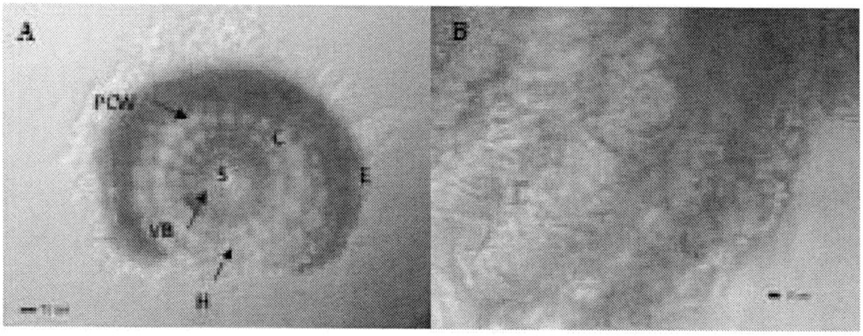

Figure 7. Rice inoculated with wild-type *Gaeumannomyces graminis* var. *graminis* isolate WT2+ and cultured in the Petri-plate assay. The transverse sections of rice roots (A. & B.) were unstained. Root morphology is labeled as follows: Plant cell walls (PCW), epidermis (E); cortex (C); stele (S); vascular bundles (V). Fungal hyphae are labeled as "H".

Azure A stained sections of WT 2+ inoculated plants showed colonizing mycelia infecting the root in an intracellular manner. Hyphae appeared to be the same diameter (6 μm) in each tissue. The melanin deficient isolate M1- could infect and colonize the epidermal and cortical cells of the root by day 28 (Figure 9). The hyphae produced by M1- during infection were hyaline in color and could not be detected without staining. Azure A stained the anticlinal plant cell walls dark purple, and fungal hyphae were stained a light purple color. Infective hyphae of M1- were produced intracellularly in the host root. At 28 days of incubation, the melanin-deficient isolate M1- was able to infect epidermal and cortical cells, but was stopped prior to entering the stele by l]lignified host tissue (lignitubers) around its hyphae (Figure 9; n=18). The hyphae produced by M2- during infection were hyaline in color and could not be detected without staining. Azure A stained the anticlinal plant cell walls dark purple, and fungal hyphae were stained a light purple color. The melanin-deficient isolate M2- was rarely able to infect single epidermal cells intercellularly (Figure 10; n=1/18).

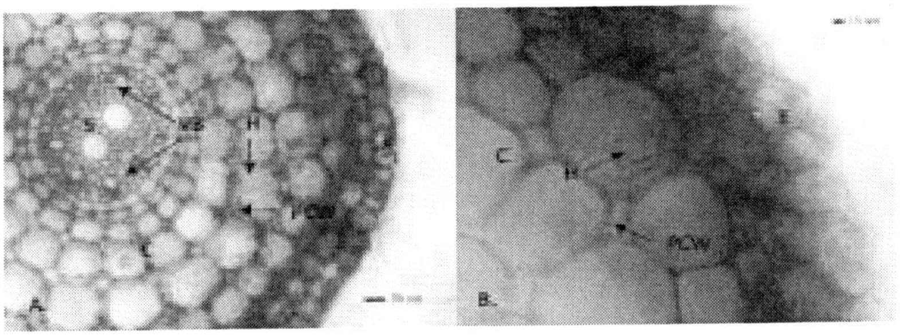

Figure 8. Rice inoculated with wild-type *Gaeumannomyces graminis* var. *graminis* isolate WT1+ and cultured in the Petri-plate assay. The transverse sections of rice roots (A. & B.) were stained with Azure A. Plant cell walls (PCW) are dark purple, fungal hyphae (H) are light purple. Root morphology is labeled as follows: epidermis (E); cortex (C); stele (S); vascular bundles (V).

Discussion

Nature of Mutations Used (Pigmentation and Morphology)

Both melanin deficient mutants (M1- and M2-) were produced from their corresponding wild-type parents using 4-nitroquinolene-1-oxide (NQO) as the mutagenic agent. Nitroquinolene oxide is an electrophile and a powerful carcinogen and mutagen (Sugimura, 1981). It mimics the mutagenic action of ultraviolet light and forms charge-transfer complexes with 5'-deoxyribonucleotides (Winkle & Tinoco, 1979). Nitroquinolene oxide (NQO) forms DNA adducts and can cause a wide range of DNA "lesions" including single-strand breaks, pyrimidine-dimer formation, abasic sites, and oxidized bases. In bacteria and yeast NQO has been shown to be a base substitution mutagen acting at guanine residues, inducing mainly guanine to adenine transitions (Fronza et al. 1992). The genetic basis for the pigmentation (melanin) changes in both M1- and M2- have not been determined. Due to the nature of NQO chemical mutagenesis, mutations in addition to conferring changes in pigmentation could have occurred, but have not been identified or characterized. For instance, the melanin mutant produced by Frederick et al. (1999) also exhibited hyphopodia and other morphological variation different from those of their parent cultures. Epstein et al. (1994) reported mutants that differed not only in hyphopodia, but pigmentation, compared to the parent culture. While the pigmentation mutations for these isolates have been characterized, it is unknown whether they possess additional DNA mutations. Epstein's isolates were selected from either Benomyl (2 of 1000 transformants) or Phleomycin (1 of 42 transformants) resistant transformants. The hyphopodial mutation was an artifact of the transformation process, not the main goal. Analysis of the transformants indicated that there was a single insertion in each case, but the exact location of the insertion in the transformants was not described. Bal et al. (1977) reported that NQO is a "good" mutagen for *Aspergillus nidulans* (Eidam) Winters because it induces mutations at a high frequency (0.5% of treated cells) and generates a broad spectrum of morphological and physiological changes.

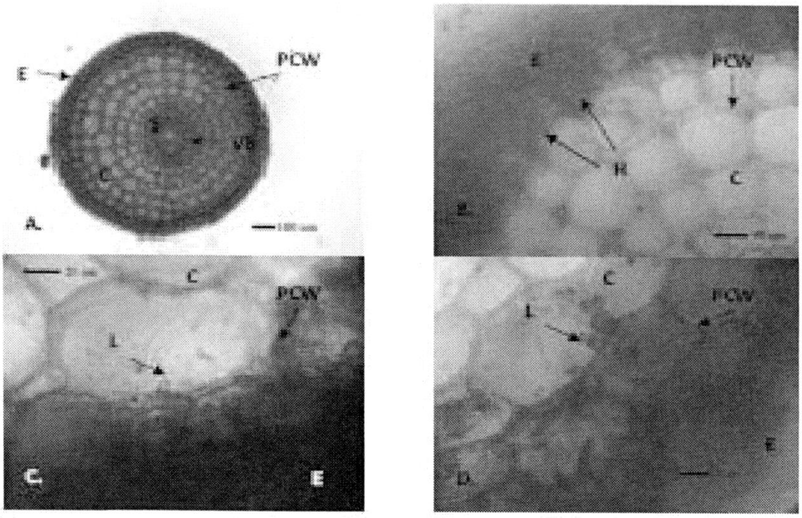

Figure 9. Rice inoculated with melanin-deficient *Gaeumannomyces graminis* var. *graminis* isolate M1- and cultured in the Petri-plate assay. The transverse sections of rice roots (A., B., C., & D.) were stained with Azure A. Plant cell walls (PCW) are dark purple, fungal hyphae (H) are light purple. Root morphology is labeled as follows: lignituber (L); epidermis (E); cortex (C); stele (S); vascular bundles (V). Fungal hyphae are labeled as "H".

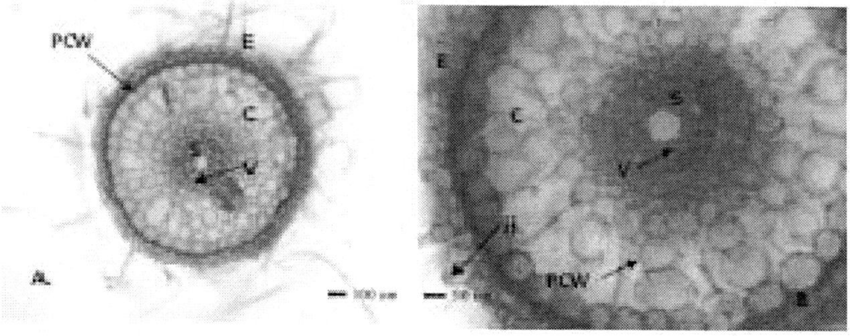

Figure 10. Rice inoculated with melanin-deficient *Gaeumannomyces graminis* var. *graminis* isolate M2- and cultured in the Petri-plate assay. The transverse sections of rice roots (A. & B.) were stained with Azure A. Plant cell walls (PCW) are dark purple. Root morphology is labeled as follows: epidermis (E); cortex (C); stele (S); vascular bundles (V). Fungal hyphae are labeled as "H".

Our mutant cultures were observed to be stable for melanin content for 36 months. M1- is similar to the hyphopodial mutant reported by Epstein et al. (1994). M1- (generated by Frederick et al. 1999) exhibited an increased frequency in production of lobed, melanized hyphopodia on the bottom of the polystyrene culture dish when cultivated on solid media as compared to its WT1+ parent culture. M2- is hyaline, and did not produce hyphopodia when cultivated on solid media, while its corresponding parent culture WT2+ is heavily pigmented and produces lobed hyphopodia under these conditions. M2- formed only simple hyaline hypal tips: M1- had hyaline mycelia and lobed, pigmented hyphopodia. Further, it appears that melanin production could be genetically segregated within a thallus of *G. graminis*. This segregation appears to be non-temporal as M2- demonstrated stable hyaline mycelia and hyphopodia for at least 36 months. Such genetic segregation could be based in the poly-nucleic nature of ascomycetes or in the N + N status of the thallus if melanin production is a dominant trait. Finally, it is very interesting that WT2+, a true *Ggg*, when transformed to M2- appears morphologically like *Gaeumannomyces graminis* var. *avenae* (*Gga*) or *Gaeumannomyces graminis* var. *tritici* (*Ggt*). This raises the question about the relationship between *Gga, Ggt* and Ggg. Fouly et al. (1997) showed genetic dissimilarities between these groups, but there was also a great deal of genetic similarity. Are these isolates really all *Ggg* sub-species, with *Gga* and *Ggt* lacking some of the functional genes of *Ggg*?

Isolate WT2+ is a wild-type isolate of *Ggg* from bermudagrass (Table 1) and a pathogen of this host. WT1+ and WT2+ both produced about the same amount of melanin in their respective hyphae. Therefore differences in their behavior as reported here (growth, hyphal width and DDB), would not be expected to be assigned to melanin content.

Effect of Melanin on Fungal Hyphal Morphology and Vegetative Growth Rate

Measurements of hyphal width were used as a means to evaluate the effect of melanin content on hyphal morphology. The basis for using hyphal width is that melanin, a wall component, is suspected of imparting a more rigid wall structure, which could allow for higher turgor pressure within a hypha. Further, it has been reported (Skou, 1981) that root-infecting hypha are melanin-less and smaller in diameter than melanized, ectotrophic hypha. This suggests that *Gaeumannomyces* species have melanin regulatory mechanisms that are environmentally sensitive. While infectious hypha appear to be devoid of melanin, it is unclear if they still are producing low levels of this pigment.

In general, the WT isolates developed hypha with similar widths, except when grown on CDA. The basis of this difference could reflect the heterogenous nature of the *Ggg* isolates as reported by Fouly and Wilkinson (2000). More interestingly, there were significant differences between the WT isolates and their respective melanin-deficient mutants in terms of hyphal width. For both isolate couplets, the WT generally displayed larger diameter hypha than the corresponding mutant. However, there were some inconsistencies in this pattern when considering behavior in different media. However the general trend toward larger hypha with melanin suggests that melanin may in fact allow hypha to grow larger while fungal walls deficient in melanin will support smaller diameter hypha. The smaller diameter of hypha for melanin-less isolates reported here supports observations that melanin-less infecting hypha are also smaller diameter. Epstein et al. (1994) reported that wild-type and corresponding single gene insertion melanin/hyphopodial mutants did not show a differences in hyphal width when cultured on dilute V8A. A reason for this difference compared to our measurements could have resulted from different experimental growth conditions. Epstein cultured isolates under thin layers of diluted V8A and measured hyphal widths after the agar layer was removed from the hypha. Both the dilution of the V8A and the sub-agar culturing could affect the osmotic and hydration conditions of the fungal environment resulting in moisture limitations. If melanin functions to control osmotic potential and/or allows for greater endogenous turgor pressure, then in a dilute osmotic medium, the loss of melanin would not be expected to correspond to a reduction in hyphal width. The comparison of our results with those of Epstein et al. (1994) are further limited by the fact that the width of wild-type and mutants reported were 6.4 +/- 0.05 μm whereas we reported that the wild-types here were 3.9 and 3.6 μm on V8A and the mutants were 3.6 and 3.1 μm, respectively.

The primary site of nutrient uptake for a fungal colony is at the thin-walled hyphal tip (Sietsma et al. 1995). This is also the only site where the fungal mycelium is actively elongating (growing) using a complicated physio-chemical process that involves hydrostatic pressure generated and controlled by osmotic regulation. The number of hyphal tips for a given thallus is determined by the frequency that hyphal branches are formed. Gaeumannomyces is characterized as having both septa, and branches. Septa are generally intercalary to the branches. In general, fungi form more branches when exposed to optimal growth conditions. The frequency of branching or distance between branches (DBB) is, in part, dependent on the physical-chemical nature of the medium, and the genetic-based ability to exploit it for growth and development (Rayner et al. 1994). As DBB increases, there are fewer hyphal tips being produced per thallus. Our results showed that WT2+ and WT1+ did not form branches at the same rate and that each formed branches at variable rates depending on the growth medium. To determine the range of DBB among Ggg isolates, a large population of isolates would be required for comparative purposes. However, the DBB data for WT and their corresponding mutants did show that the loss of melanin resulted in significantly shorter DBB compare to WT isolates. Further, this behavioral pattern was only slightly affected by WT1+ in V8A medium. Epstein et al. (1994) reported that wild-type *Ggg* and corresponding single insertion mutants also displayed no differences in hyphal DBB when cultured on dilute V8A. Their work focused on the differentiation and pigmentation of hyphal tips to form hyphopodia. Their primary objective focused on the frequency, shape, color and stimuli of hyphopodia. However their mutants all produced melanin, although in different degrees. For example, isolate JH849 produced melanized hyphopodia, but not in "sufficient quantity." Upon further examination of their work, JH849, did produce a reduced, but unquantified amount of melanin, and was the only mutant reported to branch about half as often (DBB = 158 μm) compared to wild-type or two other mutants of *Ggg* (DBB = 97, 96, and 71 μm, respectively). Mutant isolate JH2982, produced as much or more melanin than the wild-type (JH2033) and exhibited the shortest DBB (71 μm). While not statistically tested, it would appear from Epstein's work, that both hyphal width and DBB were affected similarly by reductions in melanin content of the hypha compared to the M1- and M2- mutants used in this study.

The three media (CDA, V8 and LBA) that were used in this research were also used by other researchers that investigated melanin and its role in *Ggg* morphology (Epstien et al. 1994; Frederick et al. 1999; Money et al. 1998). These media are among the most commonly used for fungal cultivation and in particular for culturing *Gaeumannomyces*. Each isolate was cultured and evaluated for hyphal width and distance between branching when grown on LBA and CDA. In general, as medium type became more defined, wild-type isolates produced narrow hyphae and with a shorter distance between branches. There was no single factor that could be attributed to the effect of medium type, melanin, and growth rate, though the data indicate that in general the more defined the medium, the slower the growth rate of isolates.

The reported effect of melanin on the vegetative growth rate of *Gaeumannomyces* is variable. High levels of DNH-melanin have been implicated in limiting the uptake of nutrients by mycelium (Frederick et al. 1999; Henson et al. 1999). A constitutive melanin producing *Ggg* mutant exhibited slower radial growth in culture than a melanin minus mutant and the corresponding wild-type (Frederick et al. 1999). In addition, the melanin deficient mutant exhibited a faster growth rate in culture as compared to the wild-type isolate of *Ggg*. Epstein et al. (1994) showed that wild-type and melanin/hyphopodial mutant *Ggg*'s, when cultured on dilute V8A on glass slides did not have different growth rates. However, the culture conditions (see above) and the incompleteness of melanin disruption preclude this work from being considered definitive in terms of the impact of melanin on vegetative growth rate.

In data presented here, melanin deficient M1- was the fastest growing isolate, growing faster than both wild-type isolates. However, the melanin deficient isolate, M2-, was the slowest growing isolate under most tested conditions. This phenomenon could be due to the presence of melanin as evidenced in the pigmented hyphopodia of this isolate. Still, the effect of melanin on growth rate based on the data collected is not definitive. Wild-type and melanin deficient isolates displayed variable responses when tested on different media. The pair consisting of WT1+ and M1- generally showed the melanin deficient M1- growing faster on different media compared to WT1+. The pair consisting of WT2+ and M2- showed the melanin deficient strain growing slower on all but the CDA medium. In the case of CDA medium, the mutant strain grows slightly faster than its melanin producing parent. The complexity of the media combined with the likely multiple mutations in both M1- and M2- preclude assigning any role of melanin in the determination of growth rate. Single insertion mutants with disrupted genes involved in the DHN-melanin synthesis pathway along with testing isolates for growth rate using defined media could allow for a determination of the role of melanin in vegetative growth rate of *Ggg*.

Melanin Quantification

The melanin content of the wild-type and mutants reported here was measured using an indirect method (Butler & LaChance, 1986). The binding of solubilized Azure A dye to hyphal melanin was used to estimate the concentration of melanin in hyphae. Wild-type isolates were not significantly different from each other in hyphal melanin content. The mutants M1- and M2- both showed very little melanin per unit mass of mycelium and the melanin content of WT isolates were considerably higher than the mutants. Melanin concentration reached a constant value after 14 days in culture. Wild-type WT1+ (JH2033) was also analyzed for melanin by Frederick, et al. (1999) who reported a concentration of 155 μg melanin/mg hyphae. The melanin concentration of the wild-type *Ggg* isolates reported here were 250 and 115 μg melanin/mg hyphae, respectively, thereby supporting the use of the Azure A method for mycelial melanin determination. While the mutants M1- and M2- reported here produced significantly less melanin compare to their respective parent cultures, they did produce an average of 65 and 30 μg melanin/mg mycelium respectively at 14-28 days of age according to the Azure A melanin assay. Bell and Wheeler (1986) and Frederick et al. (1999) also reported that melanin-deficient mutants of *Ggg* showed a similar degree of Azure A binding when compared to M1- and M2- reported here. This can perhaps be explained by cell wall components other than melanin absorbing some of the Azure A, but not an amount comparable to the binding coefficient of melanin. Hyphopodia were not produced by liquid-grown isolates, and this precludes the affect the melanin status of these appendages could produce in the assay. Furthermore, when living cultures of M1- and M2- were stained with Azure A and examined at 400X, both the cell walls and the cytoplasm absorbed some Azure A. We also immersed *Pythium aphanidermatum* (Edson) Fitzp. cultures in Azure A solution, and it absorbed stain as well. The reason for this may be due to the cell walls of *Pythium* being composed primarily of beta-glucans and cellulose, not chitin (a polymer of N–acetylglucosamine), as in filamentous fungi. These compounds may absorb Azure A to a greater extent than chitin. The melanized yeast, *Phaeococcomyces*, was reported to bind Azure A to melanin located in its cell walls (Butler & LaChance, 1986). Melanin-deficient mutants of this yeast did not take up stain at the cell wall, though dead or impaired cells showed staining.

The issues dealing with melanin as a determinant of *Ggg* morphology and vegetative growth reported here give a strong indication that melanin is important to the basic growth and development of the fungus. To further test this using a more definitive approach, single DNA insertion into one or more of the enzymes of the DHN melanin pathway should be used. Using these defined mutants would also allow non-specific binding of Azure A to be assigned to mycelial components other than melanin.

The Effect of Melanin on the Histopathology of Gaeumannomyces Graminis

The location and quantification (+/-) of hyphal melanin in sectioned tissues during pathogenesis was difficult to determine. Melanized runner hyphae were readily seen on rice plants inoculated with a wild-type isolatein the conetainer assay. In the conetainer assay, the wild-type exhibited no discernable melanization of hyphae when it had gained entry to the plant. Re-melanization of hyphae prior to infection of the stele, as seen by Wilkinson (personal communication) in regard to *Ggt* was not observed. Yet, it is common knowledge that *Gaeumannomyces* form melanized hyphae in necrotic plants at the later stages of pathogenesis. One aspect not included in these studies was induction ofphysical/physiological stress applied to the host. It is possible that had heat or drought stress been applied to the colonized host, the hyphae might have reacted differently.

Staining of fungal elements (macro and micro-hyphae, infection pegs, hyphopodia) was investigated though several methods in order to determine if stains would enhance observation of fungal melanin. Some staining procedures were not useful due to their interference with the visual detection of melanin. Melanin specific stains such as Masson-Fontana and Schmorl's used to stain these samples precluded enhanced observations of melanin deposition on hyphae because they stain all fungal tissues black and therefore obscure melanin. This was also reported by Masatomo *et al.* (1998) and Gupta *et al.* (1985). Periodic acid-Shiff staining was attempted to contrast melanized and non-melanized hyphae, but was discarded as it stained all tissues bright crimson and did not enhance the visualization of hyphal melanin. Azure A, a melanin specific stain, was also found not to be useful in selectively staining for melanin. Azure A stained plant tissues as well as fungal elements and proved valuable for enhancing observation of the fungus in rice roots inoculated in Petri-plate assay. This is interesting because infection hyphae are hyaline in appearance. It was recorded (see Chapter 1) that melanin-deficient strains of *Ggg* can show a degree of Azure A binding. The staining of hyaline infection hyphae by Azure A appears to support this finding. Fluorescence microscopy was also investigated. Melanin will fluoresce if oxidized (Kyatz *et al.*, 2001). It was postulated that by inducing fluorescence, melanin could be pinpointed as to where it was being deposited by the fungus. Unfortunately, oxidizing melanin with hydrogen peroxide to enhance visualization was not useful because plant tissues fluoresced brightly as well, and melanin in hyphae could not be discerned.

It has been stated that there are three phases for fungal nutrition during plant infection (Solomon et al, 2003). These phases are germination, proliferation, and sporulation. These phases can be compared to the seven stages of pathogenesis and are useful as a context for studying the production of melanin by *Ggg in situ.* The first, or germination, phase can be compared to melanized *Ggg* hyphae growing towards a host from the tissues they have overwintered upon (dissemination, stage 2). During this time, external nutrient sources are likely to be in short supply, and the fungus is at a disadvantage to compete with host defenses and competitive microorganisms. The production of melanin at this time may assist the pathogen in survival during inoculation (stage 3) and pre-penetration (stage 4), penetration (stage 5), and infection, (stage 6). The second phase, proliferation, takes place after the fungus has gained entry to the host. At this stage, nutrients are not limiting, and competing microorganisms will be reduced, if not eliminated, compared to stage one. After this stage, compatibility (stage 7) is determined, and melanin may not be necessary for the advance of the fungus throughout the rest of the host. At this time, the production of melanin may either hinder the progress of disease or be unnecessary for pathogenesis. This may be why *Ggg* is at first hyaline when it invades the cortex and stele of infected plants. The production of spores (sporulation, stage 3) by *Ggg* is not thought to be a major determinant in the spread of *Gaeumannomyces* (Skou, 1981). Instead, the re-melanization of hyphae in host tissues *post-mortem* is most likely most comparable to this stage of pathogenic nutritional requirements. At this point, the protective role melanin biosynthesis serves may be necessary for the pathogen in order for it to complete the disease cycle. In this case, melanin will protect the fungus as it competes with other organisms in the soil for nutrient sources, and aid in the overwintering process, thus completing the disease cycle. This is why it remains to be determined when *Ggg* resumes melanin production between colonization of the stele and necrosis.

Effect of Melanin on Fungal Pathogenicity

Pathogenicity of *Ggg* isolates was affected by their ability to produce melanin. It has been shown that melanin is necessary for Ggt to cause disease (Kelly, 1997). *Gaeumannomyces graminis* var. *tritici* may have to re-melanize upon encounter of the stele in order to penetrate vascular tissue (disease), while *Ggg* may not. Frederick *et al.* (1999) showed that melanin was not necessary for *Ggg* to cause disease in rice, but did not examine infected plants histopathologically to determine melanin status of infective hyphae, or where they were produced. Infected plants may have been colonized by the fungi they were inoculated with, and not actually diseased. Here, melanized wild type isolates were pathogenic, and isolates lacking in melanin were reduced in their ability to infect and colonize the host. Melanin can bind to and inactivate chemical agents (Hill, 1992). The inability of melanin deficient strains to colonize all tissues of host roots (parasitic vs. pathogenic) may be a result of failure to resist host-defense chemical mechanisms. This phenomenon has been described in rice (Datta et al., 2001; Nishizawa et al., 1999). Also, since melanin has an effect on hyphal turgor pressure (Brush and Money, 1999), it may be that non-melanized isolates could not produce the necessary mechanical force to penetrate through the lignified host response (lignitubers) in the epidermal and cortical layers. In contrast to this, melanized isolates were able to infect all tissues of rice roots by 28 days. Genetic analysis of the mutations in the mutant isolates would help to characterize the mutation of the mutant *Ggg* strains and perhaps their influence on the infection process.

It is important to point out that there were differences in the way the fungus behaved between the conetainer and plate assay. In conetainer assay, the wild-type produced runner hyphae, infection pegs, and non-melanized infection hyphae. This differentiation of hyphae is consistent with those found in "naturally" infected plants in the field. In Petri plate assay, only one type of hyphae was seen. These hyphae were distinguishable from those that proliferated on the culture medium only by the fact that they were produced in the roots of plants. Some researchers (Frederick et al., 1999) have stated that since melanin serves in a protective role for hyphae, unmelanized strains would be at a disadvantage in a natural setting. This may be true since M2- did not infect in conetainer assay, where the environment is not as conducive to the survival of the fungus as it is in culture (Petri-plate assay). While melanin deficient (M1- & M2-) *Ggg* strains were able to parasitize roots in plate assay, designation of these fungi as parasites may be correct only in an environment where the host is at an extreme disadvantage to repel the fungus. In a more natural setting, it appears that melanin may be required not only as a determinant of pathogenism, but for survival outside of culture.

This research indicates that the common rating system of virulence (i.e., darkening of roots) may not be adequate for assessing whether a particular fungus is a parasite or a pathogen. Rating roots for infection by *Ggg* based solely on epidermal darkening may not illustrate the actual relationship between host and fungus. When acting as parasites, melanin-deficient strains did not induce characteristic blackening of host roots. This interaction of host/pathogen would not be properly characterized by using this traditional scale.

It is undisputed that the fungus will at some point re-melanize in host tissues (Skou, 1981.). This has been previously documented in the fact that wild type fungi will often develop "cessation structures" if they are unable to advance past a certain point in host roots. This is often seen in another melanized monocot root pathogen, *Magnaporthe poae*. These structures are also produced, seemingly at random, in compromised host roots by *Ggg* (Skou, 1981). While their function remains unknown, it is postulated that they may function as survival structures (overwintering) for the fungus in temperate zones (Skou, 1981). It may be that the time-frame involved in both assays reported here are too short for this phenomenon to be evidenced and that re-melanization takes a longer amount of time than we used. Frederick et al. (1999) reported that a non-melanized mutant derived from WT1+ (JH4300) was pathogenic 28 days post-inoculation. Unfortunately, this isolate is no longer living and thus is precluded from our studies. It should be noted that their conditions for host/pathogen interaction was rated by root dry weights, at a time of incubation at 25C for 28D. Melanized wild-type isolates were capable, under our conditions, of colonizing the stele (i.e., causing disease) by 28 days and melanin-deficient isolates were not. It may be that after six months the non-melanized isolates might be able to compromise host defenses, but the apparent advantage that melanin confers to the fungi that synthesize it are clear: melanin assists in the ability of *Ggg* to cause disease.

The objective of this research was to determine if melanin plays a role in the pathogenicity of *Ggg*. The evidence presented here indicates that the ability of wild-type isolates to produce melanin has a marked effect on their ability to produce disease symptoms on rice roots. This effect on disease severity caused by *Ggg* is uniform over the plants evaluated. Melanin producing wild-types caused extensive root rotting in most host roots, while melanin-deficient strains did not. Melanin-deficient strain WT1- caused slight discoloration of inoculated oats, wheat and rice roots (data not presented). This differed from the coloration caused by wild-type isolates. Wild-type *Ggg* caused characteristic blackening of host roots. In some cases, wild-types were able to completely kill and rot host roots into an unrecognizable state. In contrast, melanin-deficient strain WT1- induced a light brown, rather than black color to inoculated roots, a phenomenon especially noticed in rice. These lesions macroscopically appeared to be limited in their deleterious effect on the roots (Wilkinson, personal communication).

The effect of melanin on the pathogenicity of *Gaeumannomyces graminis var. graminis* based solely on symptoms of host roots as indicated by this research is that melanin is required by *Ggg* to induce disease symptoms in host roots. This research shows a dependence on melanin by *Ggg* in order to cause characteristic blackened and rotted roots in host plants. In conetainer assay conducted with melanized wild-type fungi and their melanin-deficient counterparts, there was a significant difference in the ability of wild-type and melanin-mutant isolates to colonize rice plants.

References

Bal, J., Kajtaniak, E.M., & Pieniazek, N.J. 1977. 4-Nitroquinoline-1-oxide: a good mutagen for *Aspergillus nidulans*. *Mutat Res Fund Mol Mech Mutagen.* 56: 153-156.

Bell, A. A., and Wheeler, M.H. 1986. Biosynthesis and Functions of Fungal Melanins. *Ann. Rev. Phytopathology.* 24: 411-51.

Brush, L, and N.P. Money. 1999. Invasive hyphal growth in *Wangiella dermatitidis* is induced by stab inoculation and shows dependence upon melanin biosynthesis. *Fungal Genetics and Biology* 20:190-200.

Butler, M.J., and Lachance, M.A. 1986. Quantitative binding of azure A to melanin of the black yeast *Phaeococcomyces. Exp. Mycol.* 10: 166-170.

Caesar-Tonthat, T., Kloeke, F.V.O., Geesey, G.G. and Henson, J.M. 1998. Melanin production by a filamentous soil fungus in response to copper and localization of copper sulfide by sulfide-silver staining. *Appl. Environ. Microbiol.* 61: 1968-1975.

Datta, K., J.M. Tu, N. Oliva, I. Ona, R. Velazhahan, T.W. Mew, S. Muthukrishnan, and S.K. Datta. 2001. Enhanced resistance to sheath blight by constitutive expression of infection-related rice chitinase in transgenic elite indica rice cultivars. *Plant Science* v. 160, p. 405-414.

Elliot, M.L. 1991. Determination of an etiological agent of Bermudagrass decline. *Phytopathology.* 83: 414-418.

Elliot, M.L., Hagan, A.K., and Mullen, J.M.. 1993. Association of *Gaeumannomyces graminis var. graminis* with St. Augustine grass root rot disease. *Plant Dis.* 77: 206-209.

Epstein, L., Kaur, S., Goins, T., Kwon, Y.H., and Henson, J.M. 1994. Production of hyphopodia by wild-type and three transformants of *Gaeumannomyces graminis var. graminis*. *Mycologia.* 86: 72-81.

Fouly, H. M., Wilkinson, H. T. & Chen, W. 1997. Restriction analysis of internal transcribed spacers and the small subunit gene of ribosomal DNA among four *Gaeumannomyces* species. *Mycologia.* 89: 590-597.

Fouly, H.M., & Wilkinson, H.T. 2000. Detection of *Gaeumannomyces graminis* varieties using polymerase chain reaction with variety-specific primers. *Plant Dis.* 84, 947-951.

Frederick, B., T. Caesar-TonThat, M.H. Wheeler, K.B. Sheehan, W.A. Edens, and J.M Henson. 1999. Isolation and characterization of *Gaeumannomyces graminis var. graminis* melanin mutants. *Mycological Research* 103: 99-110.

Fronza, G., Campomenosi, P., Iannone, R., & Abbondandolo, A. 1992. The 4-nitroquinoline 1-oxide mutational spectrum in single stranded DNA is characterized by guanine to pyrimidine transversions. *Nucleic acids res. 20, 1283-1287.*

Hawksworth, D.L., Kirk, P.M., Sutton, B.C., & Pegler, D.N. *(Editors)*.1995. *Ainsworth and Bisby's Dictionary of the Fungi.* CAB International, Wallingford.

Henson, J., Butler, M.J., & Day A.W. 1999. The dark side of the mycelium: melanins. *Annu. Rev. Phytopathology.* 37: 47-71.

Hill, H.Z. 1992. The Function of melanin or six blind people examine an elephant. *BioEssays.* 14: 49-56.

Hornby, D. 1998. *Take-all Disease of Cereals, a Regional Perspective.* CAB International, New York. 384 pp.

Jones, D.G. & Clifford, B.C. 1978. *Cereal Diseases: Their Pathology and Control.* John Wiley & Sons, New York.

Kelly, C. 1997. Genetics of pigmentation and pathogenicity in *G. graminis. PhD thesis,* University of Birmingham, UK.

Money, N. P., Caesar-Ton That, T., Frederick, B., & Henson, J. M. 1998. Melanin synthesis is associated with changes in hyphopodial permeability, wall rigidity, and turgor pressure in *Gaeumannomyces graminis var. graminis*. *Fungal Genet. Biol.* 24: 240-251.

Nishizawa, Y., Z. Nishio, K. Nakazono, M. Soma, E. Nakajima, M. Ugaki, and T. Hibi. 1999. Enhanced resistance to blast (*Magnaporthe grisea*) in transgenic *Japonica* rice by constitutive expression of rice chitinase. *Theoretical Applied Genetics v.* 99 p. 383-390.

Rayner, A.D.M., Griffith, G.S., & Ainsworth, A.M. 1994. *Mycelial Interconnectedness. in* The Growing Fungus. *Edited by* N.A.R. Gow &.G.M. Gadd Chapman & Hall, London. pp. 21-37.

Sietsma, J.H., Wosten, H.A.B., & Wessels, J.G.H. 1995. Cell wall growth and protein secretion in fungi. *Can. J. Bot.,* 73: 388-395.

Skou, J.P. 1981. *Morphology and Cytology of the Infection Process. in Biology and Control of Take-all. Edited by* M.J.C. Asher & P.J. Shipton. Academic Press, London. pp. 175-196.

Solomon , P. S., Tan, K. C. & Oliver, R. P. 2003. The nutrient supply of phytopathogenic fungi; a fertile field for study. *Mol Plant Pathol* 4: 203–210.

Sugimura, T. 1981. *Carcinogenesis: A Comprehensive Survey.* Vol. 6. Raven, New York.

Walker, J. 1981. *Taxonomy of take-all fungi and related genera and species. in Biology and Control of Take-all. Edited by* M.J.C. Asher & P.J. Shipton. Academic Press, London. pp. 15-74.

Wilkinson, H.T. 1994. Root rot of centipedegrass (*Eremochloa ophinroides* (Munro) Hack.) caused by *Gaeumannomyces graminis* ((Sacc.) Arx & Olivier) var. *graminis*. *Plant Dis.* 78: 1220.

Wilkinson, H.T., & Kane, R.T. 1993. *Gaeumannomyces graminis* infecting zoysiagrass in Illinois. *Plant Dis.* 77: 100.

Wilkinson, H.T., J.R. Alldredge, and R.J. Cook. 1985. Estimated distance for infection of wheat roots by *Gaeumannomyces graminis var. tritici* in soils suppressive and conducive to take-all. *Phytopathology* 75: 557-559.

Winkle, S. A. & Tinoco, I., Jr. 1979. Interactions of 4-nitroquinoline 1-oxide with four deoxyribonucleotides. *Biochemistry* 18: 3833-3839.

In: Melanin: Biosynthesis, Functions and Health Effects
Editors: Xiao-Peng Ma and Xiao-Xiao Sun
ISBN: 978-1-62100-991-7

Chapter V

Skin Anatomy and Physiology Research Developments in Melanocytes

Naoki Oiso * ***and Akira Kawada***
Department of Dermatology, Kinki University Faculty of Medicine, Osaka-Sayama, Osaka, Japan

Abstract

In mice models of pigment anomalies, over 800 phenotypic alleles are known. This indicates that skin color is distinctly regulated by more than 800 genes. This requires several steps; (i) distribution of melanoblasts into skin in embryo, (ii) construction of melanosomes in melanocytes, (iii) production of melanin granules in melanosomes, (iv) translocation of melanosomes from perinuclear to peripheral region in melanocytes, (v) transfer of melanosomes from melanocytes to keratinocytes and (vi) translocation of transferred melanin granules from a peripheral to a supranuclear region in keratinocytes. The damage in each step induces pigment anomalies. We summarize biogenesis and function of melanin granules with pigment anomalies; piebaldism and Waadenburg syndrome caused by inadequate distribution of melanoblasts in embryo; Hermansky-Pudlak syndrome, Chediak-Higashi syndrome, and oculocutaneous albinism type 2 and 4 by improper biogenesis of melanosomes and melanin granules; and Griscelli syndrome by inappropriate intercellular translocation of melanosomes. Aberrant intercellular transfer of melanin granules is shown in a case of pediatric erythema dyschromicum perstans (ashy dermatosis). Aberrant translocation inside keratinocytes is present in Dowling-Degos disease. Unregulated melanogenesis is present in disorders affected in KITLG-KIT signaling and RAS-MAPK signaling. The loss or decreased enzymatic function in melanogenesis induces oculocutaneous albinism types 1 and 3. Pheomelanin-dominant production is present in red hair color phenotypes showing fair skin, poor tanning ability and elevated risk of freckles, malignant melanoma, basal cell carcinoma and squamous cell carcinoma. This section will provide the current findings to recognize

---

* Address correspondence to: Naoki Oiso, MD., PhD. Department of Dermatology, Kinki University Faculty of Medicine, 377-2 Ohno-Higashi, Osaka-Sayama, Osaka 589-8511, Japan. Tel: +81 72 366 0221. Fax: +81 72 368 2120. Email: naoiso@med.kindai.ac.jp.

the function and the health effect of melanin granules as well as the pathogenesis of pigmentation-associated disorders.

1. Introduction

More than 800 phenotypic alleles are now identified in mice models of pigment anomalies [1]. This indicates that skin, hair and eye color is distinctly regulated by multiple genes. The melanocyte-precursor melanoblasts derived from the neural crest migrate and localize as melanocytes in the basal layer of the epidermis in embryo. Melanocytes contain melanosomes where melanin granules are produced. During maturing from melanosome stage I to stage IV via stage II and III in melanocytes, melanosomes shift from perinuclear region to peripheral dendritic processes. The matured melanosomes containing melanin granules are transferred from the tip of the process of melanocytes to the peripheral region of keratinocytes. The transferred melanin granules are transported from peripheral to a supranuclear region in the same keratinocytes or are transferred to the other keratinocyts. Both intrinsic and extrinsic factors influence production of melanin granules, eumelanin and pheomelanin. Genetic and environmental factors influence melanogenesis. This chapter summarizes human pigment anomalies in the view of biosynthesis, functions and health effects of melanin granules.

2. The Disorders in Aberrant Migration of Melanoblasts

Hereditary disorders in aberrant migration of melanoblasts include piebaldism and Waadenburg syndrome (WS). Piebaldism is a rare autosomal dominantly inherited disorder, characterized by congenital leukoderma, most commonly involving the forehead, abdomen, and knees. Patients with piebaldism have mutations of the *KIT* gene, which encodes stem cell growth factor (KIT ligand (KITLG)) receptor, a type III transmembrane receptor tyrosine kinase with an extracellular domain that binds KITLG [2-9]. The complete depigmented patches in piebaldism represent regions lacking in melanocytes, the result of defective melanoblast differentiation, migration, proliferation, or survival during embryonic development [10]. KITLG acts as a chemokinetic factor for melanoblast migration, and KIT promotes melanocyte movement and acts as a chemokinetic or motogenic receptor [11].

Waardenburg syndrome (WS) is syndromatic disorder and is sub-classified into type 1 to 4. WS is characterized by localized pigment abnormalities of the hair, skin, and eyes, and congenital sensorineural hearing loss with or without other symptoms.

The association of hearing loss and pigment abnormalities results from an abnormal proliferation, survival, migration, or differentiation of neural crest-derived melanocytes [12].

WS type 1 (WS1) is characterized by the presence of dystopia canthorum: WS type 2 (WS2) is the absence of dystopia canthorum; WS type 3 (WS3) is the presence of dystopia canthorum and musculoskeletal abnormalities of the upper limbs, and WS type 4 (WS4) have the complication of Hirschsprung disease [12].

Heterochromia and white forelock may be present in WS1 and WS2. WS1 is caused by mutations in *PAX3* [13, 14]; WS2 by *MITF* [15-17], *SLUG* [18], *SOX10* [19] and PAX3 [13]; WS3 by *PAX3* [20, 21]; and WS4 by *EDB3* [22, 23], *EDNRB* [24, 25], and *SOX10* [26, 27].

A mutation in *SOX10* may cause severest phenotype of PCWH including peripheral neuropathy, mental retardation, cerebellar ataxia, and spasticity [28]. *SLUG*-associated WS2 shows an autosomal recessive inheritance, and PAX3-associateed WS3 shows both autosomal dominant and recessive forms. Others are autosomal dominant forms.

3. The Disorders in Biogenesis of Melanosomes in Melanocytes

Biogenesis of melanosomes in melanocytes is distinctly regulated. Abnormal biogenesis of melanosomes is present in Hermansky-Pudlak syndrome (HPS), Chediak-Higashi syndrome (CHS), possibly oculocutaneous albinism (OCA) type 2 (OCA2) and OCA type 4 (OCA4). Melanosomes belong to cell-specific lysosome-related organelles (LROs). LROs include lytic granules in cytotoxic T lymphocytes and natural killer cells, MHC class II compartments (MIICs) in antigen presenting cells, dense granules in platelets, lamellar bodies in lung epithelial type II cells, azurophil granules observed in neutrophils, and others [29, 30]. HPS and CHS have OCA and specific features because of the dysfunction of affected LROs. In HPS, prolonged bleeding times related to platelet dysfunction is caused by absence of platelet-dense granules [31], and pulmonary dysfunction related to lung epithelial type II cells is possibly caused by decreased secretion from lamellar bodies [32, 33]. In CHS, repeated infections related to immunological deficiency is caused by enlargement of lytic granules, MIICs and azurophil granules [31].

Human HPS is autosomal recessive disorder which has been sub-classified into 9 types. The function of HPS-assciated proteins has been studied with mice, rats, *Caenorhabditis elegans*, and yeast *Saccharomyces cerevisae*. HPS-associated proteins assemble heteromeric complexes except Rab38 [34]. Two of five complexes, adaptor protein (AP)-3 and homotypic vacuolar protein sorting (HOPS) or the class C VPS complex, are conserved from yeast to humans, whereas the remaining three complexes, biogenesis of lysosome-related organelles complex (BLOC)-1, BLOC-2, and BLOC-3, seem not to be conserved in unicellular eukaryotes [35, 36]. AP-3 complex is composed of α (a mutation identified in mouse *mocha* [37]), β3A (mouse *pearl* [38] and human HPS-2 [39]), σ3, and μ3A subunit; HOPS is composed of Vps33a (mouse *buff* [40]), Vps11, Vps16, Vps18, Vps39 and Vps41; BLOC-1 is composed of dysbindin (mouse *sandy* and human HPS-7 [41]), BLOS3 (mouse reduced pigmentation [42] and human HPS-8 [43]), pallidin (mouse *pallid* [44] and human HPS-9 [45]), cappuccino (mouse cappuccino [46]), muted (mouse *muted* [47]), snapin [42], BLOS1 [42] and BLOS2 [42]; BLOC-2 contains HPS3 (mouse *cocoa* [48] and human HPS-3 [49]), HPS5 (mouse *ruby-eye-2* [50] and human HPS-5 [50]) and HPS6 (mouse *ruby-eye* [50] and human HPS-6 [50]) and BLOC-3 contains HPS1 (mouse *pale ear* [51] and human HPS-1 [52]) and HPS4 (mouse *light ear* [53] and human HPS-4 [53]).

CHS is autosomal recessive syndromatic disorder caused by mutations in the lysosomal trafficking regulator (*LYST*) gene [54-57]. As LYST proteins act as negative regulators of fusion by limiting the heterotypic fusion of early endosomes with post-lysosomal compartments, the loss of function inducts excess fusion and large LROs [58].

Non-syndromatic autosomal recessive OCA is a heterogeneous disease with hypopigmented skin, hair, and eyes [59]. It is sub-classified into 4 types caused by mutations of four genes; the *tyrosinase* gene (*TYR*) for OCA type 1 (OCA1), the *P* gene for OCA2, the *TYRP1* (tyrosinase-related protein 1) gene for OCA type 3 (OCA3), and the *MATP* (membrane-associated transporter protein) or SLC45A2 (solute carrier family 45, member 2) gene for OCA4 [59]. The function of the products encoded by the *P* and *MATP* gene is still unknown. Recently, genetic interaction was studied between mutant alleles causing deficiency in OCA2 (*pink-eyed dilution unstable*), AP-3 (*pearl*), BLOC-1 (*pallid*), and BLOC-2 (*cocoa*) in C57BL/6J mice [60]. The study suggested that functional links between OCA2 and these three protein complexes (AP-3, BLOC-1, and BLOC-2) involved in melanosome biogenesis [59]. SLC45A2 (MATP), a solute carrier family member, and P proteins may implicate in the control of eye, hair, and skin pigmentation via the regulation of melanosome pH [61].

4. The Disorders in the Translocation of Melanosomes in Melanocytes

The defect of melanosome transport in melanocytes is present in Griscelli syndrome (GS). It is a rare autosomal recessive disorder caused by mutations in either the myosin 5A (*MYO5A*) in GS type 1 (GS1) [62], *RAB27A* in GS type 2 (GS2) [63] or melanophilin (*MLPH*) in GS type 3 (GS3) [64]. It is characterized by pigment dilution of the skin and hair color because of perinuclear accumulation of melanosomes in melanocytes and presence of large clumps of pigment in hair shafts. GS1 represents cutaneous albinism with a primary neurologic deficit [62]; GS2 dose cutaneous albinism with immune impairment [63]; and GS3 dose only cutaneous albinism [64].

In melanocytes, the RAB27A-MLPH-MYO5A tripartite protein complex is involved in the intramelanocytic melanosome transport [65]. Mature melanosomes connecting activated Rab27a move to the cell periphery on microtubules via the motor protein kinesin [65]. At the cell peripherally, Rab27a-Mlph-Myo5a tripartite protein complex is formed that captures the melanosomes in the actin-rich dendritic tips [65]. The loss of function of Rab27a-Mlph-Myo5a tripartite induces the accumulation of melanosomes at the perinuclear regions and induces cutaneous albinism.

The transportation of synaptic vesicles in a neuron is shown to be regulated by Rab3a-Rabphilin3A-Myo5a tripartite protein complex. The loss of function in myosin 5A is therefore associated with a primary neurological deficit [66].

A variety of Rab27 effector proteins have been identified:

Exophilin1/Rabphilin-3a,
Exophilin2/Granuphilin-a/Slp4-a,
Exophilin3/Melanophilin/Slac2-a,
Exophilin4/Slp2-a,
Exophilin5/Slac2-b,
Exophilin6/Slp3,

Exophilin7/JFC1/Slp1,
Exophilin8/MyRIP/Slac2-c,
Exophilin9/Slp5, Noc2, and Munc13-4 [67-69]. GS2 is characterized by defects in melanosome transport in melanocytes, defects in granule secretion by cytotoxic T lymphocytes [63, 69, 70] and excessive phagocytosis in macrophages [71]. As phenotypic diversity and different binding ability for myosin 5A and melanophilin is present in each mutation in Rab27a [72], further functional investigation would be needed for elucidating the relationship between immunologic impairment and the binding ability to various Rab27a effector proteins in each mutation in Rab27a.

5. The Disorders in the Transfer of Melanosomes via Intercellular Spaces

The precise mechanism of melanosome transfer from melanocytes to keratinocytes and between keratinocytes has not been completely elucidated. However, possible mechanisms have been suggested; (i) pinching off of melanocyte dendrites containing melanosomes by keratinocytes; (ii) direct inoculation of melanosomes into keratinocytes via keratinocyte-melanocyte membrane fusions through nanotubular filopodia; and/ or(iii) melanosome release into the extracellular space followed by their phagocytosis by keratinocytes [73]. Protease-activated receptor-2 (PAR-2), a seven-transmembrane G-protein coupled receptor expressing in keratinocytes but not in melanocytes, is a key regulator of melanosome transfer via keratinocyte phagocytosis [74].

We examined electron microscopic features in erythema dyschromicum perstans (ashy dermatosis) in a Japanese pediatric patient [75]. It showed melanosomes transferred from a melanocyte to a keratinocyte following a forced curve resembling a filopodial-phagocytosis model [76, 77], but did not identify melanosomes transferred between keratinocytes, possibly because of the intercellular spaces and the retracted melanosomes [75]. Some acquired pigment disorders may be caused by the improper transfer of melanin granules [78].

6. The Disorders in the Translocation of Melanosomes in Keratinocytes

The mechanism of intracellular distribution of melanosome in keratinocytes is poorly understood. Dowling-Degos disease (DDD) may be caused by aberrant translocation in keratinocytes. It is a rare autosomal dominant keratinocyte pigmentation disorder, and is caused by haploinsufficiency by a mutation in the keratin 5 (*KRT5*) gene [79]. The mutation in *KRT5* affects melanosome distribution in keratinocytes but not the integrity of the keratin cytoskeleton [79, 80]. Keratin 5 is a component of the intermediate filament (IF) cytoskeleton in the basal layer of the keratinocytes. Dysfunction of the IF cytoskeleton causes aberrant distribution of melanin granules in keratinocytes [79, 81]. Further study will shed light on the accurate mechanism of translocation of melanin granules from peripheral to supranuclear region in keratinocytes.

7. The Disorders of Unregulated Melanogenesis

Skin pigmentation is controlled by a complex melanogenic paracrine network between mesenchymal and epithelial cells, which regulates melanocyte survival, proliferation, and melanogenesis [82, 83]. Keratinocyte-derived factors that act as activators of melanocytes include KITLG, basic fibroblast growth factor, hepatocyte growth factor, granulocyte-macrophage colony-stimulating factor, nerve growth factor, α-melanocyte stimulating hormone (α-MSH), adrenocorticotropic hormone, endorphin, endothelin-1, prostaglandin (PG) E2/PGF2α and leukemia inhibitory factor [84, 85]. Among melanogenic growth factors, KITLG and its receptor KIT signaling that triggers RAS-MAPK (mitogen-activated protein kinase) signaling pathway plays crucial roles in the control of physiological and pathological skin pigmentation [82, 83]. The unregulated melanogenesis is present in disorders affected in KITLG-KIT signaling and RAS-MAPK signaling. The disorders in aberrant KITLG-KIT signaling include familial progressive hyper- and hypopigmentation (FPHH), familial progressive hyperpigmentation (FPH), and possibly dyschromatosis universalis hereditaria type 2 (DUH2) [82, 83]. The disorders in anomalous RAS-MAPK signaling (neuro-cardio-facial-cutaneous syndrome) comprise (i) pigment anomaly-related Leopard syndrome type 1 to 3, neurofibromatosis type 1, neurofibromatosis type 1-Noonan syndrome, and neurofibromatosis type 1-like syndrome (Legius syndrome) and (ii) pigment anomaly-unrelated Noonan syndrome, cardio-facial-cutaneous syndrome and Costello syndrome.

FPHH is autosomal dominantly inherited disorder. It is characterized by diffuse, progressive hyperpigmentation that begins at an early age [82, 83, 86]. It may show café-au-lait macules and generalized lentiginosis intermixed with larger hypopigmented ash-leaf macules [82, 83, 86]. FPHH is caused by a gain-of-function mutation in *KITLG* [83]. FPH is an uncommon dominantly inherited disorder characterized by progressive hyperpigmentation similar to that seen in FPHH, but without hypopigmented lesions [83]. FPH is linked to two loci on chromosome 19p13-pter and on 12q21.31-q23.1 [87, 88]. A six-generated family with FPH is caused by a gain-of-function mutation in *KITLG* [88]. DUH, characterized by depigmented and hyperpigmented features on the trunk and extremities, is mapped on two loci on chromosome 6q24.2-q25.2 (initially reported as dyschromatosis symmetrica hereditaria) and on chromosome 12q21-q23 where *KITLG* is located [89, 90].

RAS genes are cancer-related genes due to their frequent activation in human cancers and play a central role in the RAS-MAPK signaling cascade, which has a pivotal role in cell proliferation, differentiation, survival, and cell death [91, 92].

Neuro-cardio-facial-cutaneous (NCFC) syndrome is proposed for disorders caused by mutations in the genes involved in the RAS-MAPK signaling pathway. NCFC syndrome includes several phenotypically overlapping, but clinically distinct disorders [93].

Leopard syndrome (LS) is a rare multiple congenital anomalies condition, mainly characterized by skin, facial and cardiac anomalies [94]. LEOPARD is an acronym for the major features including multiple Lentigines, ECG conduction abnormalities, Ocular hypertelorism, Pulmonic stenosis, Abnormal genitalia, Retardation of growth, and sensorineural Deafness [94]. LS type 1 (LS1) is caused by a mutation in *PTPN11* [95]; LS2 in ***RAF1*** [96]; and LS3 in *BRAF* [97]. LS mutants in *PTPN11* are catalytically defective and act as dominant negative mutations [98] and are associated with multiple granular cell tumors [99].

Noonan syndrome (NS), characterized by short stature, congenital heart defect, and developmental delay and related disorders such as cardio-facio-cutaneous syndrome (CFCS) and Costello syndromes, are caused by a mutation in genes involving in the RAS- MAPK signaling cascade [92]. Mutations in *PTPN11* are identified in NS [100]; *RAF1* in NS [101]; and *BRAF* in NS [97] and CFCS [102].

Neurofibromatosis type 1 (NF1) is autosomal dominant disorder caused by a loss-of-function mutation in neurofibromin encoded by the *NF1* gene [103-107].

It is characterized by café-au-lait spots, axillary freckling, Lisch nodules in the eye, and multiple neurofibromas on the skin. The affected persons are susceptible to other benign and malignant tumors. The incidence of NF1 is high, 1 in 2,500 to 1 in 3,000 individuals [108]. Neurofibromin acts as RAS-GTPase, catalyzing RAS-GTP into RAS-GDP. The loss-of-function of neurofibromin induces excess presence of RAS-GTP accelerating the RAS-MAPK signaling cascade [109, 110].

Neurofibromatosis type 1-Noonan syndrome (NFNS) is an entity characterized by the presence of features of NS in individuals in NF1 [111-113]. Most cases are caused by a mutation in *NF1* [114-116] and rare in both *PTPN11* and *NF1* [117].

Neurofibromatosis type 1-like syndrome or Legius syndrome is an autosomal dominant disorder caused by inactivating sprouty-related EVH1 domain-containing protein 1 (*SPRED1*) mutations, which is initially identified in individuals presenting mainly with café-au-lait macules, axillary freckling, and macrocephaly [118].

Subsequent studies identify that a high *SPRED1* mutation detection rate is present in NF1 mutation-negative families with an autosomal dominant phenotype of café-au-lait macules with or without freckling, and no other NF1 features including neurofibromas [119-122].

Legius syndrome is not associated with the peripheral and central nervous system tumors seen in NF1 [121]. As SPRED-1 negatively regulates RAS-MAPK activation [123-125], the loss-of-function of SPRED-1 inducts the activation of RAS-MAPK signaling cascade.

8. The Disorders of No or Decreased Melanogenesis

Melanin granules are produced in melanosomes with tyrosine as a substrate and tyrosinase (TYR), tyrosinase-related protein 1 (TYRP1)/ 5,6-dihydroxyindol-2-carboxylic acids (DHICA) oxidase, and dopachrome tautomerase/ 5,6-dihidroxyindole (DCT) as enzymes. Tyrosine is converted into dopaquinone via dopa by tyrosinase. Eumelanins are constructed from dopaquinone without glutathione or cysteine. Pheomelanin is produced from dopaquinone with glutathione or cysteine. Eumelanin are defined as black or brown nitrogeneous pigments and are insoluble in all solvents. Pheomelanins are yellow to reddish brown pigments and are soluble in alkali solvents.

The decreased or non-enzymatic function in TYR and TYRP1 results in OCA1 and OCA3, respectively. OCA1 is autosomal recessive pigment disorder caused by mutations in *TYR* [126-128] and subclassified into tyrosinase-negative OCA1A, tyrosinase-positive OCA1B. Individuals with OCA1A are the most severe phenotype, because they cannot produce any melanin granules. The clinical features are (i) white skin without tanning, (ii) white hair, eyelashes and eyebrows, and (iii) light blue to almost pink and fully translucent irises with severe photophobia and decreased visual acuity [129]. Persons with OCA1B are a milder phenotype, because they can produce a few melanin granules. The clinical characteristics are gradual pigmentation of the skin and hair to some extent during growing, and the gradual color change of irises from blue to green or brown. Temperature-sensitive variants manifest as having depigmented body hairs, and pigmented hairs on hands and feet due to lower temperatures [129]. OCA3 is autosomal recessive pigment disorder caused by mutations in *TYRP1* [130, 131]. OCA3 is present mostly in African individuals as rufous or red OCA [130, 131] and rarely in Caucasian [132] and Asian [133, 134]. African individuals with rufous or red OCA have red hair and reddish brown skin [129]. The synergic effect in *P* and *TYRP1* is present in a family, suggesting both are modifier genes of each other [135].

9. The Variants in Hair, Eyes and Skin Color and Associated Disorders

Hair, eyes and skin color are different between African individuals, Asian and Caucasian. The determinants of hair, eyes and skin color have been investigated. Variants of the MSH receptor gene (*MC1R*) are shown to be associated with red hair and fair skin with a poor tanning response in Caucasian [136]. The loss-of-functional variants are associated with production of pheomelanin in Caucasian. Subsequently, variants in *MC1R* are identified as a susceptibility gene of malignant melanoma [137-139], squamous cell carcinoma [140, 141], basal cell carcinoma [140, 141], and freckles [142]. So far, red hair color phenotype having specific variants in *MC1R* shows the association between red hair and increased risk of melanoma and skin cancer [143].

Using genomewide association study for hair, eyes and skin color determinants in the European population, variants located in six loci are identified; MC1R associated with red hair color, blond hair color, fair skin, skin sensitivity to sun, and freckles; 6p25.3 with freckles; tyrosinase with eye color and freckles; SLC24A4 with eye and hair color; OCA2 (P) with eye, hair and skin color; and KITLG with hair color [144]. Another study identified variants in TPCN2 associated with hair color and a variant at the ASIP locus associated with skin sensitivity to sun, freckling and red hair [145]. With genetic studies, melanoma susceptibility genes have been identified; *MC1R* [137-139, 148], *ASIP* [146], *TYR* [146, 148], *MATP/SLC45A2* [147], *CDKN2A* [148], and common sequence variants on 20q11.22 [149]. The combination of susceptible variants in *MC1R* and mutations in *BRAF* [150] or *CDKN2A* [151] are associated with the high frequent development of melanoma. Similarly, basal cell carcinoma susceptibility genes have been identified; *MC1R* [140, 141], *ASIP* [146], *TYR* [146], *KRT5* [152], *CDKN2A* [152], *CDKN2B* [152], *KLF14* [152], *MATP/SLC45A2* [152], and the TERT-CLPTM1L locus [152].

10. Other Disorders

(1) Dyschromatosis Symmetrica Hereditaria

Dyschromatosis symmetrica hereditaria (DSH) (or reticulate acropigmentation of Dohi) is a pigmentary genodermatosis of autosomal dominant inheritance. It is characterized by a mixture of hyperpigmented and hypopigmented macules on the dorsal aspects of the hands and feet [153]. It is caused by a heterozygous mutation of the adenosine deaminase acting on RNA 1 (ADAR1, previously called double-stranded RNA-specific adenosine deaminase (DSRAD)) gene [154]. The precise pathogenesis is still unknown, even though adenosine-to-inosine (A-to-I) RNA editing is a widespread modification of the transcriptome [155].

Dermoscopy to the hyper- and hypopigmented macules on the dorsal hands showed round and variously pigmented spots 0.5-1.5 mm in diameter connected to each other [156]. The different and unregulated A-to-I RNA editing may induct different melanocytes function in each pigmented spots.

(2) Reticulate Acropigmentation of Kitamura

Reticulate acropigmentation of Kitamura (RAK) is autosomal dominant dermatosis. It is characterized by pigmented and irregular freckle-like lesions with atrophy on the surface, arranged in a reticular pattern on the dorsa of the hands and feet [157]. As some cases overlap clinical and histological features of both DDD and RAK, these disorders may be phenotypic diversity to DDD and RAK [158, 159].

11. Function and Health Effect

The production of melanin granules by melanosomes in melanocytes is important for humans to survive in the sun-exposed surroundings. The adequate quality and quantity of melanin granule is needed for hair, eyes and skin function. The production of melanin granules in the eyes prevents photophobia and decreased visual acuity, and the synthesis in the skin protects sun-burn and damage of DNA from ultraviolet exposure.

Conclusion

The melanin synthesis, translocation, and transfer are distinctly regulated by various proteins. The genetic and environmental factors influence not only the quantity but also the quality of melanin granule. Syndromatic symptoms are present in disorders caused by mutations in the genes having the function in other cells, tissues or organs. As over 800 phenotypic alleles are known in mice models of pigment anomalies, more players will be identified. Studies in melanocytes will give a gift to humans to reduce the mobility and the mortality of malignant melanoma and skin cancers.

References

[1] Bennett, D. C., and Lamoreux, M. L. (2003). The color loci of mice--a genetic century. *Pigment Cell Res.*, 16, 333-344.

[2] Giebel, L. B., and Spritz, R.A. (1991). Mutation of the KIT (mast/stem cell growth factor receptor) proto-oncogene in human piebaldism. *Proc. Natl. Acad. Sci. U.S.A.*, 88, 8696-8699.

[3] Spritz, R. A., Giebel, L. B., and Holmes, S. A. (1992). Dominant negative and loss of function mutations of the c-kit (mast/stem cell growth factor receptor) proto-oncogene in human piebaldism. *Am. J. Hum. Genet.*, 50, 261-269.

[4] Spritz, R. A., Holmes, S. A., Ramesar, R., Greenberg, J., Curtis, D., and Beighton, P. (1992). Mutations of the KIT (mast/stem cell growth factor receptor) proto-oncogene account for a continuous range of phenotypes in human piebaldism. *Am. J. Hum. Genet.,* 51, 1058-1065.

[5] Richards, K. A., Fukai, K., Oiso, N., and Paller, A. S. (2001). A novel KIT mutation results in piebaldism with progressive depigmentation. *J. Am. Acad. Dermatol.,* 44, 288-292.

[6] Murakami, T., Fukai, K., Oiso, N., Hosomi, N., Kato, A., Garganta, C., Barnicoat, A., Poppelaars, F., Aquaron, R., Paller, A. S., and Ishii. M. (2004). New KIT mutations in patients with piebaldism. *J. Dermatol. Sci.*, 35, 29-33.

[7] Murakami, T., Hosomi, N., Oiso, N., Giovannucci-Uzielli, M. L., Aquaron, R., Mizoguchi, M., Kato, A., Ishii, M., Bitner-Glindzicz, M., Barnicoat, A., Wilson, L., Tsukamoto, K., Ueda, H., Mancini, A. J., Suzuki, T., Riley, J., Miertus, J., Camargo, M., Santoro-Zea, A., Atkin, J., and Fukai, K. (2005). Analysis of KIT, SCF, and initial screening of SLUG in patients with piebaldism. *J. Invest. Dermatol.*, 124, 670-672.

[8] Oiso, N., Kishida, K., Fukai, K., Motokawa, T., Hosomi, N., Suzuki, T., Mitsuhashi, Y., Tsuboi, R., and Kawada, A. (2009). A Japanese piebald patient with auburn hair color associated with a novel mutation p.P832L in the KIT gene and a homozygous variant p.I120T in the *MC1R* gene. *Br. J. Dermatol.*, 161, 468-469.

[9] Narita, T., Oiso, N., Fukai, K., Motokawa, T., Hayashi, M., Yokoyama, K., Hozumi, Y., Kawada, A., and Suzuki, T. Two children with a mild or moderate piebaldism phenotype and a father without leukoderma in a family with the same recurrent missense mutation in the kinase domain of KIT. *Eur. J. Dermatol.*, in press.

[10] Spritz, R. A., Ho, L., and Strunk, K. M. (1994). Inhibition of proliferation of human melanocytes by a KIT anti-sense oligodeoxynucleotide: implications for human piebaldism and mouse dominant white spotting (W). *J. Invest. Dermatol.*, 103, 148-150.

[11] Jordan, S. A., and Jackson, I. J. (2000). MGF (KIT ligand) is a chemokinetic factor for melanoblast migration into hair follicles. *Dev. Biol.*, 225, 424-436.

[12] Pingault, V., Ente, D., Dastot-Le Moal, F., Goossens, M., Marlin, S., and Bondurand, N. (2010). Review and update of mutations causing Waardenburg syndrome. *Hum. Mutat.*, 31, 391-406.

[13] Tassabehji, M., Read, A. P., Newton, V. E., Patton, M., Gruss, P., Harris, R., and Strachan, T. (1993) Mutations in the PAX3 gene causing Waardenburg syndrome type 1 and type 2. *Nat. Genet.*, 3, 26-30.

[14] Hoth, C. F., Milunsky, A., Lipsky, N., Sheffer, R., Clarren, S. K., and Baldwin, C. T. (1993) Mutations in the paired domain of the human PAX3 gene cause Klein-Waardenburg syndrome (WS-III) as well as Waardenburg syndrome type I (WS-I). *Am. J. Hum. Genet.*, 52, 455-462.
[15] Hughes, A. E., Newton, V. E., Liu, X. Z., and Read, A. P. (1994). A gene for Waardenburg syndrome type-2 maps close to the human homologue of the microphthalmia gene at chromosome 3p12-p14.1. *Nat. Genet.*, 7, 509-512.
[16] Tassabehji, M., Newton, V. E., and Read, A. P. (1994). Waardenburg syndrome type 2 caused by mutations in the human microphthalmia (MITF) gene. Nat. Genet., 8, 251-255.
[17] Steingrímsson, E., Moore, K. J., M. Lamoreux, L, Ferré-D'Amaré A. R., Burley, S. K., Sanders Zimring, D. C., Skow, L. C., Hodgkinson, C. A., Arnheiter, H., Copeland, N. G. and Jenkins, N. A. (1994). Molecular basis of mouse microphthalmia (mi) mutations helps explain their developmental and phenotypic consequences. *Nat. Genet.*, 8, 256-263.
[18] Sánchez-Martín, M., Rodríguez-García, A., Pérez-Losada, J., Sagrera, A., Read, A. P., and Sánchez-García, I. (2002). SLUG (SNAI2) deletions in patients with Waardenburg disease. *Hum. Mol. Genet.*, 11, 3231-3236.
[19] Bondurand, N., Dastot-Le Moal, F., Stanchina, L., Collot, N., Baral, V., Marlin, S., Attie-Bitach, T., Giurgea, I., Skopinski, L., Reardon, W., Toutain, A., Sarda, P., Echaieb, A., Lackmy-Port-Lis, M., Touraine, R., Amiel, J., Goossens, M., and Pingault, V. (2007). Deletions at the SOX10 gene locus cause Waardenburg syndrome types 2 and 4. *Am. J. Hum. Genet.*, 81, 1169-1185.
[20] Tassabehji, M., Read, A. P., Newton, V. E., Harris, R., Balling, R., Gruss, P., and Strachan, T. (1992). Waardenburg's syndrome patients have mutations in the human homologue of the Pax-3 paired box gene. *Nature*, 355, 635-636.
[21] Baldwin, C. T., Hoth, C. F., Amos, J. A., da-Silva, E. O., and Milunsky, A. (1992). An exonic mutation in the HuP2 paired domain gene causes Waardenburg's syndrome. *Nature*, 355, 637-638.
[22] Edery, P., Attié, T., Amiel, J., Pelet, A., Eng, C., Hofstra, R. M. , Martelli, H., Bidaud, C., Munnich, A., and Lyonnet, S. (1996). Mutation of the endothelin-3 gene in the Waardenburg-Hirschsprung disease (Shah-Waardenburg syndrome). *Nat. Genet.*, 12, 442-444.
[23] Hofstra, R. M., Osinga, J., Tan-Sindhunata, G., Wu, Y., Kamsteeg, E. J., Stulp, R. P., van Ravenswaaij-Arts, C., Majoor-Krakauer, D., Angrist, M., Chakravarti, A., Meijers, C., and Buys, C. H. (1996). A homozygous mutation in the endothelin-3 gene associated with a combined Waardenburg type 2 and Hirschsprung phenotype (Shah-Waardenburg syndrome). *Nat. Genet.*, 12, 445-447.
[24] Attie, T., Till, M., Pelet, A., Amiel, J., Edery, P., Boutrand, L., Munnich, A., and Lyonnet, S. (1995). Mutation of the endothelin-receptor B gene in Waardenburg-Hirschsprung disease. *Hum. Mol. Genet.*, 4: 2407-2409.
[25] Syrris, P., Carter, N. D., and Patton, M. A. (1999). Novel nonsense mutation of the endothelin-B receptor gene in a family with Waardenburg-Hirschsprung disease. *Am. J. Med. Genet.*, 87, 69-71.
[26] Pingault, V., Bondurand, N., Kuhlbrodt, K., Goerich, D. E., Préhu, M. O., Puliti, A., Herbarth, B., Hermans-Borgmeyer, I., Legius, E., Matthijs, G., Amiel, J., Lyonnet, S.,

Ceccherini, I., Romeo, G., Smith, J. C., Read, A. P., Wegner, M., and Goossens, M. (1998). SOX10 mutations in patients with Waardenburg-Hirschsprung disease. *Nat. Genet.*, 18, 171-173.

[27] Herbarth, B., Pingault, V., Bondurand, N., Kuhlbrodt, K., Hermans-Borgmeyer, I., Puliti, A., Lemort, N., Goossens, M., and Wegner, M. (1998). Mutation of the Sry-related Sox10 gene in Dominant megacolon, a mouse model for human Hirschsprung disease. *Proc. Natl. Acad. Sci. USA.*, 95, 5161-5165.

[28] Inoue, K., Khajavi, M., Ohyama, T., Hirabayashi, S., Wilson, J., Reggin, J. D., Mancias, P., Butler, I. J., Wilkinson, M. F., Wegner, M., and Lupski, J. R. (2004). Molecular mechanism for distinct neurological phenotypes conveyed by allelic truncating mutations. *Nat. Genet.*, 36, 361-369.

[29] Raposo, G., Marks, M. S., and Cutler, D. F. (2007). Lysosome-related organelles: driving post-Golgi compartments into specialization. *Curr. Opin. Cell Biol.*, 19, 394-401.

[30] Raposo, G., and Marks, M. S. (2007). Melanosomes--dark organelles enlighten endosomal membrane transport. *Nat. Rev. Mol. Cell Biol.*, 8, 786-797.

[31] Spritz, R. A., Chiang, P. W., Oiso, N., and Alkhateeb A. (2003). Human and mouse disorders of pigmentation. *Curr. Opin. Genet. Dev.*, 13, 284-9.

[32] Guttentag, S. H., Akhtar, A., Tao, J. Q., Atochina, E., Rusiniak, M. E., Swank, R. T., and Bates, S. R. (2005). Defective surfactant secretion in a mouse model of Hermansky-Pudlak syndrome. *Am. J. Respir. Cell Mol. Biol.*, 33, 14-21.

[33] Osanai, K., Higuchi, J., Oikawa, R., Kobayashi, M., Tsuchihara, K., Iguchi, M., Huang, J., Voelker, D. R., and Toga, H. (2010). Altered lung surfactant system in a Rab38-deficient rat model of Hermansky-Pudlak syndrome. *Am. J. Physiol. Lung Cell Mol.* Physiol., 298, L243-251.

[34] Oiso, N., Riddle, S. R., Serikawa, T., Kuramoto, T., and Spritz, R. A. (2004). The rat Ruby (*R*) locus is Rab38: identical mutations in Fawn-hooded and Tester-Moriyama rats derived from an ancestral Long Evans rat sub-strain. *Mamm. Genome*, 15, 307-314.

[35] Di Pietro, S. M., and Dell'Angelica, E. C. (2005). The cell biology of Hermansky-Pudlak syndrome: recent advances. *Traffic,* 6, 525-533.

[36] Oiso, N. (2007). Recent advance I Hermansky-Pudlak syndrome. *Acta. Med. Kinki Univ.*, 32, 9-17.

[37] Kantheti, P., Qiao, X., Diaz, M. E., Peden, A. A., Meyer, G. E., Carskadon, S. L., Kapfhamer, D., Sufalko, D., Robinson, M. S., Noebels, J. L., and Burmeister, M. (1998). Mutation in AP-3 delta in the mocha mouse links endosomal transport to storage deficiency in platelets, melanosomes, and synaptic vesicles. *Neuron,* 21, 111-122.

[38] Feng, L., Seymour, A. B., Jiang, S., To, A., Peden, A. A., Novak, E. K., Zhen, L., Rusiniak, M. E., Eicher, E. M., Robinson, M. S., Gorin, M. B., and Swank, R. T. (1999). The beta3A subunit gene (Ap3b1) of the AP-3 adaptor complex is altered in the mouse hypopigmentation mutant pearl, a model for Hermansky-Pudlak syndrome and night blindness. *Hum. Mol. Genet.*, 8, 323-330.

[39] Dell'Angelica, E. C., Shotelersuk, V., Aguilar, R. C., Gahl, W. A., and Bonifacino, J. S. (1999). Altered trafficking of lysosomal proteins in Hermansky-Pudlak syndrome due to mutations in the beta 3A subunit of the AP-3 adaptor. *Mol. Cell, 1999*, 3, 11-21.

[40] Suzuki, T., Oiso, N., Gautam, R., Novak, E. K., Panthier, J. J., Suprabha, P. G., Vida, T., Swank, R. T., Spritz, R. A. (2003). The mouse organellar biogenesis mutant buff results from a mutation in Vps33a, a homologue of yeast vps33 and Drosophila carnation. *Proc. Natl. Acad. Sci. USA.*, 100, 1146-1150.
[41] Li, W., Zhang, Q., Oiso, N., Novak, E. K., Gautam, R., O'Brien, E. P., Tinsley, C. L., Blake, D. J., Spritz, R. A., Copeland, N. G., Jenkins, N. A., Amato, D., Roe, B. A., Starcevic, M., Dell'Angelica, E. C., Elliott, R. W., Mishra, V., Kingsmore, S. F., Paylor, R. E., and Swank, R. T.. (2003). Hermansky-Pudlak syndrome type 7 (HPS-7) results from mutant dysbindin, a member of the biogenesis of lysosome-related organelles complex 1 (BLOC-1a). *Nat. Genet.*, 35, 84-89.
[42] Starcevic, M., and Dell'Angelica, E. C. (2004). Identification of snapin and three novel proteins (BLOS1, BLOS2, and BLOS3/reduced pigmentation) as subunits of biogenesis of lysosome-related organelles complex-1 (BLOC-1). *J. Biol. Chem.*, 279, 28393-28401.
[43] Morgan, N. V., Pasha, S., Johnson, C. A., Ainsworth, J. R., Eady, R.A., Dawood, B., McKeown, C., Trembath, R. C., Wilde, J., Watson, S. P., and Maher, E. R. (2006). A germline mutation in BLOC1S3/reduced pigmentation causes a novel variant of Hermansky-Pudlak syndrome (HPS8). *Am. J. Hum. Genet.*, 78, 160-166.
[44] Huang, L., Kuo, Y. M., and Gitschier, J. (1999). The pallid gene encodes a novel, syntaxin 13-interacting protein involved in platelet storage pool deficiency. *Nat. Genet.*, 23, 329-332.
[45] Cullinane, A. R., Curry, J. A., Carmona-Rivera, C., Summers, C. G., Ciccone, C., Cardillo, N. D., Dorward, H., Hess, R. A., White, J. G., Adams, D., Huizing, M., and Gahl, W. A. (2011). A BLOC-1 mutation screen reveals that PLDN is mutated in Hermansky-Pudlak syndrome type 9. *Am. J. Hum. Genet.*, 88, 778-787.
[46] Ciciotte, S. L., Gwynn, B., Moriyama, K., Huizing, M., Gahl, W. A., Bonifacino, J. S., and Peters, L. L. (2003). Cappuccino, a mouse model of Hermansky-Pudlak syndrome, encodes a novel protein that is part of the pallidin-muted complex (BLOC-1). *Blood* 2003, 101, 4402-4407.
[47] Zhang, Q., Li, W., Novak, E. K., Karim, A., Mishra, V. S., Kingsmore, S. F., Roe, B. A., Suzuki, T., and Swank, R. T. (2002). The gene for the muted (mu) mouse, a model for Hermansky-Pudlak syndrome, defines a novel protein which regulates vesicle trafficking. *Hum. Mol. Genet.*, 11, 697-706.
[48] Suzuki, T., Li, W., Zhang, Q., Novak, E. K., Sviderskaya, E. V., Wilson, A., Bennett, D. C., Roe, B. A., Swank, R. T., and Spritz, R. A. (2001). The gene mutated in cocoa mice, carrying a defect of organelle biogenesis, is a homologue of the human Hermansky-Pudlak syndrome-3 gene. *Genomics*, 78, 30-37.
[49] Anikster, Y., Huizing, M., White, J., Shevchenko, Y.O., Fitzpatrick, D.L., Touchman, J.W., Compton, J.G., Bale, S.J., Swank, R.T., Gahl, W.A., Toro, J.R. (2001). Mutation of a new gene causes a unique form of Hermansky-Pudlak syndrome in a genetic isolate of central Puerto Rico. *Nat. Genet.*, 28, 376-80.
[50] Zhang, Q., Zhao, B., Li, W., Oiso, N., Novak, E. K., Rusiniak, M. E., Gautam, R., Chintala, S., O'Brien, E. P., Zhang, Y., Roe, B. A., Elliott, R. W., Eicher, E. M., Liang, P., Kratz, C., Legius, E., Spritz, R. A., O'Sullivan, T. N., Copeland, N. G., Jenkins, N. A., and Swank, R. T. (2003). Ru2 and Ru encode mouse orthologs of the genes mutated in human Hermansky-Pudlak syndrome types 5 and 6. *Nat. Genet.*, 33, 145-153.

[51] Feng, G. H., Bailin, T., Oh, J., and Spritz, R. A. (1997). Mouse pale ear (ep) is homologous to human Hermansky-Pudlak syndrome and contains a rare 'AT-AC' intron. *Hum. Mol. Genet.*, 6, 793-797.

[52] Oh, J., Bailin, T., Fukai, K., Feng, G. H., Ho, L., Mao, J. I., Frenk, E., Tamura, N., and Spritz, R. A. (1996). Positional cloning of a gene for Hermansky-Pudlak syndrome, a disorder of cytoplasmic organelles. *Nat. Genet.*, 14, 300-306.

[53] Suzuki, T., Li, W., Zhang, Q., Karim, A., Novak, E. K., Sviderskaya, E. V., Hill, S. P., Bennett, D. C., Levin, A. V., Nieuwenhuis, H. K., Fong, C. T., Castellan, C., Miterski, B., Swank, R. T., and Spritz, R. A. (2002). Hermansky-Pudlak syndrome is caused by mutations in HPS4, the human homolog of the mouse light-ear gene. *Nat. Genet.*, 30, 321-324.

[54] Barbosa, M. D., Nguyen, Q. A., Tchernev, V. T., Ashley, J. A., Detter, J. C., Blaydes, S. M., Brandt, S. J., Chotai, D., Hodgman, C., Solari, R. C., Lovett, M., and Kingsmore, S. F. (1996). Identification of the homologous beige and Chediak-Higashi syndrome genes. *Nature*, 382, 262-265.

[55] Nagle, D. L., Karim, M. A., Woolf, E. A., Holmgren, L., Bork, P., Misumi, D. J., McGrail, S. H., Dussault, B. J. Jr, Perou, C. M., Boissy, R. E., Duyk, G. M., Spritz, R. A., and Moore, K. J. (1996). Identification and mutation analysis of the complete gene for Chediak-Higashi syndrome. *Nat. Genet.*, 14, 307-311.

[56] Karim, M. A., Nagle, D. L., Kandil, H. H., Bürger, J., Moore, K. J., and Spritz, R. A. (1997). Mutations in the Chediak-Higashi syndrome gene (CHS1) indicate requirement for the complete 3801 amino acid CHS protein. *Hum. Mol. Genet.*, 6, 1087-1089.

[57] Barbosa, M. D., Barrat, F. J., Tchernev, V. T., Nguyen, Q. A., Mishra, V. S., Colman, S. D., Pastural, E., Dufourcq-Lagelouse, R., Fischer, A., Holcombe, R. F., Wallace, M. R., Brandt, S. J., de Saint Basile, G., and Kingsmore, S. F. (1997). Identification of mutations in two major mRNA isoforms of the Chediak-Higashi syndrome gene in human and mouse. *Hum. Mol. Genet.*, 6, 1091-1098.

[58] Kypri, E., Schmauch, C., Maniak, M., and De Lozanne, A. (2007). The BEACH protein LvsB is localized on lysosomes and postlysosomes and limits their fusion with early endosomes. *Traffic,* 8, 774-783.

[59] Li, H., Meng, S., Zheng, H., Wei, H., and Zhang, Y. (2008). A Chinese case of oculocutaneous albinism type 4 with two novel mutations. *Int. J. Dermatol.*, 47, 1198-1201.

[60] Hoyle, D. J., Rodriguez-Fernandez, I. A., and Dell'angelica, E. C. (2011). Functional interactions between OCA2 and the protein complexes BLOC-1, BLOC-2, and AP-3 inferred from epistatic analyses of mouse coat pigmentation. *Pigment Cell Melanoma Res.*, 24, 275-281.

[61] Cheli, Y., Luciani, F., Khaled, M., Beuret, L., Bille, K., Gounon, P., Ortonne, J. P., Bertolotto, C., Ballotti, R. (2009). {alpha}MSH and Cyclic AMP elevating agents control melanosome pH through a protein kinase A-independent mechanism. *J. Biol. Chem.*, 284, 18699-18706.

[62] Pastural, E., Barrat, F. J., Dufourcq-Lagelouse, R., Certain, S., Sanal, O., Jabado, N., Seger, R., Griscelli, C., Fischer, A., and de Saint Basile, G. (1997). Griscelli disease maps to chromosome 15q21 and is associated with mutations in the myosin-Va gene. *Nature Genet.*, 16, 289-292.

[63] Ménasché, G., Pastural, E., Feldmann, J., Certain, S., Ersoy, F., Dupuis, S., Wulffraat, N., Bianchi, D., Fischer, A., Le Deist, F., and de Saint Basile, G. (2000). Mutations in RAB27A cause Griscelli syndrome associated with hemophagocytic syndrome. *Nat. Genet.*, 25, 173-176.

[64] Ménasché, G., Ho, C. H., Sanal, O., Feldmann, J., Tezcan, I., Ersoy, F., Houdusse, A., Fischer, A., and de Saint Basile, G. (2003). Griscelli syndrome restricted to hypopigmentation results from a melanophilin defect (GS3) or a MYO5A F-exon deletion (GS1). *J. Clin. Invest.*, 112,450-456.

[65] van Gele, M., Dynoodt, P., and Lambert, J. (2009). Griscelli syndrome: a model system to study vesicular trafficking. Pigment Cell Melanoma Res., 22, 268-282.

[66] Wöllert, T., Patel, A., Lee, Y. L., Provance, D. W. Jr, Vought, V. E., Cosgrove, M. S., Mercer, J. A., and Langford, G. M. (2011). Myosin5a tail associates directly with Rab3A-containing compartments in neurons. J. Biol. Chem., 286, 14352-14361.

[67] Fukuda, M. (2006). Rab27 and its effectors in secretory granule exocytosis: a novel docking machinery composed of a Rab27 effector complex. *Biochem. Soc. Trans.*, 8, 691-695.

[68] Izumi, T. (2007). Physiological roles of Rab27 effectors in regulated exocytosis. *Endocr. J.*, 54, 649-657.

[69] Chavas, L. M., Ihara, K., Kawasaki, M., Torii, S., Uejima, T., Kato, R., Izumi, T., and Wakatsuki, S. (2008). Elucidation of Rab27 recruitment by its effectors: structure of Rab27a bound to Exophilin4/Slp2-a. *Structure*, 16, 1468-1477.

[70] Seabra, M. C., Mules, E. H., and Hume, A. N. (2002). Rab GTPases, intracellular traffic and disease. *Trends Mol. Med.*, 8, 23-30.

[71] Yokoyama, K., Kaji, H., He, J., Tanaka, C., Hazama, R., Kamigaki, T., Ku, Y., Tohyama, K., and Tohyama, Y. (2011). Rab27a negatively regulates phagocytosis by prolongation of the actin-coating stage around phagosomes. *J. Biol. Chem.*, 286, 5375-5382.

[72] Ohbayashi, N., Mamishi, S., Ishibashi, K., Maruta, Y., Pourakbari, B., Tamizifar, B., Mohammadpour, M., Fukuda, M., and Parvaneh, N. (2010). Functional characterization of two RAB27A missense mutations found in Griscelli syndrome type 2. *Pigment Cell Melanoma Res.*, 23, 365-374.

[73] Ando, H., Niki, Y., Yoshida, M., Ito, M., Akiyama, K., Kim, J. H., Yoon, T. J., Lee, J. H., Matsui, M. S., and Ichihashi, M. (2010). Keratinocytes in culture-accumulated phagocytosed melanosomes in the perinuclear area. *Pigment Cell Melanoma Res.*, 23, 129-133.

[74] Boissy, R. (2003). Melanosome transfer to and translocation in the keratinocyte. *Exp. Dermatol.* 12, 5-12.

[75] Oiso N, Tsuruta D, Imanishi H, Kobayashi H, and Kawada A. (*in press*). Erythema dyschromicum perstans in a Japanese pediatric patient. *Pediatr. Dermatol.*

[76] Scott, G., Leopardi, S., Printup, S., and Madden, B. C. (2002). Filopodia are conduits for melanosome transfer to keratinocytes. *J. Cell Sci.*, 115, 1441-1451.

[77] Singh, S. K., Kurfurst, R., Nizard, C., Schnebert, S., Perrier, E., and Tobin, D. J. (2010). Melanin transfer in human skin cells is mediated by filopodia-a model for homotypic and heterotypic lysosome-related organelle transfer. *FASEB J.*, 24, 3756-3769.

[78] Choi, E. J., Kang, Y. G., Kim, J., and Hwang, J. K. (2011). Macelignan inhibits melanosome transfer mediated by protease-activated receptor-2 in keratinocytes. *Biol. Pharm. Bull.*, 34, 748-754.

[79] Betz, R.C., Planko, L., Eigelshoven, S., Hanneken, S., Pasternack, S. M., Bussow, H., Bogaert, K. V., Wenzel, J., Braun-Falco, M., Rutten, A., Rogers, M. A., Ruzicka, T., Nothen, M. M., Magin, T. M., and Kruse, R. (2006). Loss-of-function mutations in the keratin 5 gene lead to Dowling-Degos disease. *Am. J. Hum. Genet.*, 78, 510-519.

[80] Liao, H., Zhao, Y., Baty, D.U., McGrath, J.A., Mellerio, J.E., and McLean, W.H. (2007). A heterozygous frameshift mutation in the V1 domain of keratin 5 in a family with Dowling–Degos disease. *J. Invest. Dermatol.*, 127, 298-300.

[81] Oiso, N., Tsuruta, D., Ota, T., Kobayashi, H., and Kawada, A. (2007). Spotted and rippled reticulate hypermelanosis: a possible variant of Dowling-Degos disease. *Br. J. Dermatol.*, 156, 196-198.

[82] Picardo, M., and Cardinali, G. (2011). The genetic determination of skin pigmentation: KITLG and the KITLG/c-Kit pathway as key players in the onset of human familial pigmentary diseases. *J. Invest. Dermatol.*, 131, 1182-1185.

[83] Amyere, M., Vogt, T., Hoo, J., Brandrup, F., Bygum, A., Boon, L., and Vikkula, M. (2011). KITLG mutations cause familial progressive hyper- and hypopigmentation. *J. Invest. Dermatol.*, 131, 1234-1239.

[84] Hirobe, T. (2005). Role of keratinocyte-derived factors involved in regulating the proliferation and differentiation of mammalian epidermal melanocytes. *Pigment Cell Res.*, 18, 2-12.

[85] Yamaguchi, Y., and Hearing, V. J. (2005). Physiological factors that regulate skin pigmentation. *Biofactors,* 35, 193-199.

[86] Zanardo, L., Stolz, W., Schmitz, G., Kaminski, W., Vikkula, M., Landthaler, M., and Vogt, T. (2004). Progressive hyperpigmentation and generalized lentiginosis without associated systemic symptoms: a rare hereditary pigmentation disorder in south-east Germany. *Acta. Derm. Venereol.*, 84, 57-60.

[87] Zhang, C., Deng, Y., Chen, X., Wu, X., Jin, W., Li, H., Yu, C., Xiong, Y., Zhou, L., and Chen, Y. (2006) Linkage of a locus determining familial progressive hyperpigmentation (FPH) to chromosome 19p13.1-pter in a Chinese family. *Eur. J. Dermatol.,* 16, 246-250.

[88] Wang, Z. Q., Si, L., Tang, Q., Lin, D., Fu, Z., Zhang, J., Cui, B., Zhu, Y., Kong, X., Deng, M., Xia, Y., Xu, H., Le, W., Hu, L., and Kong, X. (2009). Gain-of-function mutation of KIT ligand on melanin synthesis causes familial progressive hyperpigmentation. *Am. J. Hum. Genet.*, 84, 672-677.

[89] Xing, Q. H., Wang, M. T., Chen, X. D. Feng, G. Y., Ji, H. Y., Yang, J. D., Gao, J. J., Qin, W., Qian, X. Q., Wu, S. N., and He, L. (2003). A gene locus responsible for dyschromatosis symmetrica hereditaria (DSH) maps to chromosome 6q24.2-q25.2. *Am. J. Hum. Genet.*, 73, 377-382.

[90] Stuhrmann, M., Hennies, H. C., Bukhari, I. A., Brakensiek, K., Nürnberg, G., Becker, C., Huebener, J., Miranda, M. C., Frye-Boukhriss, H., Knothe, S., Schmidtke, J., El-Harith, E. H. (2008). Dyschromatosis universalis hereditaria: evidence for autosomal recessive inheritance and identification of a new locus on chromosome 12q21-q23. *Clin. Genet.*, 73, 566-572.

[91] Giehl, K. (2005). Oncogenic Ras in tumor progression and metastasis. *Biol. Chem.*, 386, 193-205.

[92] Aoki, Y., Niihori, T., Narumi, Y., Kure, S., and Matsubara, Y. (2008). The RAS/MAPK syndromes: novel roles of the RAS pathway in human genetic disorders. *Hum. Mutat.*, 29, 992-1006.

[93] Bentires-Alj, M., Kontaridis, M. I., and Neel, B. G. (2006). Stops along the RAS pathway in human genetic disease. Nat. Med., 12, 283-285.

[94] Sarkozy, A., Digilio, M. C., and Dallapiccola, B. (2008). Leopard syndrome. *Orphanet. J. Rare Dis.*, 3, 13.

[95] Digilio, M. C., Conti, E., Sarkozy, A., Mingarelli, R., Dottorini, T., Marino, B., Pizzuti, A., and Dallapiccola, B. (2002). Grouping of multiple-lentigines/LEOPARD and Noonan syndromes on the PTPN11 gene. *Am. J. Hum. Genet.*, 71, 389-394.

[96] Pandit, B., Sarkozy, A., Pennacchio, L. A., Carta, C., Oishi, K., Martinelli, S., Pogna, E. A., Schackwitz, W., Ustaszewska, A., Landstrom, A., Bos, J. M., and Ommen, S. R., Esposito, G., Lepri, F., Faul, C., Mundel, P., López Siguero, J. P., Tenconi, R., Selicorni, A., Rossi, C., Mazzanti, L., Torrente, I., Marino, B., Digilio, M. C., Zampino, G., Ackerman, M. J., Dallapiccola, B., Tartaglia, M., and Gelb, B. D. (2007). Gain-of-function RAF1 mutations cause Noonan and LEOPARD syndromes with hypertrophic cardiomyopathy. *Nat. Genet.*, 39: 1007-1012.

[97] Sarkozy, A., Carta, C., Moretti, S., Zampino, G., Digilio, M. C., Pantaleoni, F., Scioletti, A. P., Esposito, G., Cordeddu, V., Lepri, F., Petrangeli, V., Dentici, M. L., Mancini, G. M., Selicorni, A., Rossi, C., Mazzanti, L., Marino, B., Ferrero, G. B., Silengo, M. C., Memo, L., Stanzial, F., Faravelli, F., Stuppia, L., Puxeddu, E., Gelb, B. D., Dallapiccola, B., and Tartaglia, M. (2009). Germline BRAF mutations in Noonan, LEOPARD, and cardiofaciocutaneous syndromes: molecular diversity and associated phenotypic spectrum. *Hum. Mutat.*, 30, 695-702.

[98] Kontaridis, M. I., Swanson, K. D., David, F. S., Barford, D., and Neel, B. G. (2006). PTPN11 (Shp2) mutations in LEOPARD syndrome have dominant negative, not activating, effects. *J. Biol. Chem.*, 281, 6785-6792.

[99] Schrader, K. A., Nelson, T. N., De Luca, A., Huntsman, D. G., McGillivray, B. C. (2009). Multiple granular cell tumors are an associated feature of LEOPARD syndrome caused by mutation in PTPN11. *Clin. Genet.*, 75, 185-189.

[100] Tartaglia, M., Mehler, E. L., Goldberg, R., Zampino, G., Brunner, H. G., Kremer, H., van der Burgt, I., Crosby, A. H., Ion, A., Jeffery, S., Kalidas, K., Patton, M. A., Kucherlapati, R. S., and Gelb, B. D. (2011). Mutations in PTPN11, encoding the protein tyrosine phosphatase SHP-2, cause Noonan syndrome. *Nat. Genet.*, 29, 465-468.

[101] Razzaque, M.A., Nishizawa, T., Komoike, Y., Yagi, H., Furutani, M., Amo, R., Kamisago, M., Momma, K., Katayama, H., Nakagawa, M., Fujiwara, Y., Matsushima, M., Mizuno, K., Tokuyama, M., Hirota, H., Muneuchi, J., Higashinakagawa, T., and Matsuoka, R. (2007). Germline gain-of-function mutations in RAF1 cause Noonan syndrome. *Nat. Genet.*, 39, 1013-1017.

[102] Niihori, T., Aoki, Y., Narumi, Y., Neri, G., Cavé, H., Verloes, A., Okamoto, N., Hennekam, R. C., Gillessen-Kaesbach, G., Wieczorek, D., Kavamura, M. I., Kurosawa, K., Ohashi, H., Wilson, L., Heron, D., Bonneau, D., Corona, G., Kaname, T., Naritomi, K., Baumann, C., Matsumoto, N., Kato, K., Kure, S., and Matsubara, Y. (2006).

Germline KRAS and BRAF mutations in cardio-facio-cutaneous syndrome. *Nat. Genet.*, 38, 294-296.

[103] Xu, G. F., O'Connell, P., Viskochil, D., Cawthon, R., Robertson, M., Culver, M., Dunn, D., Stevens, J., Gesteland, R., White, R., and Weiss, R. (1990). The neurofibromatosis type 1 gene encodes a protein related to GAP. *Cell,* 62, 599-608.

[104] Xu, G. F., Lin, B., Tanaka, K., Dunn, D., Wood, D., Gesteland, R., White, R., Weiss, R., and Tamanoi, F. (1990). The catalytic domain of the neurofibromatosis type 1 gene product stimulates ras GTPase and complements ira mutants of S. cerevisiae. *Cell,* 63, 835-841.

[105] Martin, G. A., Viskochil, D., Bollag, G., McCabe, P. C., Crosier, W. J., Haubruck, H., Conroy, L., Clark, R., O'Connell, .P, Cawthon, R. M., Innis M. A., and McCormick, F. (1990). The GAP-related domain of the neurofibromatosis type 1 gene product interacts with ras p21. *Cell,* 63, 843-849.

[106] Ballester, R., Marchuk, D., Boguski, M., Saulino, A., Letcher, R., Wigler, M., and Collins, F. (1990). The NF1 locus encodes a protein functionally related to mammalian GAP and yeast IRA proteins. *Cell,* 63, 851-859.

[107] Huynh, D. P., Lin, C. T., and Pulst, S. M. (1992). Expression of neurofibromin, the neurofibromatosis type-1 gene product: studies in human neuroblastoma cells and rat brain. Neurosci. Lett., 143, 233-236.

[108] Williams, V. C., Lucas, J., Babcock, M. A., Gutmann, D. H., Korf, B., and Maria, B. L. (2009). Neurofibromatosis type 1 revisited. *Pediatrics* 123: 124-133.

[109] Lau, N., Feldkamp, M. M., Roncari, L., Loehr, A. H., Shannon, P., Gutmann, D. H., and Guha, A. (2000). Loss of neurofibromin is associated with activation of RAS/MAPK and PI3-K/AKT signaling in a neurofibromatosis type-1 astrocytoma. *J. Neuropathol. Exp. Neurol.*, 59, 759-767.

[110] Phillips, R. A., Hunter, J. L., Eccleston, J. F., and Webb, M. R. (2003). The mechanism of Ras GTPase activation by neurofibromin. *Biochemistry*, 42, 3956-3965.

[111] Allanson, J. E., Hall, J. G., and Van Allen, M. I. (1985). Noonan phenotype associated with neurofibromatosis. *Am. J. Med. Genet.*, 21, 457-462.

[112] Mendez, H. M. The neurofibromatosis-Noonan syndrome. (1985). *Am. J. Med. Genet.*, 21, 471-476.

[113] Opitz, J. M., and Weaver, D. D. (1985). The neurofibromatosis-Noonan syndrome. *Am. J. Med. Genet.*, 21, 477-490.

[114] Baralle, D., Mattocks, C., Kalidas, K., Elmslie, F., Whittaker, J., Lees, M., Ragge, N., Patton, M. A., Winter, R. M., and ffrench-Constant, C. (2003). Different mutations in the NF1 gene are associated with neurofibromatosis-Noonan syndrome (NFNS). *Am. J. Med. Genet.*, 119A, 1-8.

[115] De Luca, A., Bottillo, I., Sarkozy, A., Carta, C., Neri, C., Bellacchio, E., Schirinzi, A., Conti, E., Zampino, G., Battaglia, A., Majore, S., Rinaldi, M. M., Carella, M., Marino, B., Pizzuti, A., Digilio, M. C., Tartaglia, M., and Dallapiccola, B. (2005). NF1 gene mutations represent the major molecular event underlying neurofibromatosis-Noonan syndrome. *Am. J. Hum. Genet.*, 77, 1092-1101.

[116] Nyström, A. M., Ekvall, S., Allanson, J., Edeby, C., Elinder, M., Holmström, G., Bondeson, M. L., and Annerén, G. (2009). Noonan syndrome and neurofibromatosis type I in a family with a novel mutation in NF1. *Clin. Genet.*, 76, 524-534.

[117] Bertola, D. R., Pereira, A. C., Passetti, F., de Oliveira, P. S., Messiaen, L., Gelb, B. D., Kim, C. A., and Krieger, J. E. (2005). Neurofibromatosis-Noonan syndrome: molecular evidence of the concurrence of both disorders in a patient. *Am. J. Med. Genet., A*, 136, 242-245.

[118] Brems, H., Chmara, M., Sahbatou, M., Denayer, E., Taniguchi, K., Kato, R., Somers, R., Messiaen, L., De Schepper, S., Fryns, J. P., Cools, J., Marynen, P., Thomas, G., Yoshimura, A., and Legius, E. (2007). Germline loss-of-function mutations in SPRED1 cause a neurofibromatosis 1-like phenotype. *Nat. Genet.*, 39, 1120-1126.

[119] Pasmant, E., Sabbagh, A., Hanna, N., Masliah-Planchon, J., Jolly, E., Goussard, P., Ballerini, P., Cartault, F., Barbarot, S., Landman-Parker, J., Soufir, N., Parfait, B., Vidaud, M., Wolkenstein, P., Vidaud, D., and France, R. N. (2009). SPRED1 germline mutations caused a neurofibromatosis type 1 overlapping phenotype. *J. Med. Genet.*, 46, 425-430.

[120] Spurlock, G., Bennett, E., Chuzhanova, N., Thomas, N., Jim, H. P., Side, L., Davies, S., Haan, E., Kerr, B., Huson, S. M., and Upadhyaya, M. (2009). SPRED1 mutations (Legius syndrome): another clinically useful genotype for dissecting the neurofibromatosis type 1 phenotype. *J. Med. Genet.*, 46, 431-437.

[121] Messiaen, L., Yao, S., Brems, H., Callens, T., Sathienkijkanchai, A., Denayer, E., Spencer, E., Arn, P., Babovic-Vuksanovic, D., Bay, C., Bobele, G., Cohen, B. H., Escobar. L., Eunpu, D., Grebe, T., Greenstein, R., Hachen, R., Irons, M., Kronn, D., Lemire, E., Leppig, K., Lim, C., McDonald, M., Narayanan, V., Pearn, A., Pedersen, R., Powell, B., Shapiro, L. R., Skidmore, D., Tegay, D., Thiese, H., Zackai, E. H., Vijzelaar, R., Taniguchi, K., Ayada, T., Okamoto, F., Yoshimura, A., Parret, A., Korf, B., and Legius, E. (2009). Clinical and mutational spectrum of neurofibromatosis type 1-like syndrome. *JAMA*, 302, 2111-2118.

[122] Denayer, E., Chmara, M., Brems, H., Kievit, A. M., van Bever, Y., Van den Ouweland, A. M., Van Minkelen, R., de Goede-Bolder, A., Oostenbrink, R., Lakeman, P., Beert, E., Ishizaki, T., Mor,i T., Keymolen, K., Van den Ende, J., Mangold, E., Peltonen, S., Brice, G., Rankin, J., Van Spaendonck-Zwarts, K. Y., Yoshimura, A., and Legius, E. (2011). Legius syndrome in fourteen families. *Hum. Mutat.*, 32, E1985-1998.

[123] Wakioka, T., Sasaki, A., Kato, R., Shouda, T., Matsumoto, A., Miyoshi, K., Tsuneoka, M., Komiya, S., Baron, R., and Yoshimura, A. (2001). Spred is a Sprouty-related suppressor of Ras signaling. *Nature*, 412, 647-651.

[124] Nonami, A., Kato, R., Taniguchi, K., Yoshiga, D., Taketomi, T., Fukuyama, S., Harada, M., Sasaki, A., and Yoshimura, A. (2004). Spred-1 negatively regulates interleukin-3-mediated ERK/mitogen-activated protein (MAP) kinase activation in hematopoietic cells. J. Biol. Chem., 279, 52543-52551.

[125] Quintanar-Audelo, M., Yusoff, P., Sinniah, S., Chandramouli, S., and Guy, G. R. (2011). Sprouty-related ena/vasodilator-stimulated phosphoprotein homology 1-domain-containing protein (SPRED1), a tyrosine-protein phosphatase non-receptor type 11 (SHP2) substrate in the Ras/extracellular signal-regulated kinase (ERK) pathway. *J. Biol. Chem.*, 286, 23102-23112.

[126] Tomita, Y., Takeda, A., Okinaga, S., Tagami, H., and Shibahara, S. (1989). Human oculocutaneous albinism caused by single base insertion in the tyrosinase gene. *Biochem. Biophys. Res. Commun.*, 164, 990-996.

[127] Giebel, L. B., Strunk, K. M., King, R. A., Hanifin, J. M., andSpritz, R. A. (1990). A frequent tyrosinase gene mutation in classic, tyrosinase-negative (type IA) oculocutaneous albinism. *Proc. Natl. Acad. Sci. U. S. A.*, 187, 3255-3258.

[128] Spritz, R. A., Strunk, K. M., Giebel, L. B., and King, R. A., (1990). Detection of mutations in the tyrosinase gene in a patient with type IA oculocutaneous albinism. *N. Engl. J. Med.*, 322, 1724-1728.

[129] Grønskov, K., Ek, J., and Brondum-Nielsen, K. (2007). Oculocutaneous albinism. Orphanet. *J. Rare Dis.*, 2, 43.

[130] Boissy, R. E., Zhao, H., Oetting, W. S., Austin, L. M., Wildenberg, S. C., Boissy, Y. L., Zhao, Y., Sturm, R. A., Hearing, V. J., King, R. A., and Nordlund, J. J. (1996). Mutation in and lack of expression of tyrosinase-related protein-1 (TRP-1) in melanocytes from an individual with brown oculocutaneous albinism: a new subtype of albinism classified as "OCA3". *Am. J. Hum. Genet.*, 58, 1145-1156.

[131] Manga, P., Kromberg, J. G., Box, N. F., Sturm, R. A., Jenkins, T., and Ramsay, M. (1997). Rufous oculocutaneous albinism in southern African Blacks is caused by mutations in the TYRP1 gene. *Am. J. Hum. Genet.*, 61, 1095-1101.

[132] Rooryck, C., Roudaut, C., Robine, E., Müsebeck, J., and Arveiler, B. (2006). Oculocutaneous albinism with TYRP1 gene mutations in a Caucasian patient. *Pigment Cell Res.*, 19, 239-242.

[133] Chiang, P. W., Spector, E., and Scheuerle, A. (2009). A case of Asian Indian OCA3 patient. *Am. J. Med. Genet. A*, 149A, 1578-1580.

[134] Zhang, K. H., Li, Z., Lei, J., Pang, T., Xu, B., Jiang, W. Y., and Li, H. Y. (in press). Oculocutaneous albinism type-3 (OCA3): analysis of two novel mutations in TYRP1 gene in two Chinese patients. *Cell Biochem. Biophys.*

[135] Chiang, P. W., Fulton, A. B., Spector, E., and Hisama, F. M. (2008). Synergistic interaction of the OCA2 and OCA3 genes in a family. *Am. J. Med. Genet.*, A, 146A, 2427-2430.

[136] Valverde, P., Healy, E., Jackson, I., Rees, J. L., and Thody, A. J. (1995). Variants of the melanocyte-stimulating hormone receptor gene are associated with red hair and fair skin in humans. *Nat. Genet.*, 11, 328-30.

[137] Valverde, P., Healy, E., Sikkink, S., Haldane, F., Thody, A. J., Carothers, A., Jackson, I. J., and Rees, J. L. (1996). The Asp84Glu variant of the melanocortin 1 receptor (MC1R) is associated with melanoma. *Hum. Mol. Genet.*, 5, 1663-1666.

[138] Ichii-Jones, F., Lear, J. T., Heagerty, A. H., Smith, A. G., Hutchinson, P. E., Osborne. J., Bowers, B., Jones, P. W., Davies, E., Ollier, W. E., Thomson, W., Yengi, L., Bath, J., Fryer, A. A., and Strange, R. C. (1998). Susceptibility to melanoma: influence of skin type and polymorphism in the melanocyte stimulating hormone receptor gene. *J. Invest. Dermatol.*, 111, 218-221.

[139] Palmer, J. S., Duffy, D. L., Box, N. F., Aitken, J. F., O'Gorman, L. E., Green, A. C., Hayward, N. K., Martin, N. G., and Sturm, R. A. (2000). Melanocortin-1 receptor polymorphisms and risk of melanoma: is the association explained solely by pigmentation phenotype? *Am. J. Hum. Genet.*, 66, 176-186.

[140] Box, N. F., Duffy, D. L., Irving, R. E., Russell, A., Chen, W., Griffyths, L. R., Parsons, P. G., Green, A. C., and Sturm, R. A. (2001). Melanocortin-1 receptor genotype is a risk factor for basal and squamous cell carcinoma. *J. Invest. Dermatol.*, 116, 224-229.

[141] Bastiaens, M.T., ter Huurne, J.A., Kielich, C., Gruis, N.A., Westendorp, R.G., Vermeer, B.J., Bavinck, J.N.; Leiden Skin Cancer Study Team. (2001). Melanocortin-1 receptor gene variants determine the risk of non-melanoma skin cancer independently of fair skin and red hair. *Am. J. Hum. Genet.*, 68, 884-894.

[142] Bastiaens, M., ter Huurne, J., Gruis, N., Bergman, W., Westendorp, R., Vermeer, B. J., and Bouwes Bavinck, J. N. (2001). The melanocortin-1-receptor gene is the major freckle gene. *Hum. Mol. Genet.*, 10, 1701-1708.

[143] Beaumont, K. A., Shekar, S. N., Newton, R. A., James, M. R., Stow, J. L., Duffy, D. L., and Sturm, R. A. (2007). Receptor function, dominant negative activity and phenotype correlations for MC1R variant alleles. *Hum. Mol. Genet.*, 16, 2249-2260.

[144] Sulem, P., Gudbjartsson, D.F., Stacey, S. N., Helgason, A., Rafnar, T., Magnusson, K. P., Manolescu, A., Karason, A., Palsson, A., Thorleifsson, G., Jakobsdottir, M., Steinberg, S., Pálsson, S., Jonasson, F., Sigurgeirsson, B., Thorisdottir, K., Ragnarsson, R., Benediktsdottir, K. R., Aben, K. K., Kiemeney, L. A., Olafsson, J. H., Gulcher, J., Kongm, A., Thorsteinsdottir, U., and Stefansson, K. (2007). Genetic determinants of hair, eye and skin pigmentation in Europeans. *Nat. Genet.*, 39, 1443-1452.

[145] Sulem, P., Gudbjartsson, D. F., Stacey, S. N., Helgason, A., Rafnar, T., Jakobsdottir, M., Steinberg, S., Gudjonsson, S. A., Palsson, A., Thorleifsson, G., Pálsson, S., Sigurgeirsson, B., Thorisdottir, K., Ragnarsson, R., Benediktsdottir, K. R., Aben, K. K., Vermeulen, S. H., Goldstein, A. M., Tucker, M. A., Kiemeney, L. A., Olafsson, J. H., Gulcher, J., Kong, A., Thorsteinsdottir, U., and Stefansson, K. (2008). Two newly identified genetic determinants of pigmentation in Europeans. *Nat. Genet.*, 40, 835-837.

[146] Gudbjartsson, D.F., Sulem, P., Stacey, S.N., Goldstein, A.M., Rafnar, T., Sigurgeirsson, B., Benediktsdottir, K.R., Thorisdottir, K., Ragnarsson, R., Sveinsdottir, S.G., Magnusson, V., Lindblom, A., Kostulas, K., Botella-Estrada, R., Soriano, V., Juberías, P., Grasa, M., Saez, B., Andres, R., Scherer, D., Rudnai, P., Gurzau, E., Koppova ,K., Kiemeney, L.A., Jakobsdottir, M., Steinberg, S., Helgason, A., Gretarsdottir, S., Tucker, M.A., Mayordomo, J.I., Nagore, E., Kumar, R., Hansson, J., Olafsson, J.H., Gulcher, J., Kong, A., Thorsteinsdottir, U., and Stefansson, K. (2008). ASIP and TYR pigmentation variants associate with cutaneous melanoma and basal cell carcinoma. *Nat. Genet.*, 40, 886-891.

[147] Guedj, M., Bourillon, A., Combadières, C., Rodero, M., Dieudé, P., Descamps, V., Dupin, N., Wolkenstein, P., Aegerter, P., Lebbe, C., Basset-Seguin, N., Prum, B., Saiag, P., Grandchamp, B., Soufir, N.; MelanCohort Investigators. (2008). Variants of the MATP/SLC45A2 gene are protective for melanoma in the French population. *Hum. Mutat.*, 29, 1154-1160.

[148] Bishop, D. T., Demenais, F., Iles, M. M., Harland, M., Taylor, J. C., Corda, E., Randerson-Moor, J., Aitken, J. F., Avril, M. F., Azizi, E., Bakker, B., Bianchi-Scarrà, G., Bressac-de Paillerets, B., Calista, D., Cannon-Albright, L. A., Chin-A-Woeng, T., Debniak, T., Galore-Haskel, G., Ghiorzo, P., Gut, I., Hansson, J., Hocevar, M., Höiom, V., Hopper, J. L., Ingvar, C., Kanetsky, P. A., Kefford, R. F., Landi, M. T., Lang, J., Lubiński, J., Mackie, R., Malvehy, J., Mann, G. J., Martin, N. G., Montgomery, G. W., van Nieuwpoort, F. A., Novakovic, S., Olsson, H., Puig, S., Weiss, M., van Workum, W., Zelenika, D., Brown, K. M., Goldstein, A. M., Gillanders, E. M., Boland, A., Galan, P., Elder, D. E., Gruis, N. A., Hayward, N. K., Lathrop, G. M., Barrett, J. H.,

and Bishop, J. A. (2009). Genome-wide association study identifies three loci associated with melanoma risk. *Nat. Genet.*, 41, 920-925.

[149] Brown, K. M., Macgregor, S., Montgomery, G. W., Craig, D. W., Zhao, Z. Z., Iyadurai, K., Henders, A. K., Homer, N., Campbell, M. J., Stark, M., Thomas, S., Schmid, H., Holland, E. A., Gillanders. E. M., Duffy, D. L., Maskiell, J. A., Jetann, J., Ferguson, M., Stephan, D. A., Cust, A. E., Whiteman, D., Green, A., Olsson, H., Puig, S., Ghiorzo, P., Hansson, J., Demenais, F., Goldstein, A. M., Gruis, N. A., Elder, D. E., Bishop, J. N., Kefford, R. F., Giles, G. G., Armstrong ,B. K., Aitken, J. F., Hopper, J. L., Martin, N. G., Trent, J. M., Mann, G. J., Hayward, N. K. (2008). Common sequence variants on 20q11.22 confer melanoma susceptibility. *Nat. Genet.*, 40, 838-840.

[150] Fargnoli, M. C., Pike, K., Pfeiffer, R. M., Tsang, S., Rozenblum, E., Munroe, D. J., Golubeva, Y., Calista, D., Seidenari, S., Massi, D., Carli, P., Bauer, J., Elder, D. E., Bastian, B. C., Peris, K., and Landi, M. T. (2008). MC1R variants increase risk of melanomas harboring BRAF mutations. *J. Invest. Dermatol.*, 128, 2485-2490.

[151] Cuéllar, F., Puig, S., Kolm, I., Puig-Butille, J., Zaballos, P., Martí-Laborda, R., Badenas, C., and Malvehy, J. (2009). Dermoscopic features of melanomas associated with MC1R variants in Spanish CDKN2A mutation carriers. *Br. J. Dermatol.*, 160, 48-53.

[152] Stacey, S. N., Sulem, P., Masson, G., Gudjonsson, S. A., Thorleifsson, G., Jakobsdottir, M., Sigurdsson, A., Gudbjartsson, D. F., Sigurgeirsson, B., Benediktsdottir, K. R., Thorisdottir, K., Ragnarsson, R., Scherer, D., Hemminki, K., Rudnai, P., Gurzau, E., Koppova, K., Botella-Estrada, R., Soriano, V., Juberias, P., Saez, B., Gilaberte, Y., Fuentelsaz, V., Corredera, C., Grasa, M., Höiom, V., Lindblom, A., Bonenkamp, J. J., van Rossum, M. M., Aben, K. K., de Vries, E., Santinami, M., Di Mauro, M. G., Maurichi, A., Wendt, J., Hochleitner, P., Pehamberger, H., Gudmundsson, J., Magnusdottir, D. N., Gretarsdottir, S., Holm, H., Steinthorsdottir, V., Frigge, M. L., Blondal, T., Saemundsdottir, J., Bjarnason, H., Kristjansson, K., Bjornsdottir, G., Okamoto, I., Rivoltini, L., Rodolfo, M., Kiemeney, L. A., Hansson, J., Nagore, E., Mayordomo, J. I., Kumar, R., Karagas, M. R., Nelson, H. H., Gulcher, J. R., Rafnar, T., Thorsteinsdottir, U., Olafsson, J. H., Kong, A., and Stefansson, K. (2009). New common variants affecting susceptibility to basal cell carcinoma. *Nat. Genet.*, 41, 909-914.

[153] Miyamura, Y., Suzuki, T., Kono, M., Inagaki, K., Ito, S., Suzuki, N., and Tomita, Y. (2003). Mutations of the RNA-specific adenosine deaminase gene (DSRAD) are involved in dyschromatosis symmetrica hereditaria. Am. *J. Hum. Genet.*, 73, 693-699.

[154] Murata, I., Hayashi, M., Hozumi, Y., Fujii, K., Mitsuhashi, Y., Oiso, N., Fukai, K., Kuroki, N., Mori, Y., Utani, A., Tomita, Y., Fujita, Y., and Suzuk,i T. (2010). Mutation analyses of patients with dyschromatosis symmetrica hereditaria: five novel mutations of the ADAR1 gene. *J. Dermatol. Sci.,* 58, 218-220.

[155] Paz-Yaacov, N., Levanon, E.Y., Nevo, E., Kinar, Y., Harmelin, A., Jacob-Hirsch, J., Amariglio, N., Eisenberg, E., and Rechavi, G. (2010). Adenosine-to-inosine RNA editing shapes transcriptome diversity in primates. *Proc. Natl. Acad. Sci. U.S.A.* 2010, 107, 12174-12179.

[156] Oiso, N., Murata, I., Hayashi, M., Amatsu, A., Yoshida, M., Suzuki, T., and Kawada, A. (2011). Dermoscopic features in a case of dyschromatosis symmetrica hereditaria. *J. Dermatol.*, 38, 91-93.

[157] Sharma, R., Sharma, S. C., Radotra, B. D., and Kaur, S. (1989). Reticulate acropigmentation of Kitamura. *Clin. Exp. Dermatol.*, 14, 302-303.

[158] Lestringant, G. G., Masouyé, I., Frossard, P. M., Adeghate, E., and Galadari, I. H. (1997). Co-existence of leukoderma with features of Dowling-Degos disease: reticulate acropigmentation of Kitamura spectrum in five unrelated patients. *Dermatology,* 195, 337-343.

[159] Al Hawsawi, K., Al Aboud, K., Alfadley, A., and Al Aboud, D. (2002). Reticulate acropigmentation of Kitamura-Dowling Degos disease overlap: a case report. *Int. J. Dermatol.*, 41, 518-520.

In: Melanin: Biosynthesis, Functions and Health Effects
Editors: Xiao-Peng Ma and Xiao-Xiao Sun
ISBN: 978-1-62100-991-7

Chapter VI

Optical Spectroscopy and Structural Properties of Synthetic and Natural Eumelanin

Giuseppe Perna and Vito Capozzi
Dipartimento di Scienze Biomediche, Università degli Studi di Foggia,
Viale L. Pinto, I-71100 Foggia, Italy

Abstract

Optical properties of synthetic and natural eumelanin are presented and compared, in order to investigate the structural organization of eumelanin, which is related to the function of this biopolymer. Synthetic eumelanin is produced by oxidation of tyrosine with hydrogen peroxide, whereas natural eumelanin is extracted from *Sepia Officinalis* and from *Rana Esculenta*. Vibrational spectroscopy techniques (as Raman scattering and infrared absorption) show that both types of biopolymer include chemical functional groups characteristic of the monomeric units of eumelanin, although natural eumelanin includes also protein-related groups, proportionally to the protein content. X-ray diffraction spectra are in agreement with the hypothesis that eumelanin monomers assembly themselves and form protomolecules consisting of stacked layers (distant 3 – 4 Å each other) of indolic sheets. Absorption measurements, characterized by a monotonic increase of optical density from near-IR to UV range, support the model that eumelanin consists of a distribution of aggregates of oligomeric structures having different size and chemical composition. The estimated values of the optical gap indicate that the natural eumelanins are characterized by a larger structural disorder than the synthetic one. Fluorescence spectra confirm that the biopolymer consists of ensembles of chemically distinct oligomer systems, which can be selectively excited. This result is also supported by Dynamic Light Scattering measurements, which permit to visualize the distribution of particles size. In fact, the nanoaggregate systems of natural eumelanin have a larger size than those of synthetic eumelanin. This might be related to the biological functions of such a biopolymer, particularly as far as photoprotective action is concerned.

Introduction

The melanins are a class of biological pigments that provide coloration to animals and plants [1]. In particular, eumelanin (a brown-black pigment containing nitrogen) and pheomelanin (a brown-red pigment containing also sulphur) are the predominant forms of melanin in humans. Eumelanin, the most diffuse form, is formed inside specialized organelles called melanosomes. The key enzyme of melanogenic pathway is the tyrosinase [2]. This enzyme catalyzes the first rate-limiting steps of melanogenesis, the hydroxylation of L-tyrosine and the subsequent oxidation of the intermediate L-dopa to yield L-dopaquinone. Several other proteins located in the melanosomes are involved in melanogenesis process. Therefore, eumelanins are considered to be firmly bound to proteinaceous components, through covalent or ionic bonds [3]. In fact, purification processes can be used to isolate eumelanin from the protein component, although a complete separation is hardly achievable. A method to prepare eumelanin without protein is to synthesize it non-enzymatically, for example through a process starting from oxidation of tyrosine with hydrogen peroxide. The sample obtained in this way is called synthetic eumelanin.

In humans, eumelanin pigment is found in skin, hair and eyes, where it acts mainly as an excellent photoprotectant [4], because it largely absorbs UV and visible light by converting the light energy into heat. However, eumelanin plays a dual role with respect to the sunlight's UV radiation: on one hand, it is beneficial because it absorbs the UV radiation, thereby reducing the UV damage in skin cells [5]; on the other hand, it is deleterious by acting as a photosensitizer that generates active oxygen species capable of causing DNA strand breaks, although such a role occurs mostly in pheomelanin [5]. The balance of these two processes determines whether a beneficial action or a malignant transformation activated by the oxygen species occurs.

Eumelanin, besides its important biological role, has very attractive physical properties for material science applications. In view of such applications, synthetic eumelanin has been widely investigated [4, 6, 7–11]. It exhibits broad UV and visible absorption spectra [4, 7, 8], electrical conductivity similar to that of amorphous silicon [9], strong non radiative relaxation [6] and photoconductivity [10], as it occurs for amorphous semiconductors; therefore, it has been proposed for photovoltaic and optoelectronic applications. Recently, hysteresis behaviour of the current–voltage characteristic of synthetic eumelanin-based structures allows to foresee the possible integration of eumelanin in memory devices [11].

The properties of synthetic eumelanin, although interesting for technological applications, cannot be directly generalized for the natural pigment, because of the presence of protein component in the latter. Instead, the investigation of synthetic eumelanin can be used as starting point to study the physical properties of natural eumelanin and the role of proteins in the structural organization of the natural biopolymer, which is partly debated yet. In fact, it is accepted that eumelanin is a biopolymer resulting from aggregation of indolic monomers, such as 5,6-dihydroxyindole (DHI), 5,6-dihydroxyndole-2-carboxylic acid (DHICA), 5,6-indolequinone (IQ) and semiquinone (SQ). A schematic representation of these monomers is shown in Fig. 1. Nonetheless, it is still not well known how these monomer units are connected together to form eumelanin pigment. Until the last decades of the XX century, it was still unclear whether eumelanin was actually a highly cross-linked extended heteropolymer [1] or it was composed of much smaller oligomers condensed into nanoaggregates [12]. In the last decade, several theoretical [8, 13] and experimental [14, 15] studies have been published to support the structural model of eumelanin as consisting of stacked oligomeric nanoaggregates. In particular, it has been recently confirmed that both synthetic and natural eumelanin are organized according to planar sheets of varying dimensions which stack each other with inter-sheet spacing values between 3.7 and 4.0 Å [16]. Furthermore, it has been established that the lateral extension of the indolic sheets in synthetic eumelanin is less than 10 nm, whereas it is about one order of magnitude larger in natural eumelanin (from bovine epithelium and ink sacks of *Sepia officinalis*) [16].

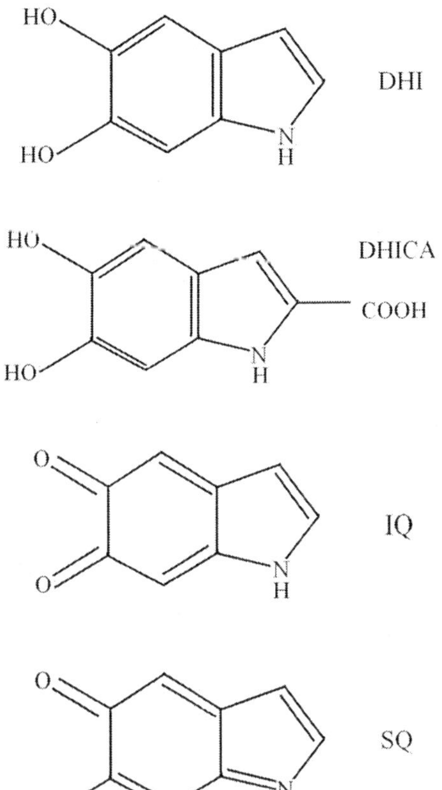

Figure 1. Schematic representation of the structure of the basic monomeric building blocks of eumelanin: 5,6-dihydroxyindole (DHI), 5,6-dihydroxyndole-2-carboxylic acid (DHICA) and the redox forms 5,6-indolequinone (IQ) and semiquinone (SQ).

An accurate investigation of the structural organization of eumelanin can be provided by optical spectroscopy techniques. In fact, such techniques are non destructive (and, consequently, the same sample can be analysed by different techniques) and they require a very small amount of material for such analysis. In particular, vibrational, absorption and fluorescence spectroscopy are useful analytical tools to investigate the presence of monomer and oligomer components inside the eumelanin biomolecules. This can be accomplished by means of a comparison with theoretical models and calculations about the eumelanin structure.

In fact, Raman and Fourier Transform Infrared (FTIR) spectra provide information about the energy of vibrational modes of the chemical bonds involved in the structure of the investigated sample: therefore, the spectral position of Raman and FTIR features of eumelanin spectra allows to identify the functional groups present in the structure of eumelanin components. Several works exist about Raman [17-19] and FTIR [17, 20-24] investigation of the melanin. In particular, the article from Powell et al. [17] reports a first principles density-functional calculation of the Raman and FTIR spectrum of the eumelanin monomers. These calculated spectra consist of several very narrow peaks, because they are related to gaseous phase monomers. Nonetheless, such calculated spectra can be compared with the experimental ones in order to attribute the spectral peaks, even if the broadening and shifting effects should be considered as well when a solid biopolymer is formed.

The absorption properties of all types of melanin is characterized by a very broad absorption, whose intensity increases from visible to UV [6, 25]. In addition, such absorption band is structureless, i.e. it includes no resolved absorption peaks related to some specific component of the biopolymer. Some authors have remarked that melanins are indeed disordered organic semiconductors [26, 27], because of such similar absorption properties (and also electrical conductivity and photoconductivity [28]). Therefore, absorption spectra are not sensitive probes to reveal specific components of the eumelanin structure. Nevertheless, several attempts have been performed to simulate the monotonic behaviour of eumelanin absorption spectra. This was achieved by the convolution of a basis set of numeric atomic functions [8, 13] or several broadened Gaussian functions [4], each with different peak position and intensity, related to highest occupied molecular orbital–lowest unoccupied molecular orbital (HOMO-LUMO) gaps of distinct eumelanin monomers and/or oligomers. The good agreement of calculated absorption spectra with the experimental ones have suggested that an ensemble of similar but chemically distinct species can explain the observed monotonic, broad band absorbance. Linh Tran et al. [29] introduced the term "chemical disorder model" to explain the eumelanin structure as consisting of many chemically distinct oligomers, each with a different HOMO–LUMO energy gap. According to this model, the broadband absorption characteristics is due to overlapping of a large number of HOMO-LUMO transitions associated with each of the eumelanin components.

Fluorescence (FL) spectroscopy technique has been widely used to investigate the structural organization of eumelanin [6, 30–33], although the radiative quantum yield is extremely low [6]. The eumelanin FL spectra support the hypothesis that radiative emission in synthetic eumelanin is related to chemically distinct oligomeric units that are selectively excited, in agreement with the chemical disorder model. So, the emission bands are due to the convolution of many different narrower features, each one corresponding to the FL of a different eumelanin component. However, the results obtained for synthetic eumelanin cannot be directly generalized to the natural pigment, because of the presence of protein component in the latter.

In addition to optical techniques, also structural techniques as Dynamic Light Scattering (DLS), X-ray Diffraction (XRD) and Atomic Force Microscopy (AFM) can be properly applied to investigate the size of the structural components of the biopolymer. In fact, DLS technique is usually used to determine the size distribution profile of small *particles* or polymers in *suspension*. X-ray scattering measurements [34-36] of eumelanin samples have revealed the presence of nanometric particles consisting of 3 or 4 planar layers of few indolequinone units having lateral size of 15–20 Å and stacked each other of about 3.4 Å.

Also AFM images of eumelanin samples have revealed the coexistence of nanometric particles having different sizes, from about tens nanometers to few hundred nanometers, and different shape, as spherical and filamentous ones [12, 15, 37-39]. Therefore, the structural techniques suggest a model for eumelanin structure, as consisting of nanoaggregates of different shape and size comprising several protomolecules each one formed by 3 or 4 planar layers of few monomer units having lateral size of 15–20 Å and stacked each other of about 3.4 Å.

In this article, we review our recent results concerning the optical and structural properties of the synthetic and natural eumelanin biopolymer, by focusing on important aspect such as its capability to absorb, scatter and emit light and including its molecular and supramolecular structure. We have found that several physical properties are influenced by the protein content of the biopolymer. In particular, the protein content result to influence the structural organization of eumelanin, by aiding to construct aggregates having a larger size.

Experimental

Materials

Three types of eumelanin samples have been investigated: *i)* synthetic eumelanin samples, obtained from commercial eumelanin powder produced by oxidation of tyrosine with hydrogen peroxide (Sigma-Aldrich): nominally it doesn't contain proteins; *ii)* natural eumelanin samples obtained from commercial eumelanin powder extracted from ink sacs of *Sepia Officinalis* (Sigma-Aldrich): for such samples a protein content of about 8% is reported [40]; *iii)* natural eumelanin samples extracted from liver of *Rana esculenta* according to the method of Cicero et al. [41]: for such samples a protein content larger than that of *Sepia officinalis* has been estimated [42].

Experimental Techniques

The Raman spectra were measured at room temperature by means of a Raman confocal micro-spectrometer using the 632.8 nm line of He–Ne as laser source and a notch filter (200 cm^{-1} line-with) to suppress the laser scattered light. The Raman signal was detected by means of a cooled CCD (at 223 K). The laser beam was focused, by an Olympus optical microscope with a x100 objective, on the investigated sample, obtaining an illuminated spot of few μm diameter. The laser power at the sample was about 0.1 mW, corresponding to a laser intensity of about 10^3 W/cm^2 on the surface of samples. The mean spectral resolution was 4 cm^{-1}. The samples for Raman measurements were prepared starting from eumelanin powders mixed with HPLC-grade water: a continuous melanin dispersion in water was produced, because it is well known that melanin is essentially insoluble in any solvent [37]. Such dispersions were sonicated for 15 min to improve a little solubility. Successively, a drop of each type of eumelanin dispersion was deposited on glass substrate and air dried before performing Raman measurements.

Mid-Infrared absorption spectra at room temperature were performed in a Fourier Transform Interferometer Vertex70 (Bruker Optics), operating in the wavelength range 900–4000 cm^{-1}. The samples were prepared as pellets (13 mm diameter) of eumelanin powders (4 mg) in KBr (100 mg).

UV, visible and near-IR absorption spectra in the 240–1100 nm spectral range at room temperature were measured by means of a JASCO V-530 double beam spectrophotometer, at a scan rate of 400 nm/min and with a slit band-width of 2 nm. The samples for absorption measurements consisted of synthetic and natural eumelanin solutions prepared in HPLC-grade water, obtained by sonication for 15 min and centrifugation (Heraeus sepatech "Biofuge 13") at 13000 rpm for 30 min of the starting dispersions, in order to remove large suspended aggregates. The supernatant eumelanin resulting from centrifugation was a homogeneous solution; such samples were used for optical measurements. The optical density spectrum was obtained by using the well known Lambert–Beer law.

Fluorescence spectra of eumelanin samples were measured by means of a Cary Eclipse fluorescence spectrophotometer, by using the same eumelanin solutions prepared for absorption measurements. All spectra were measured by using a 1cm x 0.5cm rectangular quartz cuvette. The measurements were performed at several excitation energies between 4.960 and 2.296 eV. A band pass width of 10 nm and an integration time of 1s were used. Background scans were performed under identical instrumental conditions using the HPLC-grade water. The fluorescence spectra have been also normalized to account for excitation beam penetration depth and emission re-absorption, according to the procedure described in the literature [32, 33].

Dynamic Light Scattering (DLS) measurements were performed using a Zetasizer-NanoS correlator from Malvern operating with a 4 mW He–Ne laser (633 nm wavelength) and a fixed detector angle of 173° (non invasive backscattering geometry NIBSTM) and with the cell holder, containing the eumelanin solutions (prepared as for absorption and fluorescence measurements) at a proper concentration, maintained at 25 °C by means of a Peltier thermostatic element. Data were collected after having optimized the instrumental parameters (attenuator, optics position and number of runs). Usually, the time Autocorrelation Function (ACF) of scattered light intensity was the average of 12–16 consecutive runs of 10 s each. The ACF of scattered light intensity was converted into the ACF of scattered electric field. From this last quantity, the fraction of the light intensity scattered by particles of different size (i.e. the size distribution by intensity) has been recovered by taking the inverse Laplace transform of the ACF using the software implemented by the manufacturer.

XRD spectra were performed by using the CuKα radiation (λ =1.5406 Å) of a θ-2θ diffractometer. Samples of synthetic eumelanin for XRD measurements consisted of pellets obtained by pressing the powders at a pressure of about 500 MPa for about 3 min, whereas the natural eumelanin samples consisted of an air-dried deposit of eumelanin extracted from *Rana esculenta* on a quartz substrate.

An atomic force microscope (Perception, by Assing S.p.A.) was used for AFM imaging. Its lower unit contains the sample holder mounted on top of a cylindrical piezoelectric scanner having a maximum *x–y* scan range of 3 × 3 μm and an *z* range of 0.6 μm. The upper unit contains a cantilever holder, the mirror deflection system and a four-sector position-sensitive photodiode, used as the deflection detector. An electronic feedback loop is used to integrate the optical signal and maintain a constant cantilever deflection during the image acquisition. The measurements were performed in air, with the microscope working in the non-contact mode. Gold-coated Si_3N_4 cantilevers with a spring constant of 40 N/m and a statistical apical radius of 5–20 nm were used. Constant force images were acquired with a scan rate of 3.0–4.0 s/row. The samples for AFM measurements were obtained by suspending 1 mg of melanin in 1 ml of HPLC-grade water. The mixture was firstly sonicated for 15 min and then centrifuged at 18000g for 30 min. 10 μl of the supernant, containing only the tiny aggregates, were dropped on freshly cleaved mica substrate and air-dried in dark at room temperature before the measurements.

Results and Discussion

Vibrational Spectroscopy: Raman and FTIR

The Raman spectra of air dried drops of synthetic, *Sepia officinalis* and *Rana esculenta* eumelanin at room temperature are shown in Fig. 2a, 2b and 2c, respectively. The spectra have been normalized by subtracting the contribution of the FL emission. Such spectra present a strong similarity to the Raman spectrum of amorphous carbon, which is dominated by two bands, centred at 1350 and 1550 cm^{-1} [43], both related to vibrational modes of the carbon atoms arranged in graphitic-like domains. Although carbon is the main constituent of the eumelanin samples, several atoms other than carbon (such as O, H and N) are bonded to the carbon atoms in the biopolymer. Therefore, the eumelanin Raman spectra can present contributions from Raman active vibrational modes involving different atoms. In fact, the three spectra in Fig. 2 are very similar: they are dominated by the two strong and broad bands centred at about 1400 and 1600 cm^{-1}, with other lower intensity bands appearing at 950 and 1200 cm^{-1}. The Raman intensity of the two main bands are similar, except for the *Rana esculenta* spectrum in Fig. 2c, where the band at 1600 cm^{-1} presents an intensity value larger than that at 1400 cm^{-1}. Moreover, the two main bands at 1400 and 1600 cm^{-1} have a larger intensity in the natural eumelanin spectra comparing with the synthetic one.

The features of the Raman spectra can be assigned to vibrational modes related to the structural units of the biopolymer; in addition, vibrational modes of the protein content should be considered when analysing the spectra of natural eumelanin samples [44, 45]. In particular, the overall shape of the Raman spectra are similar to that calculated by Powell et al. [17], so confirming the presence of the eumelanin monomers DHI, IQ and SQ inside the analysed samples. By considering the spectral position of vibrational modes inside functional groups similar to those present in eumelanin monomers, the dominant mode in the high wavenumber region, centred at about 1600 cm^{-1}, can be attributed to ring vibrations of the indole structure [46]. Moreover, the C=O stretching bond, present in the quinone structure of IQ and SQ and in the carboxylic acid group of DHICA, also weakly contributes to the high wavenumber side of the strong band at 1600 cm^{-1}. Indeed, the weak spectral feature at about 1700 cm^{-1} in Fig. 2, can be assigned to the C=O stretching vibrational mode, which is reported in the 1655-1690 cm^{-1} range for a quinone group and in the 1680-1715 cm^{-1} range for a carboxylic acid group [46]. Instead, the low wavenumber side of the band at 1600 cm^{-1} is also broadened by the C=C and C=N in plane vibrations of the pyrrole structure: indeed, such vibrational modes are reported in the 1460-1510 cm^{-1} and 1380-1430 cm^{-1} spectral ranges [46]. The main contribution to the low wavenumber region of the Raman spectrum results from the band centred at about 1400 cm^{-1}, which is due to the overlapping of several vibrational modes, mainly *i)* the C=C and C=N in plane vibrations of the pyrrole structure descrived above, *ii)* the C–N stretching mode of the pyrrole structure (reported in the 1325-1367 cm^{-1} spectral range [19, 47, 48]) and *iii)* combination bands due to C–O stretching and O–H deformation of the carboxylic acid (reported in the region of 1250 cm^{-1} [49]). Finally, the low intensity bands at about 950 and 1200 cm^{-1} are related to O-H out-of-plane deformation mode (reported at 935 cm^{-1} [49]) and C–H bending modes (reported in the 1145-1200 cm^{-1} region [50], respectively.

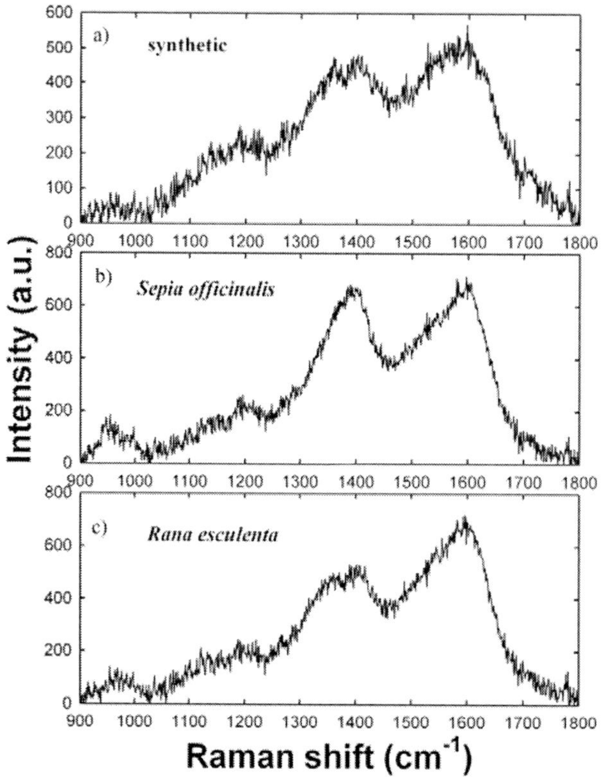

Figure 2. Micro-Raman spectra at room temperature of a air dried drop of synthetic (a), *Sepia officinalis* (b) and *Rana esculenta* eumelanin (c).

In addition to vibrational modes of the eumelanin structure, also Raman modes characteristic of functional groups of proteins contribute to spectra in Fig. 2, especially for the natural eumelanins in Fig. 2b and 2c. In fact, several vibrational modes due to protein components are reported in the spectral regions covered by the bands centred at 1400 and 1600 cm^{-1}, as CH_2 (1436-1460 cm^{-1}) and CH_3 (1335-1343 cm^{-1}) deformation modes, C-C and C-N breathing modes (1573-1582 cm^{-1}) and C=C mode (1615-1618 cm^{-1}) [51]. The contribution of such protein modes can be responsible of the intensity increase of the two main bands with respect to the other bands in the two natural eumelanins, particularly for the band at 1600 cm^{-1} in the *Rana esculenta* spectrum in Fig. 2c.

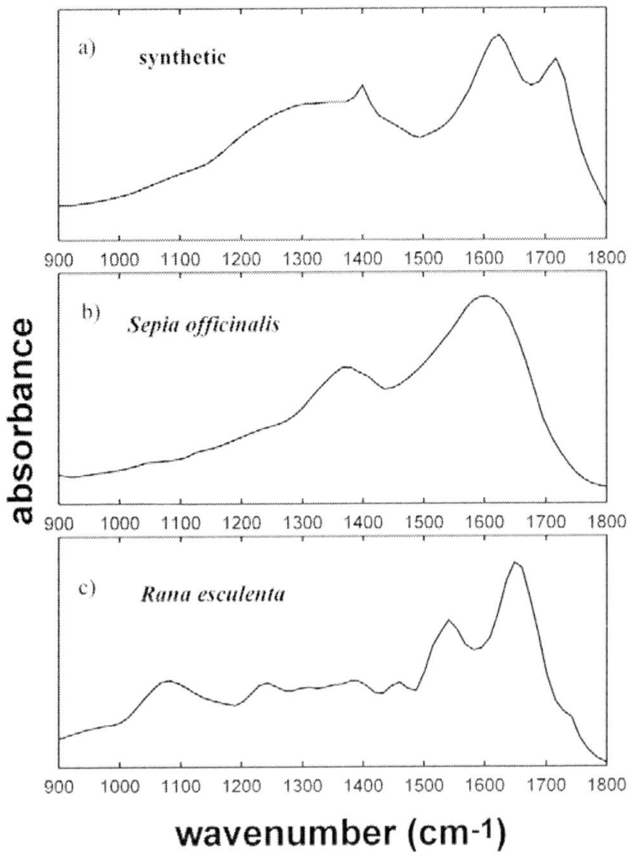

Figure 3. Absorption FTIR spectra at room temperature of a sample of synthetic (a), *Sepia officinalis* (b) and *Rana esculenta* (c) eumelanin. The samples are pellets (13 mm diameter) of eumelanin powders (4 mg) in KBr (100 mg).

These differences between synthetic and natural eumelanins are also more evident in the FTIR spectra, shown in Fig. 3. The analysis of the synthetic eumelanin spectrum in Fig. 3a provides information about the main functional groups characteristic of eumelanin structure, according to the spectral position of absorption peak, as reported in the literature [21, 22]. So, it can be deduced that the synthetic eumelanin sample includes aromatic systems (C=C stretching at about 1620 cm^{-1}), indole rings (C–N stretching at about 1360 cm^{-1}) and carboxyl groups (C=O asymmetrical stretching at about 1710 cm^{-1}, C=O symmetrical stretching at about 1400 cm^{-1} and –C–OH stretching at about 1280 cm^{-1}). In contrast, the *Sepia officinalis* eumelanin spectrum, shown in Fig. 3b, differs from the synthetic one for several features. First of all, the peaks related to carboxyl groups are much less evident, so indicating the small amount of DHICA monomers in this sample. In addition, the peak at about 1600 cm^{-1} is broader with respect to the corresponding peak in the synthetic sample; such broadening can be due to a contribution of amide II (1550 cm^{-1}) and amide I (1660 cm^{-1} [22]) vibrations, typical of protein groups. The presence of protein content is more evident in the FTIR spectrum of *Rana esculenta* sample, shown in Fig. 3c. Indeed, such spectrum is dominated by peaks related to proteins, as the amide I peak at 1650 cm^{-1} and the amide II peak at 1550 cm^{-1}: these two peaks overlaps to the C=C stretching group. The contribution of carboxyl groups is also scarcely resolved: C=O asymmetrical stretching is visible as a shoulder at about 1710 cm^{-1}, C=O symmetrical stretching overlaps to the amide III peak at about 1380 cm^{-1} and CH bending groups at about 1450 cm^{-1}, whereas the –C–OH stretching is resolved at about 1250 cm^{-1}. Moreover, the peak at about 1080 cm^{-1} is related to C-O-C groups of protein components.

Absorption Spectroscopy

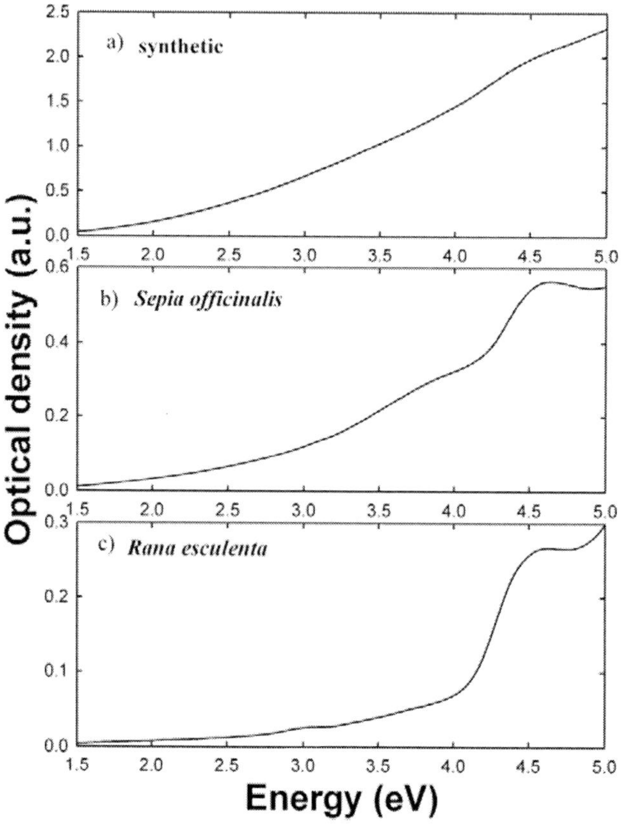

Figure 4. Optical density spectra at room temperature of synthetic (a), *Sepia officinalis* (b) and *Rana esculenta* (c) eumelanin solutions.

The absorption spectra of natural and synthetic eumelanin solutions at room temperature in the spectral region from near-IR to near-UV are reported in Fig. 4. All solutions present an increase of the optical density versus the energy, with a very strong and broad UV–visible absorption. Such a behaviour promotes the photoprotection function of the biopolymer. In particular, the absorption of synthetic melanin decreases monotonically from UV to IR energies, without any resolved peak: only a weak absorption shoulder is visible at about 4.6 eV, due to absorption on behalf of residual tyrosine in the synthetic sample. Instead, the spectra of both natural eumelanins present a broad absorption band at about 4.6 eV. Such band is due to light absorption of residual proteins, which are not completely removed during isolation and purification processes. In fact, several aromatic aminoacids, as phenylalanine, tyrosine and tryptophan, present absorption features in this spectral region [52]. Moreover, the absorption spectra of eumelanin from *Sepia officinalis* and *Rana esculenta* show weak features at about 3.9 eV and 3.1 eV, respectively. Such shoulders are also related to the protein coat, which cannot be fully removed during the preparation of the biopolymer sample.

Fluorescence Spectroscopy

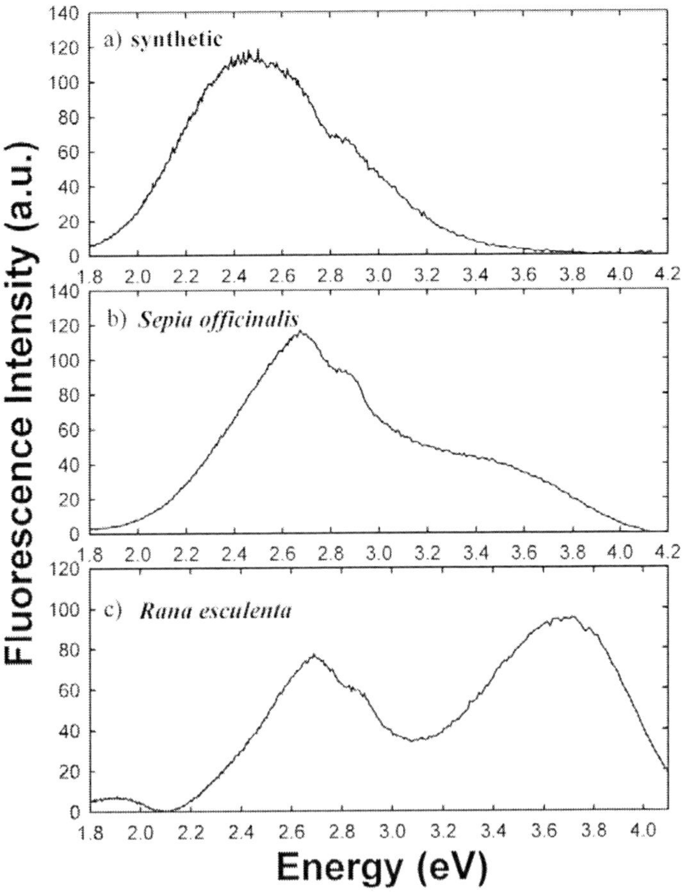

Figure 5. Fluorescence emission spectra at room temperature of synthetic (a), *Sepia officinalis* (b) and *Rana esculenta* (c) eumelanin solutions, measured by the excitation light energy of 4.960 eV.

The presence of protein components in natural eumelanins influences also the fluorescence properties, as it is evident in Fig. 5, which shows the FL spectra of the three types of eumelanin solutions measured at room temperature and with the same excitation energy (4.96 eV). The spectra show similar spectral features, except for the presence of a high energy band, at about 3.50 eV and 3.70 eV, observed in *Sepia officinalis* and *Rana esculenta* eumelanin, respectively. Such feature is lacking in synthetic eumelanin sample. According to the different chemical composition of the eumelanin samples, we can attribute such high energy bands to radiative emission of the residual protein components. In fact, some aminoacids, as tryptophan and tyrosine, when excited by UV wavelengths, have fluorescence emission in this spectral range [52]. Such attribution is also in agreement with the larger intensity of the high energy band in *Rana esculenta* with respect to *Sepia officinalis*: indeed, the protein content of the former is larger than that of the latter. A broad low energy band at 2.45 eV dominates the spectrum of the synthetic eumelanin; it is blue-shifted at 2.68 eV in the spectrum of the two natural ones. Finally, all spectra in Fig. 5 are characterized by a shoulder at about 2.85 eV. FL spectral features of eumelanin are due to radiative transitions between energy levels of the molecular groups present in the biopolymer; hence, the energy of radiative emission depends on the HOMO–LUMO transition, which is also related to the specific molecular species and the degree of delocalization of HOMO and LUMO wavefunctions. For example, when monomeric units are linked to form an oligomer, delocalization of HOMO and LUMO wavefunctions occurs if the oligomer presents a planar structure. In this case, a redshift of the HOMO–LUMO gap of the oligomer species with respect to that of the monomer units results. In addition, larger the number of coplanar monomers forming the oligomer, lower the energy of the corresponding radiative emission.

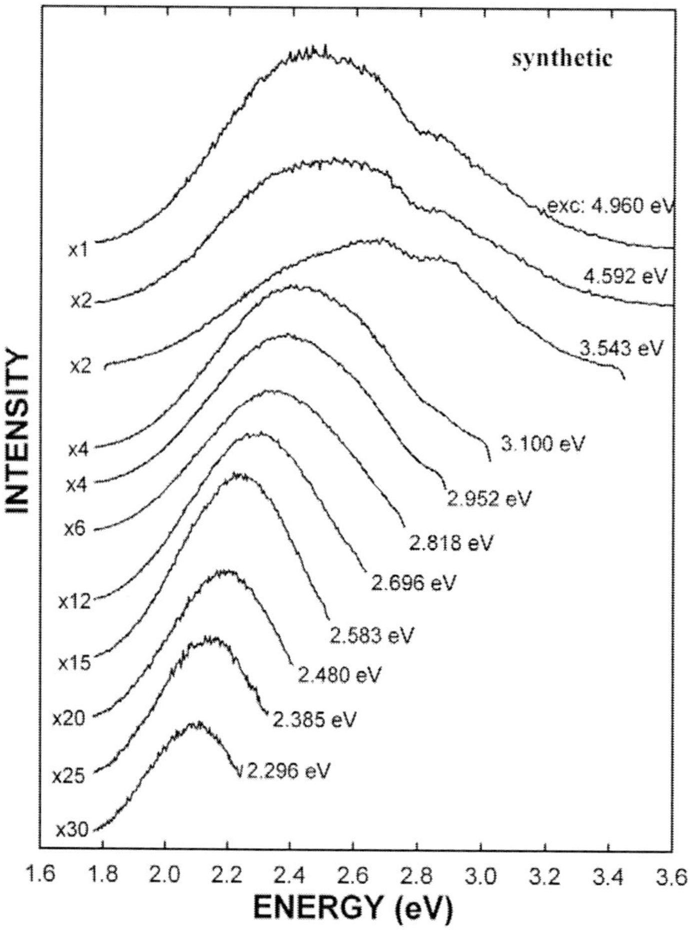

Figure 6. Fluorescence spectra at room temperature of a synthetic eumelanin solution at different excitation energies. The excitation energy value is reported on the right hand side of each spectrum and the sensitivity factor is reported on the left hand side of each spectrum.

The attribution of the FL features can be obtained by investigating the FL emission of eumelanin samples as a function of the excitation energy, shown in Figs. 6, 7 and 8 for synthetic, *Sepia officinalis* and *Rana esculenta* eumelanin, respectively [53, 54]. The FL spectra at different excitation energies have similar behaviours for the three samples. In fact, at lower (visible) excitation energies, a single broad band characterizes the FL spectra, whereas a few bands are present in the spectra at higher (near-UV) excitation energies. Furthermore, the spectral position of the FL bands does not change at higher excitation energies, whereas it red shifts as the excitation energy decreases; the intensity and full-width at half-maximum (FWHM) of the FL emission decrease with excitation energy.

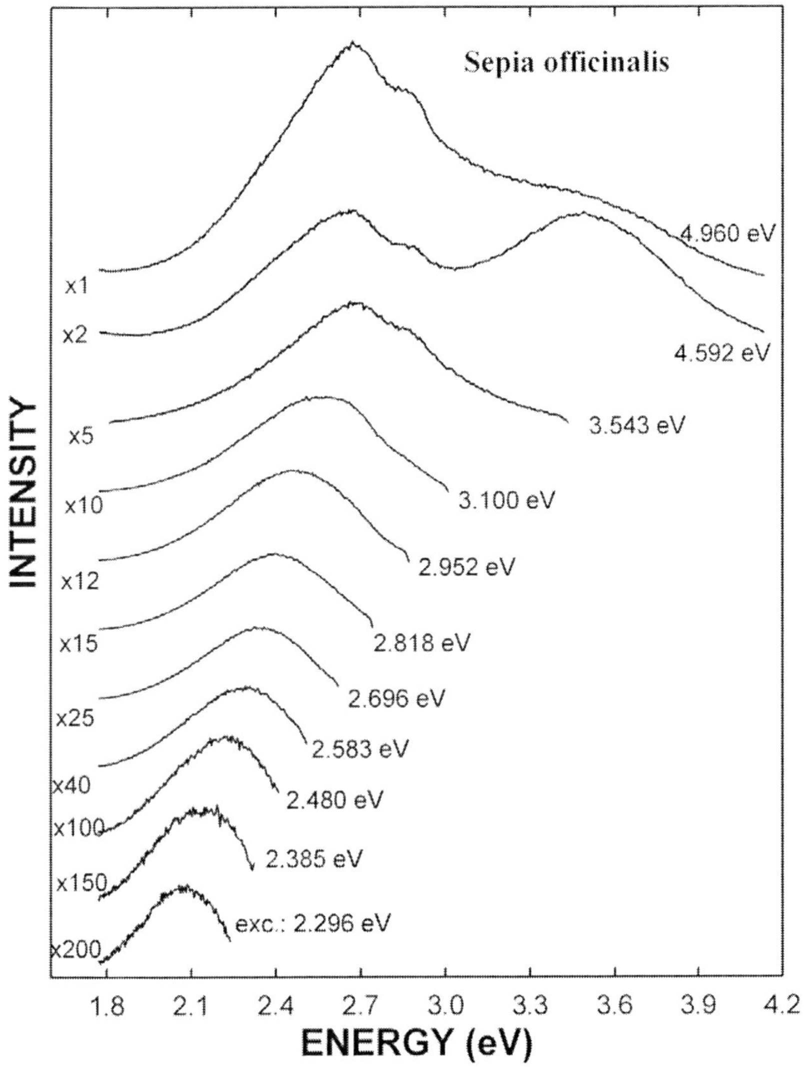

Figure 7. Fluorescence spectra at room temperature of a *Sepia officinalis* eumelanin solution at different excitation energies. The excitation energy value is reported on the right hand side of each spectrum and the sensitivity factor is reported on the left hand side of each spectrum.

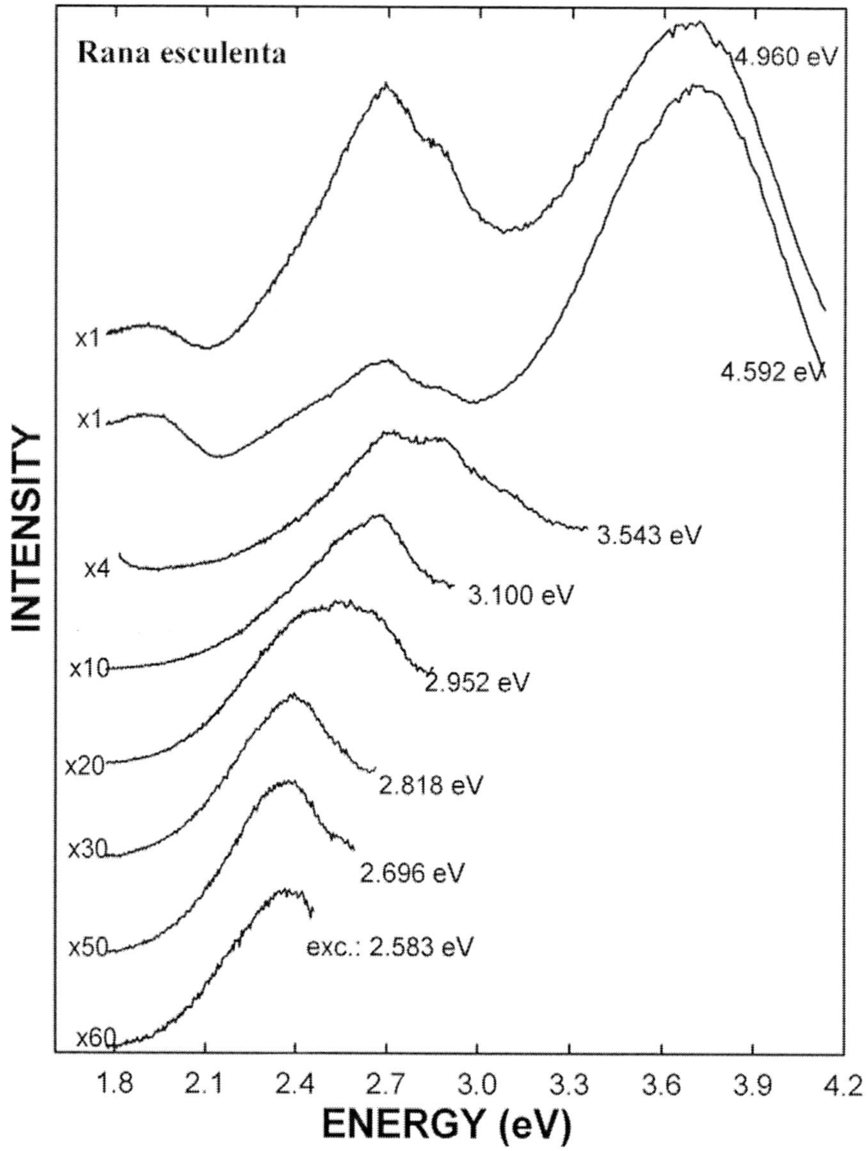

Figure 8. Fluorescence spectra at room temperature of a *Rana esculenta* eumelanin solution at different excitation energies. The excitation energy value is reported on the right hand side of each spectrum and the sensitivity factor is reported on the left hand side of each spectrum.

Such behaviour can be explained according to the "chemical disorder model" [29], which involves the presence of HOMO–LUMO radiative recombinations related to slightly different chemical species, as monomer units and oligomer groups, each one contributing to the emission process with a narrow FL peak. The overlapping of different peaks causes the broad bands observed in the FL spectra. In addition, the contribution of radiative emission due to monomeric units and small oligomer groups can be discriminated from the contribution of polymeric groups in the spectra shown in Figs. 6, 7 and 8. In particular, the FL band observed at about 2.85 eV only in the spectra measured at higher excitation energies for all the eumelanin samples is due to FL from monomers and small oligomer groups. In fact, many monomers (DHI, IQ, DHICA), with different stable tautomeric forms, can coexist in melanin aqueous solution [55]. In contrast, the FL band observed at higher excitation energies at about 2.45 eV in Fig. 6 and at about 2.68 eV in Figs. 7 and 8 arises from radiative recombination of polymeric groups, i.e. entities made of a higher number of coplanar indolic units. In fact, red-shift of the HOMO–LUMO gap occurs in the polymerization form [4].

The independence of the spectral position of FL bands on the excitation energies observed at excitation in the UV region occurs because the HOMO–LUMO gap energy of each polymeric species is lower than the energy of exciting light. Consequently, all the FL centres can absorb incident light and are involved in the emission process. Therefore, the band energy and FWHM remain almost constant, independently of the excitation energy. On the contrary, the excitation energies in the visible region are not large enough to excite all the polymeric species and their selective excitation with lower HOMO–LUMO gap occurs as the excitation energy decreases. The decrease of the number of species having larger HOMO–LUMO gap (i.e. smaller size) causes a red-shift of the peak energy and a bleaching of the peak intensity. At the same time, by lowering the excitation energy, the number of species or radiative centres that can absorb the excitation light (i.e. the centres having lower HOMO–LUMO gaps) decreases and this effect causes a narrowing of the FL band.

The spectral narrowing and shift (about 0.23 eV) of the low energy band in the natural eumelanin samples (at 2.68 eV) with respect to that of the synthetic ones (at 2.45 eV), in the spectrum obtained at the largest excitation energy can be related to the fact that natural eumelanins include oligomer systems (inside which radiative recombinations occur) whose size distribution is narrower with respect to the corresponding systems in synthetic eumelanin. In particular, a narrower size centre distribution corresponds to a narrower HOMO–LUMO gap distribution in natural eumelanin samples with respect to the synthetic one. So, since the fluorescence band results from the convolution of radiative recombinations from the distribution of the excited HOMO–LUMO gaps, a narrower fluorescence band occurs in the natural eumelanins than in the synthetic one. The shift of the low energy band in the spectra of the two kind of samples can be related to a different density of states connected to the HOMO–LUMO transitions occurring inside the chemical components of the natural and synthetic biopolymer.

Macromolecular Structure: Dynamic Light Scattering

The structural organization of the biopolymer and the role of proteins have been investigated also by means of DLS measurements, which allows to estimate the size distribution of the macromolecular components of the three eumelanin samples in solution, as shown in Fig. 9 [54]. It is evident that the distributions of eumelanin particles have slightly different modal values, i.e. 70 nm for synthetic eumelanin and 120 nm for natural eumelanins. The latter value is quite in agreement with analogous results of the macromolecule sizes of *Sepia officinalis* eumelanin as obtained by SEM, TEM and AFM techniques [12, 16]. It is also confirmed that the size of natural eumelanin nanoaggregates is larger than that of synthetic ones, as reported in [16] for indolic planar sheets, although the lateral extent of synthetic sheets was estimated to be less than 10 nm large. Although the modal value of the particle sizes obtained for synthetic eumelanin is slightly lower than that got for the natural ones, the distribution of the particle sizes for synthetic eumelanin results broader than that for natural eumelanins (full width at half maximum of about 180, 147 and 152 nm for synthetic, *Sepia officinalis* and *Rana esculenta* samples, respectively). In addition, a more intense tail towards higher size values can be observed in Fig. 9 for the distribution of the synthetic eumelanin with respect to the natural ones. Since the main difference between natural and synthetic eumelanin is the larger protein content of the former with respect to the latter, DLS results suggest that the presence of proteins modifies the chemical environment in which the indolic sheets are assembled. Further, they aid in the connection of each monomer units and build up large oligomers. Such protein control of oligomers assembly is lacking in synthetic eumelanin. Consequently, the modal value of the size distribution of the synthetic eumelanin particles is lower than the corresponding value of the natural eumelanins, as well as the size distribution is broader in the former than in the latter cases.

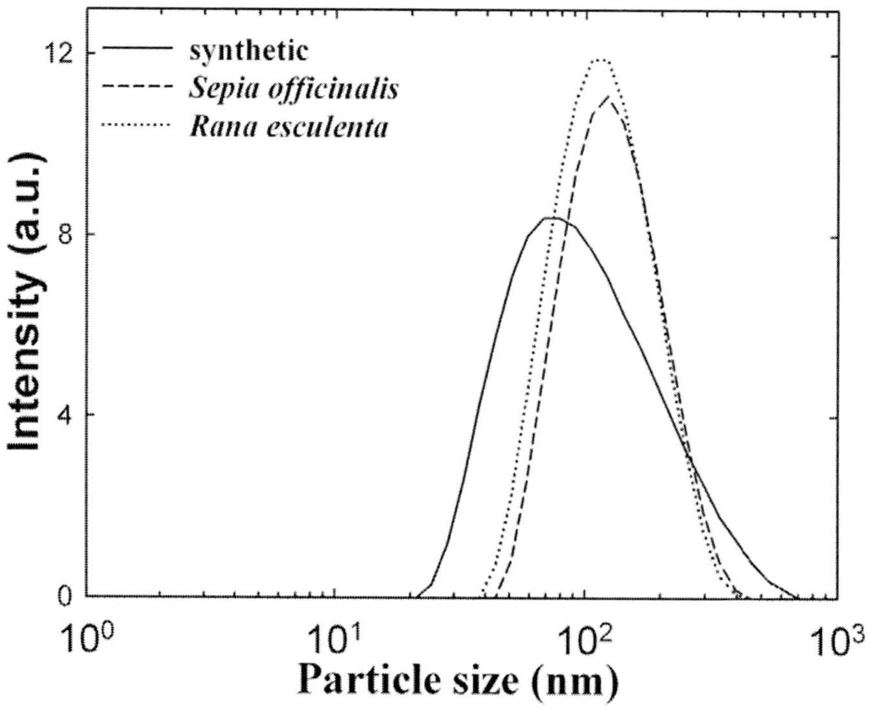

Figure 9. Distribution of particle size for synthetic (continuous line), *Sepia officinalis* (dashed line) and *Rana esculenta* (dotted line) eumelanin solutions, obtained by Dynamic Light Scattering measurements.

Macromolecular Structure: X-Ray Diffraction

The XRD spectra at room temperature of synthetic and *Rana esculenta* eumelanin are shown in Fig. 10a and 10b, respectively. Both spectra are characterised by a broad peak (as it occurs in amorphous and disordered materials), centred at about 25.6° for synthetic eumelanin and 21.5° for natural one. Such peaks are due to X-ray diffraction from parallel planar layers [56]. The peak position can give information about the interlayer spacing *d*, according to the Bragg equation:

$$2d \sin \theta = m\lambda \qquad (1)$$

where θ is the diffraction angle, m is the diffraction order and λ is the X-ray wavelength. By considering the first order diffraction (m=1) we obtain d =3.5 Å for synthetic eumelanin and d =4.0 Å for natural one. In particular, the value of 3.5 Å is in good agreement with the literature value of the interlayer spacing in the stacked sheets model of the melanin [15]. In contrast, the increase of the d distance occurring in natural eumelanin is probably due to the presence of residual molecules (e.g. proteins from the purification procedure) intercalated between the layers, which increases the interlayer distance.

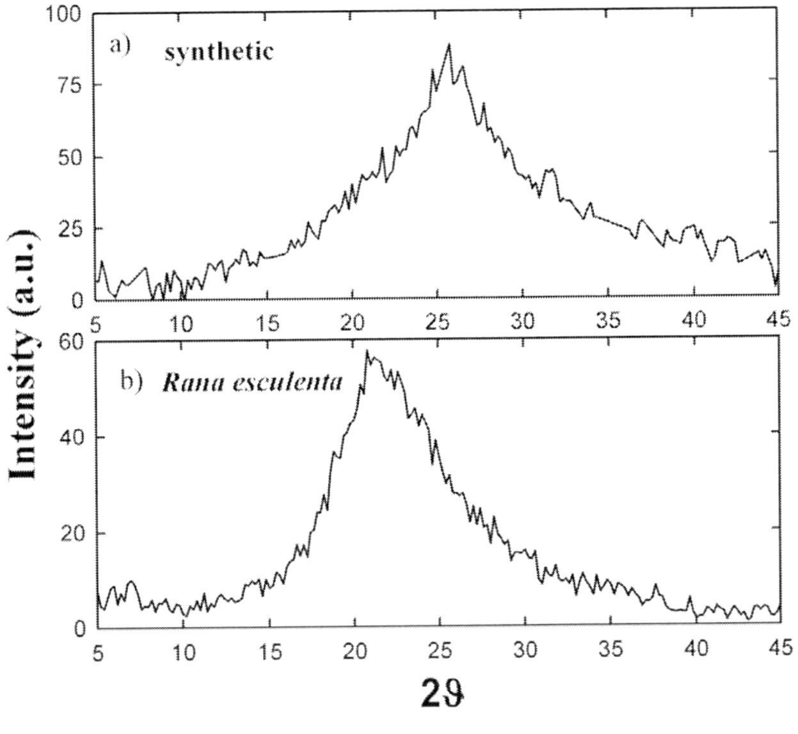

Figure 10. X-ray Diffraction spectra of a pellet of synthetic eumelanin (a) and a air dried deposit of *Rana esculenta* eumelanin (b).

An estimate of the average melanin grain size D can be obtained from the Debye–Schrerrer relationship [57]:

$$D = \frac{0.9\lambda}{(FWHM \cdot \cos\vartheta)} \qquad (2)$$

where *FWHM* is the full width at half maximum of the diffraction peak. The obtained D values are 13.5 Å for synthetic eumelanin and 10.1 Å for natural one. These values support the nanoaggregate model of eumelanin: in fact, they may correspond to the lateral or height extension of the eumelanin stacked sheets protomolecules. In particular, the value D=13.5 Å obtained for synthetic eumelanin corresponds to about four stacked sheets of planar structures. The average size of the natural eumelanin protomolecules is lower than that of synthetic eumelanin probably for the presence of proteic residual in the former: it weakens the bonding forces between the layers and, consequently, counteracts the stacking.

Macromolecular Structure: Atomic Force Microscopy

AFM images of height data for synthetic and *Rana esculenta* eumelanin samples are shown in Figs. 11 and 12, respectively. In particular, the comparison between Fig. 11 and Fig. 12 reveals that the two samples comprise aggregates having similar morphology and size, whose values range from few nanometers of height size and few tens nanometers of lateral size (see cross section 2 in Fig. 11 and cross sections 2 and 3 in Fig. 12) to about ten nanometers of height size and few hundred nanometers of lateral size (see cross section 1 in Fig. 11 and cross section 1 in Fig. 12). The main difference between the two images is that synthetic eumelanin comprises nanoaggregates more isolated than those present in natural eumelanin, i.e. the former seems less organized than the latter. Such behaviour could be related to the role of proteins, which are absent in synthetic eumelanin and largely present in *Rana esculenta* eumelanin. So we can assume that the proteins, which act either as scaffolding matrix for eumelanin deposition or as enzymes involved in melanogenic pathway, are important in defining the assembly of natural pigment.

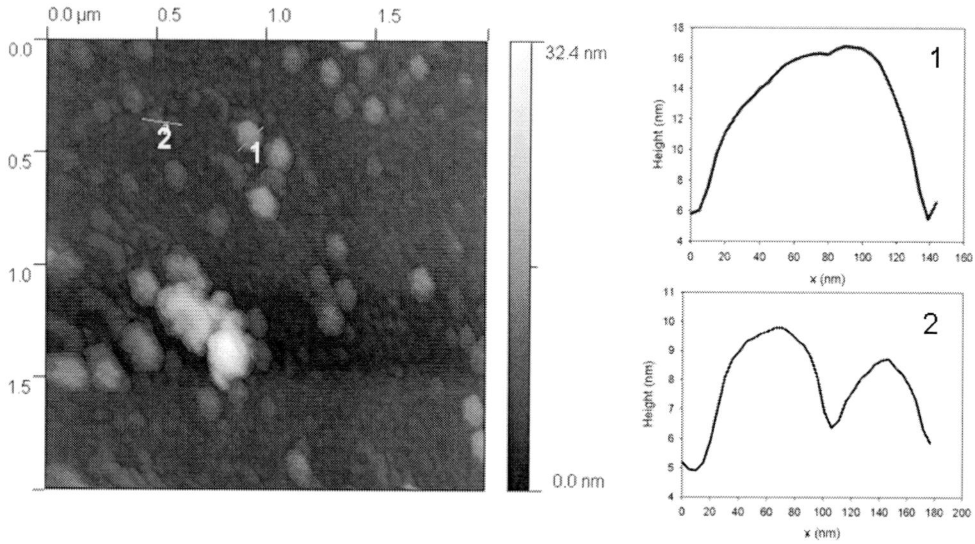

Figure 11. AFM picture measured in non-contact mode topography and cross section profiles (corresponding to the straight lines marked on the AFM images) of a synthetic eumelanin sample, obtained from a drop of eumelanin solution deposited on mica substrate and air dried. The scale bar of AFM image is reported on its right hand side.

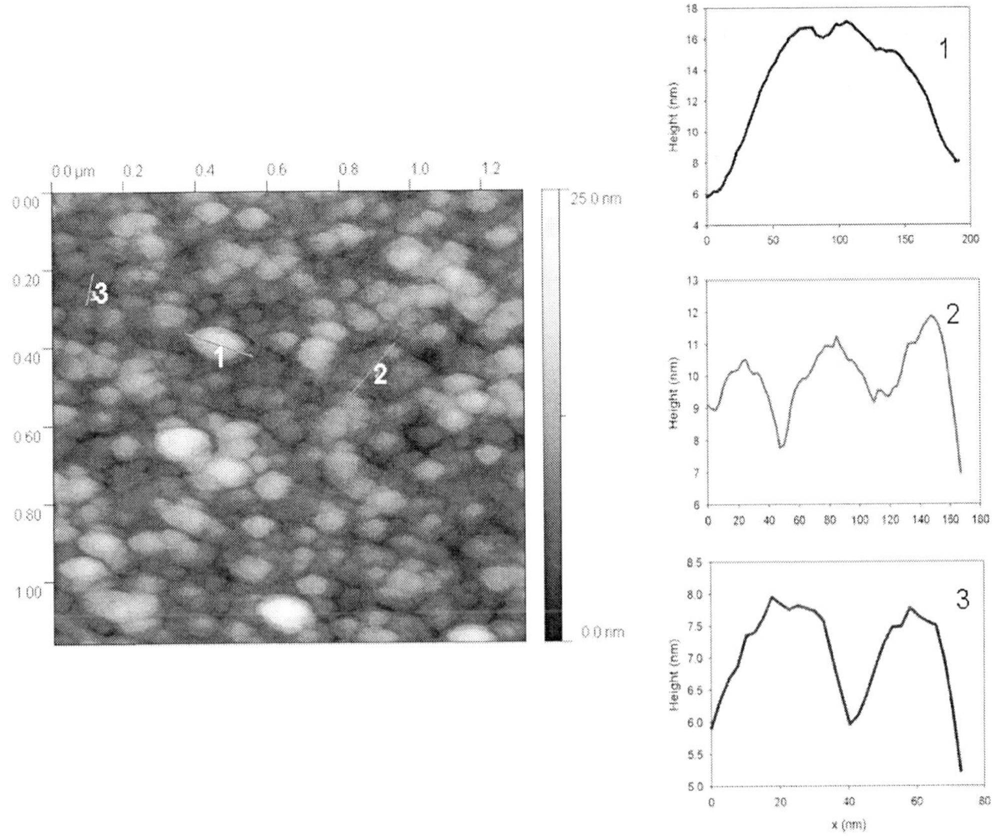

Figure 12. AFM picture measured in non-contact mode topography and cross section profiles (corresponding to the straight lines marked on the AFM images) of a *Rana esculenta* eumelanin sample, obtained from a drop of eumelanin solution deposited on mica substrate and air dried. The scale bar of AFM image is reported on its right hand side.

Conclusions

In this paper review we have described some recent results concerning the optical properties of eumelanin and the structural organization of this biopolymer. The observed properties are explained by considering eumelanin as formed by many distinct nanometric protomolecules, each one consisting of several monomer units arranged in different manner. Indeed, the vibrational spectra confirm the presence of the functional groups present in the main monomer units (DHI, DHICA, IQ and SQ) of eumelanin, whereas the optical absorption spectra evidence the overlapping contribution of many distinct HOMO-LUMO transitions. Moreover, the fluorescence spectra measured as a function of excitation energy indicate that the radiative emission is due to both ensembles of large oligomer systems and to monomers and small oligomer systems. So, a large degree of chemical heterogeneity and structural disorder characterize the nanoaggregate macromolecules building up the biopolymer. Such large degree of disorder characterizes the optical spectra of both synthetic and natural eumelanin. Therefore, it can be deduced that this structural and chemical disorder is a property of eumelanin organization, independently of the presence of proteins. Instead, the structural analysis performed by means of DLS, AFM and XRD techniques indicates that the size distribution of the natural eumelanin has a larger modal value and it is narrower than the corresponding size distribution occurring in synthetic eumelanin. Therefore, the role of protein content in the structural organization of natural eumelanin accounts for the linkage of the large oligomer systems, in order to achieve a size distribution centered at a typical value (about 120 nm in *Sepia officinalis* and *Rana esculenta* eumelanin), which is larger than the typical value of the size distribution of synthetic eumelanin (about 70 nm). This might be related to the biological functions of such a biopolymer, particularly as for its photoprotective action. Today, the physical and chemical properties of eumelanin are known enough and technical applications finalized to obtain eumelanin-based devices capable of long range absorption (from UV to IR) are currently being defined.

References

[1] G. Prota, *Melanins and Melanogenesis*, Academic Press, New York, 1992.

[2] A. Sanchez-Ferrer, J.N. Rodriguez-Lopez, F. Garcia-Canovas, F. Garcia-Carmona, Biochem. *Biophys. Acta* 1247 (1995) 1.

[3] L. Zeise, *Analytical methods for characterization and identification of eumelanins*, in: L. Zeise, M.R. Chedekel, T.B. Fitzpatrick (Eds.), *Melanin: Its Role in Human Photoprotection*, Valdenmar Publishing, Overland Park, KS, 1995.

[4] P. Meredith, B.J. Powell, J. Riesz, S.P. Nighswander-Rempel, M.R. Pederson, E.G. Moore, *Soft Matter* 2 (2006) 37.

[5] S. Takeuchi, W. Zhang, K. Wakamatsu, S. Ito, V.J. Hearing, K.H. Kraemer, D.E. Brash, *Proc. Natl. Acad. Sci.* 101 (2004) 15076.

[6] P. Meredith, J. Riesz, *Photochem. Photobiol.* 79 (2004) 211.

[7] J.B. Nofsinger, E.E. Weinert, J.D. Simon, *Biopolymers* 67 (2002) 302.

[8] K.B. Stark, J.M. Gallas, G.W. Zajac, M. Eisner, J.T. Golab, *J. Phys. Chem. B* 107 (2003) 11558.

[9] J.P. Bothma, J. de Boor, U. Divakar, P.E. Schwenn, P. Meredith, *Adv. Mat.* 9999 (2008) 1.

[10] M. Jastrzebska, A. Kocot, L. Tajber, *J. Photochem. Photobiol. B* 66 (2002) 201.

[11] M. Ambrico, A. Cardone, T. Ligonzo, V. Augelli, P.F. Ambrico, S. Cicco, G.M. Farinola, M. Filannino, G. Perna, V. Capozzi, *Org. Electr.* 11 (2010) 1809.

[12] C.M.R. Clancy, J.B. Nofsinger, R.K. Hanks, J.D. Simon, *J. Chem. Phys.* B 104 (2000) 7871.

[13] K. Bochenek, E. Gudowska-Nowak, *Chem. Phys. Lett.* 373 (2003) 532.

[14] J.M. Gallas, K.C. Littrel, S. Seifert, G.W. Zajac, P. Thiyagarajan, *Biophys. J.* 77 (1999) 1135.

[15] C.M.R. Clancy, J.D. Simon, *Biochemistry* 40 (2001) 13353.

[16] A.A.R. Watt, J.P. Bothma, P. Meredith, *Soft Matter* 5 (2009) 3754.

[17] B.J. Powell, T. Baruah, N. Bernstein, K. Brake, R.H. McKenzie, P. Meredith, M.R. Pederson, *J. Chem. Phys.* 120 (2004) 8608.

[18] Z. Huang, H. Lui, X.K. Chen, A. Alajlan, D.I. McLean, H. Zeng, *J. Biom. Opt.* 9 (2004) 1198.
[19] S.A. Centeno, J. Shamir, *J. Mol. Struct.* 873 (2008) 149.
[20] J. Stainsack, A.S. Mangrich, C.M.B.F. Maia, V.G. Machado, J.C.P. dos Santos, S. Nakagaki, *Inorg. Chim. Acta* 356 (2003) 243.
[21] B. Bilinska, *Spectrochim. Acta A* 57 (2001) 2525.
[22] M.G. Bridelli, D. Tampellini, L. Zecca, *FEBS Lett.* 457 (1999) 18.
[23] E. Harki, T. Talou, R. Dargent, *Food Chem.* 58 (1997) 69.
[24] B. Bilinska, *Spectrochim. Acta A* 52 (1996) 1157.
[25] M. L. Wolbarsht, A. W. Walsh, G. George, *Appl. Opt.* 20 (1981) 2184.
[26] J. McGinnes, P. Corry, P. *Proctor, Science* 183 (1974) 853.
[27] H. C. Longuet-Higgins, *Arch. Biochem. Biophys.* 88 (1960) 231.
[28] P. R. Crippa, V. Cristofoletti, N. Romeo, *Biochim. Biophys. Acta* 538 (1978) 164.
[29] M. Linh Tran, B.J. Powell, P. Meredith, *Biophys. J.* 90 (2006) 743.
[30] M. Gallas, M. Eisner, *Photochem. Photobiol.* 45 (1987) 595.
[31] J.B. Nofsinger, J.D. Simon, *Photochem. Photobiol.* 74 (2001) 31.
[32] S.P. Nighswander-Rempel, J. Riesz, J. Gilmore, J.P. Bothma, P. Meredith, *J. Phys. Chem.* B 109 (2005) 20629.
[33] S.P. Nighswander-Rempel, J. Riesz, J. Gilmore, P. Meredith, *J. Chem. Phys.* 123 (2005) 194901.
[34] J. Cheng, S.C. Moss, M. Eisner, P. Zschack, *Pigm. Cell. Res.* 7 (1994) 255.
[35] J. Cheng, S.C. Moss, M. Eisner, *Pigm. Cell. Res.* 7 (1994) 263.
[36] K.C. Littrel, J.M. Gallas, G.W. Zajac, P. Thiyagarajan, *Photochem. Photobiol.* 77 (2003) 115.
[37] Y. Liu, J.D. Simon, *Pigm. Cell Res.* 16 (2003) 72.
[38] Y. Liu, J.D. Simon, *Pigm. Cell Res.* 16 (2003) 606.
[39] M. Jastrzebska, I. Mroz, B. Barwinski, R. Wrzalik, S. Boryczka, *J. Mater. Sci.* 45 (2010) 5302.
[40] J.B. Nofsinger, S.E. Forest, J.D. Simon, *J. Phys. Chem.* B 103 (1999) 11428.
[41] R. Cicero, A. Mallardi, I. Maida, A. Gallone, G. Pintucci, *Pigm. Cell Res.* 2 (1989) 100.
[42] A. Gallone, A. Sagliano, G. Guida, S. Ito, K. Wakamatsu, V. Capozzi, G. Perna, P. Zanna, R. Cicero, *Histol. Histopathol.* 22 (2007) 1065.
[43] J. Robertson, *Adv. Phys.* 35 (1986) 317.
[44] G. Perna, A. Gallone, V. Capozzi, P.F. Biagi, A. Fratello, G. Guida, P. Zanna, E. Argenzio, R. Cicero, *Phys. Scripta* T118 (2005) 89.
[45] V. Capozzi, G. Perna, A. Gallone, P.F. Biagi, P. Carmone, A. Fratello, G. Guida, P. Zanna, R. Cicero, *J. Mol. Struct.* 744-747 (2005) 717.
[46] G. Socrates, *Infrared and Raman Characteristic Group Frequencies Tables and Charts*, Wiley, New York, 2001.
[47] B. Schrader, *Infrared and Raman Spectroscopy*, VCH Weinheim, New York, 1995.
[48] R.C. Lord, N.T. Yu, *J. Mol. Biol.* 50 (1970) 509.
[49] L.J. Bellamy, *The Infrared spectra of Complex Molecules*, John Wiley & Son, New York, 1962.
[50] D. Lin-Vien, N.B. Colthup, W.G. Fateley, J.G. Grasselli, *The Handbook of Infrared and Raman Characteristic Frequencies of Organic Molecules*, Academic Press, New York, 1991.

[51] Z. Movasaghi, S. Rehman, I.U. Rehman, *Appl. Spectrosc. Rev.* 42 (2007) 493.
[52] H. Du, R.A. Fuh, J. Li, A. Corkan, J.S. Lindsay, *Photochem. Photobiol.* 68 (1998) 141.
[53] G. Perna, M.C. Frassanito, G. Palazzo, A. Gallone, A. Maliardi, P.F. Biagi, V. Capozzi, *J. Lumin.* 129 (2009) 44.
[54] G. Perna, G. Palazzo, A. Mallardi, V. Capozzi, *J. Lumin.* 131 (2011) 1584.
[55] Y.V. Il'ichev, J.D. Simon, *J. Phys. Chem.* B 107 (2003) 7162.
[56] V. Capozzi, G. Perna, P. Carmone, A. Gallone, M. Lastella, E. Mezzenga, G. Quartucci, M. Ambrico, V. Augelli, P.F. Biagi, T. Ligonzo, A. Minafra, L. Schiavulli, M. Pallara, R. Cicero, *Thin Solid Films* 511 – 512 (2006) 362.
[57] H.P. Klug, L.E. Alexander, *X-ray Diffraction Procedures*, Wiley, New York, 1954.

In: Melanin: Biosynthesis, Functions and Health Effects ISBN: 978-1-62100-991-7
Editors: Xiao-Peng Ma and Xiao-Xiao Sun

Chapter VII

Melanic Pigmentation in Ectothermic Vertebrates: Occurrence and Function

***Classius de Oliveira*[1] *and Lilian Franco-Belussi*[2]**
[1] São Paulo State University – UNESP, IBILCE – São José do Rio Preto, Department of Biology. Rua Cristóvão Colombo, 2265 – São José do Rio Preto, SP, Zip code 15054-000, Brazil
[2] Post-Graduate Program in Animal Biology (UNESP/IBILCE-SJRP), SP, Brazil

Abstract

Ectotherms have specialized chromatophores whose pigments are responsible for the different colors of the epidermis. Melanocytes are one type of chromatophore that produce and store melanin in organelles called melanosomes. In ectotherms, cells containing melanin pigments occur in several organs and tissues. These cells are found in the capsule and stroma of the organs, giving it a dark coloration. The function of visceral pigment cells is poorly known, but melanomacrophages are known to perform phagocytosis in hematopoietic organs and also act against bacteria, due to melanin. In addition, the distribution of visceral melanocytes varies with physiological factors, such as age, nutritional status; and also environmental one, such as temperature and photoperiod. On the other hand, the pigmentation in some organs seems to be conservative, and may help in phylogenetic reconstructions.

Keywords*:* Chromatophores; Melanin; Melanocytes; Melanomacrophages; Extracutaneous pigmentary system

Introduction

Chromatophores are specialized cells found in invertebrates and ectothermic vertebrates that store pigments. These cells have many cytoplasmic projections, giving it a dendritic aspect. Chromatophores originate in the neural tube during embryonary development and later migrate to the skin. In the adult, chromatophores are found in the epidermis and dermis [1].

Chromatophores have many types of pigments. At least five types are described in vertebrates. The melanophores are black or brown colored cells with melanin granules. They are found in fish, amphibians, and reptiles. The erythrophores are reddish cells with pteridine pigments. The xanthophores also have pteridine, along with carotenoid pigments arranged in vesicles, which gives it a yellow color. The iridophores have a metallic color due to purine deposited in reflective crystals. As erythrophores and xanthophores, iridophores are also found in fish, amphibians, and reptiles. The leucophores are white colored cells with purine granules, and only occur in fish [1,2].

Chromatophores are found preferably in the dermis of animals. The xanthophores are the most superficial cells of this skin layer, located just below the basement membrane. Deep inside the skin there are iridophores, cells that have iridescent appearance. Even more deep, there are the melanophores. The arrangement of these pigment cells in the skin layers are closely related to their pigment type and which wavelengths they reflect or absorb [2].

In this chapter, we will discuss some hypotheses posed to explain the function of these cells in internal organs of ectothermic vertebrates.

Melanophores: Color Changes and Hormonal Control

Melanophores are found in the deepest layer of the dermis and in visceral organs of ectotherms. These cells are dendritic in shape (Figure 1A), and in dermis are responsible for the dark color and the quick color change. The arrangement of these pigment cells in the skin layers are closely related to their pigment type and which wavelengths they reflect or absorb. This feature dictates its function [2].

Some ectotherms can quickly change the body color through the regulation of chromatophores. For example, the stimulus for aggregation or dispersion of pigments in fish may come directly from innervation or alternatively from hormonal control [3]. Contrarily, pigment migration in amphibians only occurs by hormonal control [2]. This quick color change is physiological and involves numerous types of chromatophores. It is also related to camouflage and social signaling [4]. Physiological color change occurs in animals that can quickly change their coloration through the bidirectional migration of pigment granules within pigment cells. Environmental stimuli that evoke these changes are mainly associated with light intensity, background color or social context [5,6].

Color change may also happens by means of morphological change in vertebrates. It is slower but lasting than the physiological one. A change in morphological coloration is defined as a gradual color change resulting from the increase or decrease in the number of pigment cells or the amount of pigment within cells. Such a change is usually associated with ontogenetic, sexual, feeding, or seasonal changes [5,6]. Melanosomes are dispersed and transferred to skin cells in mammals and amphibians. In these animals, the dispersion of pigments also stimulates the production of new pigment cells in the long term. The morphological change in color is also modulated by hormones, although the regulation of pigment cell differentiation and the transfer of pigments are dependent on intracellular levels of cyclic AMP [6].

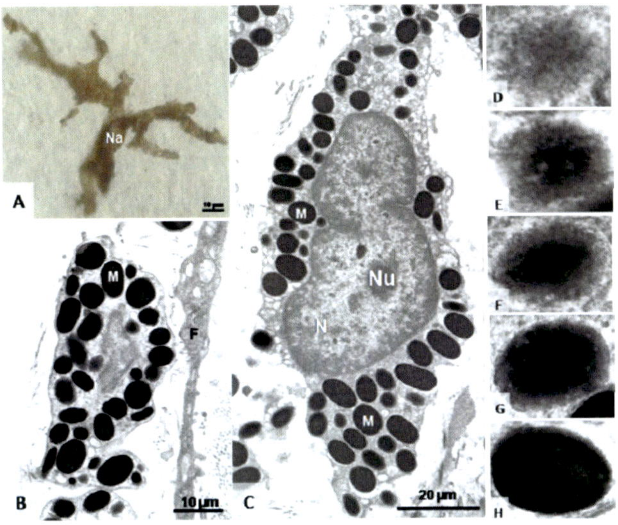

Figure 1. Visceral pigmented cells of *Eupemphix nattereri.* A: Visceral pigmented cells of parietal peritoneum showing dendritic shape. B and C: Electron micrograph of melanocyte of testicle showing association with fibroblast and presence of melanossomes in the citoplasm. D-H: Stages of melanossome development. The granules become electron dense by melanin accumulation. M: Melanossomes. N: Nuleous. Na: Nuclear area. Nu: Nucleolus.

Three main hormones modulate color change in vertebrates. The α-Melanocyte stimulating hormone (α-MSH) is among the best known of these. This hormone regulates both the cutaneous pigmentation of ectotherms and extracutaneous pigmentary system. In the cutaneous pigmentation, α-MSH regulates the dispersion of pigments in melanophores, xanthophores, and erythrophores [2]. In the extracutaneous pigmentary system, α-MSH increases the expression of tyrosinase gene, as demonstrated by Guida et al. (2004) in the liver of *Pelophylax lessonae.* The melanin-concentrating hormone (MCH), which has an antagonistic effect to α-MSH, is a cyclic neuropeptide synthesized as a pre-hormone in the hypothalamus of vertebrates [7]. As a result, MCH influences the aggregation of melanosomes [3]. Melatonin, a pineal hormone produced in darkness, is responsible for skin whitening in amphibians [8]. Melatonin also induced the aggregation of melanosomes in cultures of melanophores from fish and amphibians [9,10].

Melanossomes: An Organelle That Synthesizes and Stores Melanin

Melanosomes are organelles that produce and store melanin pigments. These organelle posses distinct stages of maturation, with different shapes, sizes an electron densities [11,23] (Figure 1B-H). The initial, or pre-melanosomes, have no pigments but distinctive features. At the Stage I, melanosomes have irregular fibrous structures and internal membranous vesicles that resemble typical late multivesicular endosomes (also known as multivesicular bodies). Stage II melanosomes are easily defined in transmission electronic microscopy due to their regular, elongated and parallel fibers. These fibers serve as a mold for the deposition of eumelanin in mature melanosomes. As a result, melanossomes at Stage III are dark and thick. The accumulation of melanin causes a masking of the intraluminal structure of melanossomes at Stage IV. Thus, the formation of melanosomes with characteristic fibers precedes the eumelanin synthesis and is an essential step in eumelanogenesis [2,11].

Melanosomes are mobile structures and move inside cells by the action of motor proteins guided by microtubules: the cytoplasmic dynein, kinesin II, and myosin V. Each protein act differently in the movement of melanosomes, and also the aggregation and dispersion of pigments. Kinesin is responsible for the centrifugal transport, dispersion of melanosomes and consequent darkening of the animal. Dynein is the antagonist of kinesin and are responsible for the centripetal transport of melanosomes, aggregation of pigment cells, and consequent bleaching of the organism [2,12]. On the other hand, actin molecules are responsible for the short or cross transport. This transport is conducted by actin molecules because this route is deslocated from the axis of microtubules. It also allows a greater dispersion of pigments throughout the cytoplasm. In this type of transport, myosin V binds to melanosomes allowing the myosin-melanosome set to slide along the actin filament [2,12].

Melanin in Ectothermic Vertebrates

Melanin is an endogenous complex polymer [13] that occurs in multifunctional forms [14,15] in both vertebrates and invertebrates. The biosynthesis of this substance is initiated by hydroxylation of L-phenylalanine into L-tyrosine or directly from L-tyrosine, which is hydroxylated to L-dihydroxyphenylalanine (L-DOPA) by the tyrosinase enzyme. Lately, L-DOPA is oxidized to dopaquinone by the tyrosinase enzyme, which diverges into the synthesis of eu- or pheomelanin [14,15]. Melanin may absorb and neutralize free radicals, cations, and other potentially toxic agents derived from the degradation of phagocytosed cellular material [16]. Melanin is also a key agent against bacterial components in ectothermic vertebrates, due to the action of hydrogen-peroxidase and their quinone precursors, which act as a bactericide [17].

A unique characteristic of ectothermic vertebrates is the presence of an extracutaneous pigmentary system [18] in various tissues and organs composed of many cells with melanin-filled cytoplasm. The melanin often present in the liver, spleen, kidneys, peritoneum, lungs, heart, blood vessels, thymus, gonads, and meninges constitute the visceral pigmentation [17,19, 20, 21,22] (Figure 2). Visceral melanocytes are localized closed to vessels and conjunctive membranes (Figure 3) and these cells are distributed in both surface and interstitium of the organs' stroma (Figure 4).

Visceral Pigmentation: Anatomical Patterns in Anurans

In anurans, visceral pigmentation is present in several organs of the abdominal cavity, we hypothesize that this pigmentation has a similar pattern of occurrence within taxonomic ranks (species, genera and families). In fishes, the presence of extracutaneous pigment is highly variable, even among closely related species [16].

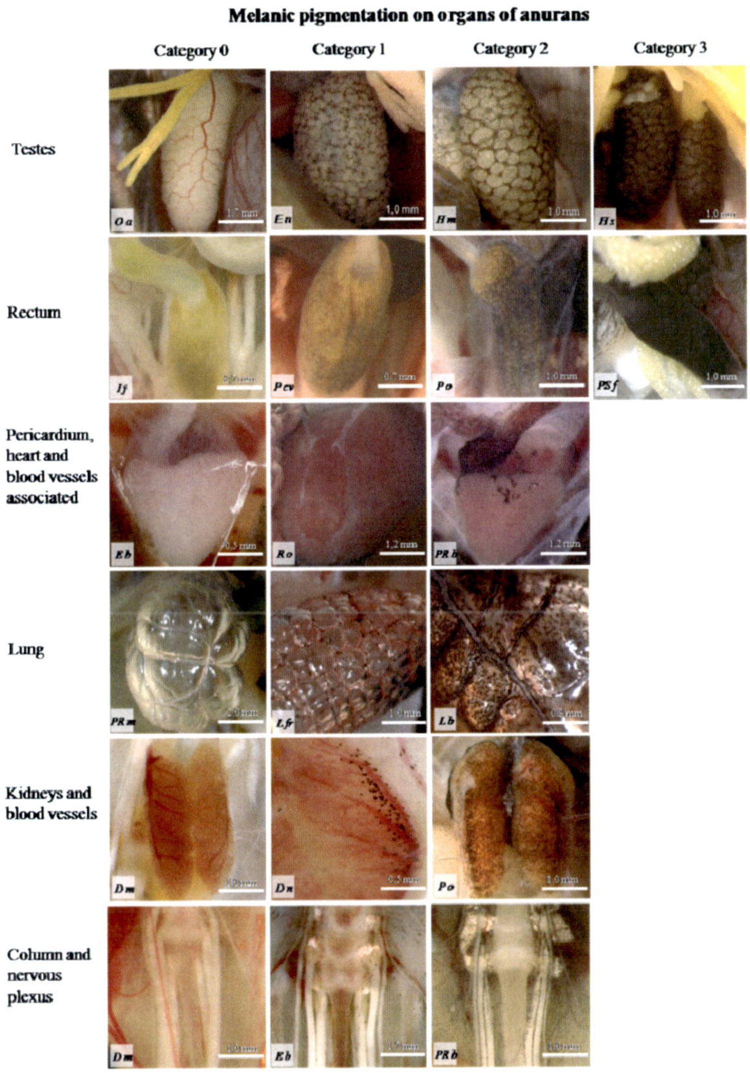

Figure 2. Organs and structures of the abdominal cavity of distinct anurans species showing variation in visceral pigmentation in categories according to Franco-Belussi *et al.* 2009. Category 0: absence of melanic pigmetnation. Category 1: Presence a few pigmented cells. Category 2: Moderated pigmentation. Category 3: Intense melanic pigmentation. *O a: Odontophrynus americanus; E n: Eupemphix nattereri; H m: Hylodes magalhaesi; H s: Hylodes sazimai, P cv: Physalaemus cuvieri; I j:* Ischnocnema juipoca*; P o: Physalaemus olfersii; PS f: Pseudopaludicola falcipes; E b: Eleutherodactylus binotatus; R o: Rhinella ornata; PR b: Proceratophrys boiei; PR m: Proceratophrys melanopogon; L fr: Leptodactylus furnarius; L b: Leptodactylus bokermanni; D m: Dendropsophus minutus; D n: Dendropsophus nanus.*

Such studies found that the pigmentation on the surface of testes of several anurans varies among species and genera. Members of genera *Adelphobates*, *Colostethus*, *Dendropsophus,* and *Leptodactylus* no present pigmentation on the testes [24,25,26]. On the other hand, members of the family Leiuperidae and other Dendrobatidae have melanic pigments on the testes in various degrees of pigmentation [24,25].

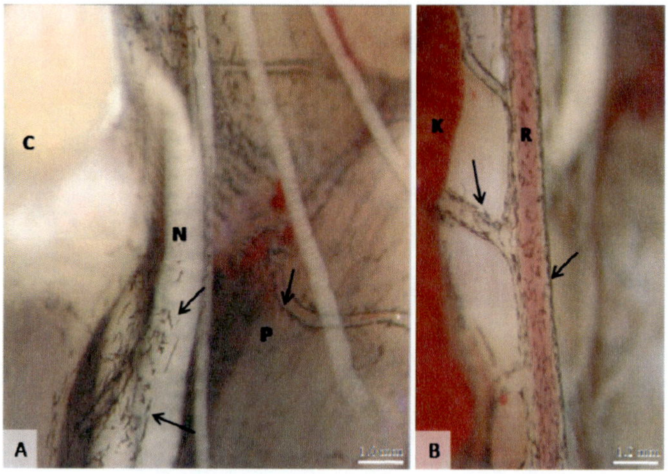

Figure 3. Presence of melanic pigmented cells in conjuntive membrane of nerves of the lumbar plexus (A) and associated with renal blood vessels (B) of *Eupemphix nattereri.* C: Vertebral column. K: Kidney. N: Nerve of the lumbar plexus. P: Lumbosacral parietal peritoneum. R:Renal blood vesels. Arrow: pigmented cells.

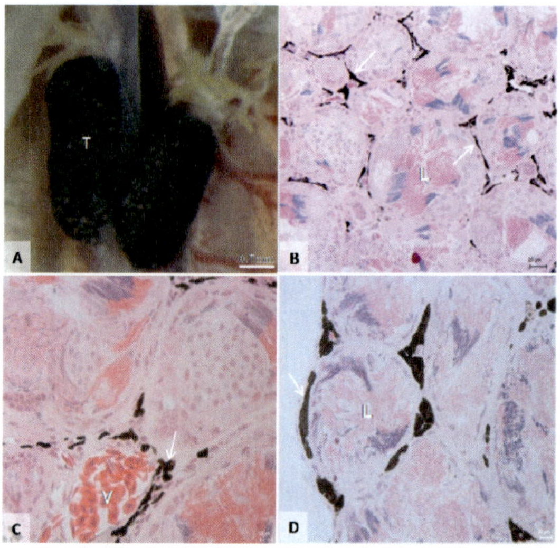

Figure 4. Melanic pigmentation in testicles of *Eupemphix nattereri* showed intense color black on the surface (A, D) and pigmented cells in interstitium of this organ (B) with associated with blood vessels (C) and presence of pigmented cells in surface (D). L: Seminiferous locule. T: Testicle. V: Blood vessel. Arrow: pigmented cells. B-D: Stained with Hematoxilin-eosin.

So, these findings suggest that the visceral pigmentation shows a phylogenetic signal. Although, studies reported that the pigmentation on testes varies. This variation is related with breeding season in the bufonids *Rhinella schneideri* [27] and *Atelopus* spp. [28]. In *Physalaemus cuvieri* testicular pigmentation is present and not varies during breeding season [27]. In the kidneys, similar to testes, the pigmentation on the dorsal surface increased from the beginning towards the end of the breeding season in *Dendropsophus nanus* [27]. On the heart, testes and kidneys pigmentation in *Eupemphix nattereri* increase following administration with *E. colli*'s lippopolysacaride [26].

Pigmented cells in the epidermis and various organs are similar to melanocytes [29,21] originated from the ectodermal neural crest [30]. These cells are able to produce and store melanin [31]. However, additional studies about its occurrence and anatomical distribution are needed in order to determine their biological functions.

The Melanin in Hematopoietic Organs

As mentioned previously, a unique feature of ectothermic vertebrates is the presence of an extracutaneous pigmentary system in various tissues and organs composed of many cells with melanin-filled cytoplasm. In hematopoietic organs, a pigmentary cell types with phagocytic activity are found. Few studies have investigated the functions of the pigmentary system in animals. The majority of studies have focused on the pigmented cells of the spleen and liver.

These macrophage-like cells [32] are derived from hematopoietic stem cells [30] and often aggregate in pigmented nodules called melanomacrophage centers [33]. These centers belong to the mononuclear phagocyte system and its main function is related to the phagocytosis of cellular material derived from catabolism [34]. This evidence suggests that melanomacrophage centers are responsible for the detoxification or recycling of both endogenous and exogenous products [35]. There are also evidences that melanomacrophage centers are involved in the resistance against bacterial pathogens, parasites, and spores [36]. The storage of iron after erythrophagocytosis is also reported [31].

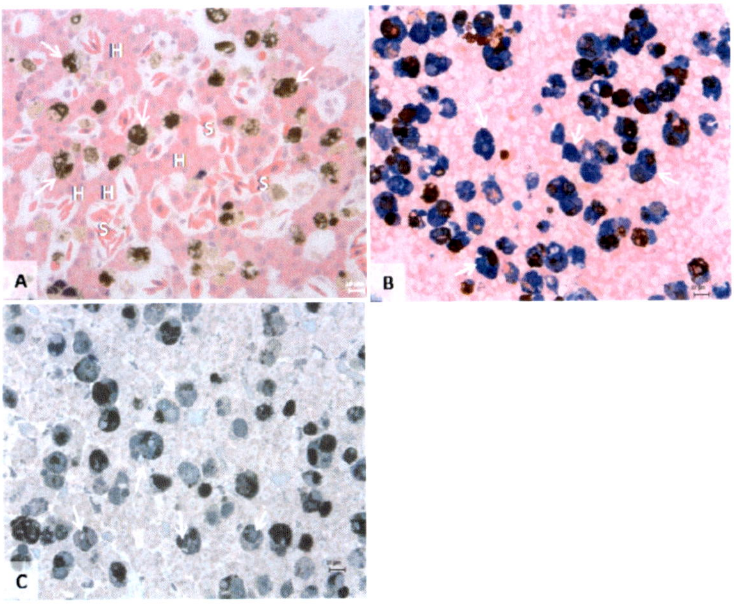

Figure 5. Liver sections showing melanomacrophages in the tissue (A) and presence of hemosiderin (B) and lipofuscin inside of pigmented cell. H: Hepatocytes. S: Sinusoids. Coloration: Acid ferrocyanide solution (B) and Schmorl's solution (C).

The presence of melanomacrophages is reported in the spleen, liver, and kidneys. These cells are known as Kupffer cells in the liver and have phagocytic activity. They can be classified as "small" or "large" Kupffer cells, according to their melanin content [37,38]. These cells have peroxidase, lipase [18], and melanin granules, along with other substances, such as hemosiderin and lipofuscin, derived from the degradation of phagocytosed cellular material (Figure 5) [21, 39,40].

Haemosiderin is a granular substance composed of iron hydroxide and proteins. It is generated in tissues saturated with iron ions and have to accumulate in granules to remain stored inside the cell [41]. The hemosiderin have protein derived from the catabolism of hemoglobin, and therefore it is an intermediate metabolite in the recycling of components in the erythropoiesis [42]. The production of granules of denatured hemoglobin occurs during the catabolism of red cells, which takes place in digestive vacuoles. These vacuoles are yellow-brownish due to iron hydroxide and bile pigments. The color tends to fade out within three to four days, although some partially digested granules may remain in the tissue, producing a yellow color due to the absorption of bilirubin [41].

Lipofuscin, also known as the age pigment, is an intra-lysosomal pigment that are neither degraded by lysosomal hydrolases nor exocitated [43]. This pigment is produced by the oxidative polymerization of polyunsaturated fatty acids and accumulates in post-mitotic cells [44]. During the normal autophagic degradation of mitochondria and iron-containing proteins in lysosomes, iron is released in lysosomes, in which it may react with hydrogen peroxide to form hydroxyl radicals. Depending on the rate of formation of these highly reactive radicals, they can bind to lysosomal material to form lipofuscin or these reactive radicals can destabilize the lysosomal membrane, inducing apoptosis and necrosis [43,45].

Some studies have described drastic structural and functional alterations in the Kupffer cells during the hibernation cycle, a period characterized by low temperatures and reduced food supply. In an experiment with three amphibian species (*Rana esculenta, Ichthyosaura alpestris*, and *Triturus carnifex*), there were much more pigments in the hepatic parenchyma in the hibernation than in the active period [46,47]. In addition, an increase in liver pigmentation may be related to hemocatereses [48,49]. For example, the activation of hepatic melanogenesis in salamanders may be related to hypoxia [50]. Accordingly, the increase of melanin pigments in melanomacrophage centers in fish has been associated with diseases [36].

The Functions of Melanin in Visceral Pigmentation

Moresco and Oliveira (2009) analyzed the extracutaneous pigmentation pattern of three species of anuran amphibians (*Dendropsophus nanus, Physalaemus cuvieri,* and *Rhinella schneideri*) during the breeding season. In that study, the change in the pigmentation of structures during the reproductive period could not be associated with or compared among species, since the occurrence of pigmentation was different for each species. The authors reported that the pigmentation varied during the reproductive period in the toad *R. schneideri.* However, the same study showed that the testicular pigmentation was evenly distributed throughout the breeding season in *P. cuvieri.*

Accordingly, the gonads of *D. nanus*, *D. minutus*, *D. elianeae*, and *D. sanborni* had no pigmentation during the reproductive period [19]. These differences between species of distinct families can be related with similar phenotypic traits, in species that lives in similar environmental conditions [51]. Ours studies showed that is possible determine a pattern for each species, and identify a relationships among within of the taxon. These description of visceral pigmentation represent helpful information to evaluate biological relations in a phylogenetic and evolutionary perspective.

Pigment cells are not found in the gonads of the majority of anuran species (e.g., Franco-Belussi et al. 2011). When present, visceral melanocytes are closely related to the vascular system, as well as blood vessels of other organs and associated conjunctive membranes. Specifically, there is an intense pigmentation in the interstitium and the tunica albuginea of the gonads of *Eupemphix nattereri*, *Physalaemus cuvieri*, and *P. marmoratus*, giving the testicle a full or mixed black color [23,52,53,54].

These cells make up the connective tissue of the organ itself or of tissues associated with it, such as the tunica adventitia or serous membranes. Pigmented cells of most organs, such as gonads and rectum have typical dendritic melanocytes, which differentiate it from melanomacrophages of organs, which have a punctuated appearance. Melanocytes are distributed in both the surface and interstitium of the organs' stroma. Its occurrence may vary from a few to a large concentration of cells, when an intense blackish color is observed on structures.

The visceral pigmentation on testes, heart, and kidneys of anurans increases after the administration of lipopolysaccharide (LPS) from *Escherichia coli* [26]. These cells responded to LPS intoxication promoting a rapid increase of pigmentation on the surface of the testes after 2 hours, followed by a decrease in the pigmentation after 24 hours of administration. These changes are probably related to the bactericide role of melanin, which neutralizes LPS effects [26].

Conclusion

Finally, the pigmentation is an anatomical feature of an organism. However there are very complex relationship between chromatophores and the organs in which they occur. Certainly melanocytes have multiple functions still waiting to be determined. Additional studies about its occurrence and anatomical distribution are needed in order to determine their biological functions.

Acknowledgments

The authors are indebted to FAPESP (São Paulo Research Foundation – grant # 02/08016-9, 05/02919-5, 09/13925-7, 06/57990-9, and 08/52389-0) and CNPq (Brazilian National Council for Scientific and Technological Development – grant # 475248/2007-4 and 473499/2010-0) for financial support and fellowships. LFB received a doctoral fellowship from FAPESP (#2011/01840-7) during the final preparation of this chapter. We would like to thank Msc. Diogo Borges Provete for suggestions in the chapter and revision of the English language, and Dr. Lia Raquel de Souza Santos, Dr. Rodrigo Zieri, Msc. Rafaela Maria Moresco for contributing for the research project.

References

[1] Wallin, M. 2002. Nature's Palette: How Animals, Incluind Humans, Produce Colours. *Bioscience Explained.* 1,1-12.

[2] Bagnara J.T. and Matsumoto, J. 2006. Comparative Anatomy and Physiology of Pigment Cells in Nonmammalian Tissues. In: Nordlund J. J.; Boissy, R.E.; Hearing, V.J.; King, R. A.; Ortonne, J-P; eds. The Pigmentary System: Physiology and Pathophysiology. New York, Oxford: Oxford University Press, 9–40.

[3] Fujii, R. 2000. The Regulation of Motile Activity in Fish Chromatophores. *Pigment Cell Research.* 13, 300-319.

[4] Aspengren, S.; Hedberg, D.; Sköld, H.N.; Wallin, M. 2009. New Insights into Melanossome Transport in Vertebrate Pigment Cells. *International Review of Cell and Molecular Biology.* 272,245-302.

[5] Bagnara, J.T.; Taylor, J. D.; Prota,G. 1973. Color changes, unusual melanosomes, and a new pigment from leaf frogs. *Science.* 182,1034–1035.

[6] Sugimoto, M. 2002. Morphological Color Changes in Fish: Regulation of Pigment Cell Density and Morphology. *Microscopy Research and Technique,.* 58, 496–503.

[7] Kawauchi, H. 2006. Functions of Melanin-Concentrating Hormone in Fish. *Journal of Experimental Zoology*, 305, 751–760.

[8] Lerner, A. B.; Case, J. D.; Takahashi, Y. 1960. Isolation of melatonin and 5-methoxyindole-3-acetic acid from bovine pineal glands. *Journal of Cell Biology*, 235, 1992–1997.

[9] Aspengren, S.; Sköld, H.N.; Martensson, L.G.E.; Quiroga, G.; Wallin, M. 2003. Noradrenaline and Melatonin-mediated Regulation of Pigment Aggregation in Fish Melanophores. *Pigment Cell Research.* 16, 59–64.

[10] Messenger, E.A. and Warner, A.E. 1977. The Action of Melatonin on Single Amphibian Pigment Cells in Tissue Culture. British *Journal of Pharmacology*, 61, 607-614.

[11] Marks, M.S. and Seabra, M.C. 2001. The Melanosome: Membrane Dynamics in Black and White. *Nature Reviews Molecular and Cell Biology.* 2, 1-11.

[12] Nascimento, A.A.; Roland, J.T.; Gelfand, V.I. 2003. Pigment cells: A Model for the Study of Organelle Transport. *Annual Review of Cell and Developmental Biology.* 19, 469–491.

[13] Césarini, J.P.1996. Melanins and their Possible Roles through Biological Evolution. *Advances in Space Research.* 18, 35-40.

[14] Hearing, V. J. 2006. The Regulation of Melanin Formation. In: Nordlund J. J.; Boissy, R.E.; Hearing, V.J.; King, R. A.; Ortonne, J-P; eds. The Pigmentary System: Physiology and Pathophysiology. New York, Oxford: Oxford University Press, 191-212.

[15] Prota, G. 1992. Melanins and Melanogenesis. Academic Press, New York. 290p.

[16] Zuasti, A.; Jara, J.R.; Ferre, C.; Solano, F. 1989. Occurrence of Melanin Granules and Melanosynthesis in the Kidney of *Sparus auratus*. *Pigment Cell Research*. 2, 93-100.

[17] Christiansen, J.L.; Grzybowski, J.M.; Kodama, R.M. 1996. Melanomacrophage Aggregations and their Age Relationships in the Yellow Mud Turtle, *Kinosternon flavescens* (Kinosternidae). *Pigment Cell Research*. 9,185-190.

[18] Gallone, A.; Guida, G.; Maida, I.; Cicero, R. 2002. Spleen and liver pigmented macrophages of *Rana esculenta* L. A new melanogenic system? *Pigment Cell Research*. 15,32-40.

[19] Franco-Belussi L. Santos LRS, Zieri R, Oliveira C. 2011. Visceral pigmentation in *Dendropsophus* (Anura: Hylidae): occurrence and comparison. *Zoologischer anzeiger*. 250,102-110.

[20] Zuasti, A.; Ferrer, C.; Aroca, P.; Solano, F. 1990. Distribution of Extracutaneous Melanin Pigment in *Sparus auratus*, *Mugil cephalus*, and *Dicentrarchus labrax* (Pisces, Teleostei). *Pigment Cell Research*. 3, 126-131.

[21] Agius, C. and Agbede, S.A. 1984. An Electron Microscopical Study on the Genesis of Lipofuscin, Melanin and Haemosiderin in the Haemopoietic Tissues of Fish. *Journal of Fish Biology*,24, 471-488.

[22] Agius, C. 1980. Phylogenetic Development of Melano-Macrophage Centers in Fish. *Journal of Zoology*. 191, 11-31.

[23] Zieri, R.; Taboga, S.R.; Oliveira, C. 2007. Melanocytes in the Testes of *Eupemphix nattereri* (Anura, Leiuperidae): Histological, Stereological and Ultrastructural Aspects. *The Anatomical Record*. 290,795-800.

[24] Franco-Belussi, L.; Zieri, R.; Santos, L.R.S.; Moresco, R.M.; Oliveira, C. 2009. Pigmentation in Anuran Testes: Anatomical Pattern and Variation. *The Anatomical Record*. 292,178-182.

[25] Grant, T.; Frost, D.R.; Caldwell, J.P.; Gagliarod, R.; Haddad, C.F.B.; Kok, P.J.R.; Means, D.B.; Noonan, B.P.; Schargel, W.E.; Wheeler, W.C. 2006. Phylogenetic Systematics of Dart-Poison Frogs and their Relatives (Amphibia: Athesphatanura: Dendrobatidae). *Bulletim of the American Museum of Natural History*. 299-362.

[26] Franco-Belussi, L. and Oliviera C. 2011. Lipopolysaccharides induce changes in the visceral pigmentation of *Eupemphix nattereri* (Anura: Leiuperidae). *Zoology*, 114, 298-305.

[27] Moresco, R.M. and Oliveira, C. 2009. A comparative study of the extracutaneous pigmentary system in three anuran amphibian species evaluated during the breeding season. *South American Journal of Herpetology*, 4,1-8.

[28] Lötters S. 1996. The Neotropical toad genus *Atelopus*: checklist, biology, and distribution. Köln: M. Vences and F. Glaw.

[29] Zuasti, A.; Jiménez-Cervantes, C., Garcia-Borrón, J.C., Ferrer, C. 1998. The Melanogenic System of *Xenopus laevis*. *Archives Histology Cytology*. 61, 305-316.

[30] Sichel, G.; Scalia, M.; Mondio, F.; Corsaro C. 1997. The Amphibian Kupffer Cells Build and Demolish Melanosomes: an Ultrastructural Point of View. *Pigment Cell Research*. 10, 271-287.

[31] Agius, C. and Roberts, R.J. 2003. Review: Melano-Macrophage Centres and their Role in Fish Pathology. *Journal of Fish Biology*. 26, 499-509.

[32] [32] Agius, C. 1980. Phylogenetic Development of Melano-Macrophage Centers in Fish. *Journal of Zoology*, 191, 11-31.

[33] Agius, C. 1981. Preliminary Studies on the Ontogeny of the Melanomacrophages of Teleost Hematopoetic Tissues and Age-Related Changes. *Developmental and Comparative Immunology.* 5, 597-606.

[34] Ellis, A.E.; Munro, A.L.S.; Roberts, R.J. 1976. Defense Mechanism in Fish: Fate of Intraperitoneally Introduced Carbon in the Plaice (*Pleuronectes platessa*). *Journal of Fish Biology.* 8,67-78.

[35] Herráez, M.P. and Zapata, A.G. 1986. Structure and Function of the Melano-Macrophage Centres of the Goldfish *Carassius auratus. Veterinary Immunology and Immunopathology.* 12,117-126.

[36] Roberts, R.J. 1975. Melanin-Containing Cells of Teleost Fish and their Relation to Disease. *In:* The Pathology of fishes (ed. By W.E. Ribelin and G. Migaki). *University of Wisconsin Press, Madisson.* W.I. 399-428.

[37] Corsaro, C.; Scalia, M.; Leotta, N.; Mondio,F.; Sichel,G. 2000. Characterization of kupffer cells in some amphibia. *Journal of Anatomy*, 196,249-261.

[38] Sichel, G.; Scalia, M.; Corsaro, C. 2002. Amphibia Kupffer cells. *Microscopy research and technique*, 57,477-490.

[39] Herráez, M.P.; Zapata, A.G. 1991. Structural Characterization of the Melanomacrophage Centres (MMC) of Goldfish *Carassius auratus. European Journal of Morphology*, 29, 89-102.

[40] Franco-Belussi, L. 2010. Efeitos do processo inflamatório sobre o sistema pigmentar extracutâneo no anuro *Eupemphix nattereri* (Anura, Leiuperidae). Dissertação de Mestrado. Universidade Estadual Paulista – Campus de São José do Rio Preto/SP. 113p.

[41] Granick, S. 1949. Iron Metabolism and Hemochromatosis. *Bulletin of the New York Academy of Medicine.* 25, 403-428.

[42] Kranz, H. 1989. Changes in Splenic Melano-Macrophages Centres of Dab, *Limanda limanda* During and After Infection with Ulcer Disease. *Disease of Aquatic Organisms.* 6, 167-173.

[43] Terman, A. and BRUNK, U. T. 2004. Lipofuscin. *The International Journal of Biochemistry and Cell Biology.* 36, 1400-1404.

[44] Pickford, G.W. 1953. Fish Endocrinology. A Study of the Hypophysectomized Male Killifish, *Fundulus heteroclitus* (L.). Bulletim of the Bingham Oceanographic Collection, *Yale University.* 14, 5-41.

[45] Kurz, T. 2008. Can Lipofuscin Accumulation be Prevented? *Rejuvenation Research.* 11, 441-443.

[46] Barni, S.; Bertone, V.; Croce, A.C.; Bottiroli, G.; Bernini, F.; Gerzeli, G. 1999. Increase in Liver Pigmentation During Natural Hibernation in some Amphibians. *Journal of Anatomy*, 195, 19-25.

[47] Barni, S.; Vaccarone, R.; Bertone, V.; Fraschini, A.; Bernini, F.; Fenoglio, C. 2002. Mechanisms of Changes to the Liver Pigmentary Component During the Annual Cycle (Activity and Hibernation) of *Rana esculenta* L. *Journal of Anatomy*, 200, 185-194.

[48] Cicero R.; Scalia M.; Sinatra F.; Zappala C. 1977. Changes in the Melanin Content in the Kupffer Cells of *Rana esculenta* L. Induced by Parenteral Administration of Heme. *Bollettino della Societa Italiana di Biologia Sperimentale.* 53,764-769.

[49] Kalashnikova, M.M. 1992. Erythrophagocytosis and Pigment Cells of the Amphibian Liver. *Bulletin of Experimental Biology and Medicine*. 113, 82-84.

[50] Frangioni, G.; Borgioli, G.; Bianche, S.; Pillozzi, S. 2000. Relationships Between Hepatic Melanogenesis and Respiratory Conditions in the Newt, *Triturus carnifex*. *Journal of Experimental Zoology*, 287, 120-127.

[51] Pavoine, S.; Vallet, J.; Dufour, A-B; Gachet, S.; Daniel, H. 2009. On the challenge of treating various types of variables: application for improving the measurement of functional diversity. Oikos, 118,391-402.

[52] Oliveira, C.; Zanetoni, C.; Zieri, R. 2002. Morphological Observations on the Testes of *Physalaemus curvieri* (Amphibia, Anura). *Revista Chilena de Anatomia*. 20, 263-268.

[53] Oliveira, C.; Sant'ana, A.C.; Omena, P.M.; Santos, L.R.S.; Zieri, R. 2003. Morphological Considerations on the Seminiferous Structures and Testes of Anuran Amphibians: *Bufo crucifer*, *Physalaemus curvieri* and *Scinax fuscovarius*. Biociências. *Porto Alegre*. 11, 39-46.

[54] Oliveira, C.; Zieri, R. 2005. Pigmentação Testicular em *Physalaemus nattereri* (Steindachner) (Amphibia, Anura) com Observações Anatômicas sobre o Sistema Pigmentar Extracutâneo. *Revista Brasileira de Zoologia*. 22, 454-460.

In: Melanin: Biosynthesis, Functions and Health Effects
Editors: Xiao-Peng Ma and Xiao-Xiao Sun
ISBN: 978-1-62100-991-7

Chapter VIII

Fairness in a Natural Way - Novel Polyherbal Ingredients Inhibiting Melanin Synthesis and Transfer

S. Gokulshankar[1], M. S. Ranjith[1], Babu[2], M. A. Deepa[3], B. K. Mohanty[1] and G. Prabhakaran[4]

[1]Faculty of Medicine, AIMST University, Semeling, Malaysia
[2]R andD Center, Cholayil Private Limited, Chennai, India
[3]Department of Life Sciences, Kristu Jayanti College, Bangalore, India
[4]Department of Biotechnology, Faculty of Applied Sciences, AIMST University, Malaysia

Abstract

Melanocytes produce melanin that determines the skin color. Skin color can be mildly manipulated by use of fairness creams with skin lightening/ whitening ingredients. Some of skin lightening ingredients are harmful to skin and health due to their deleterious effects. Yet the 'quest for fairness' is global and that puts the research on safe skin lightening products as one of the pinnacles in the billion dollar cosmetic industry. Tyrosine is the precursor in the sequels of biochemical pathways that lead to the formation of melanin pigment. Tyrosinase is the key enzyme that mediates two steps in the biochemical conversion of tyrosine to melanin. Hence most skin lightening ingredients exhibit their mode of action by tyrosinase inhibition. Melanocytes are dendritic cells and they are involved in the transfer of melanosomes to the keratinocytes. This process is aided by the dendrites in the melanocytes. Any qualitative and or quantitative changes to the dendrites in the melanocytes would effect the transfer and thereby the melanization of the skin. Besides understanding the tyrosinase modulating activity, it is also necessary to study the effect of the skin lightening agents on the dendrites in the melanocytes. The extracts of several plants such as bearberry, cranberry, mulberry or blueberry are used in the skin lightening formulations. We studied the tyrosinase inhibitory effects of the extracts of *Hemidesmus indicus*, *Decalepis hamiltonii*, *Raphanus sativus* var. *longipinnatus* (white), *Raphanus sativus* var. *sativus* (Red), *Curcuma zedoaria* and *Aloe vera* individually and in different permutation combinations. Tyrosinase inhibition assay, melanocyte cell culture assay, measurement of dendrite length and number of melanocytes were used as methods to evaluate the efficacy of the extract combinations. Tyrosinase activity was assayed spectrophotometrically by following the oxidation of DOPA to dopachrome at 475 nm. B16F10 murine melanoma cells were cultured in Eagles minimal essential medium with supplements. The extracts treated melanocytes were examined under microscope, the number and relative length of dendrites in each melanocyte were recorded at random and statistically compared with untreated control. The polyherbal extract combinations of *Curcuma zedoaria*, *Aloe vera* and *Decalepis hamiltonii* was found to be effective in inhibiting the melanin synthesis and may also have a suggestive role in preventing the melanin transfer to the keratinocytes thereby could bring about the desired skin lightening benefit.

Introduction

Melanin, a pigment which is ubiquitous in nature determines the skin colour of man. The most common form of biological melanin is Eumelanin and is produced by man, animals and certain microorganisms. In man, melanin pigments are derivatives of the amino acid tyrosine.

Skin color in man is of cosmetic significance as fairness and its perception as the symbol of beauty and the pursuit to achieve it through skin lightening cosmetics are universal. Skin color results from the transfer of the melanin-containing melanosomes, produced by the melanocytes, into the keratinocytes in the epidermis and their ensuing degradation. Interestingly, there is only a little variation in the number of epidermal melanocytes between light and dark-skinned individuals[1].

Stratum basale (also known as the stratum germinativum) is the basement layer of the skin that separates the epidermis from the dermis that consists of keratinocytes and melanocytes. The keratinocytes-melanocytes are sometimes referred as "the epidermal melanin unit". Synthesis of melanin by melanocytes, within highly organized elliptic membrane-bound organelles called melanosome, is a complex pathway[2] (Figure 1). Melanin-containing melanosomes move from the perinuclear region to the dendrite tips and are transferred to keratinocytes. It has been estimated that each melanocyte is in contact with ~40 keratinocytes[3]

Any qualitative and or quantitative changes to the dendrites in the melanocytes would affect the transfer and thereby the melanization of the skin. Besides understanding the tyrosinase modulating activity, it is also necessary to study the effect of the skin lightening agents on the dendrites in the melanocytes.

There is roughly a distribution of 2000 epidermal melanocytes/mm^2 on the head and forearm of the man and 1000 epidermal melanocytes/ mm^2 on the other parts of the body. It is also been found that these differences are usually present at birth and exist till death in the normal conditions[1]. Thus, all persons, be it either extremely dark skinned individuals or light skinned ones, have the same total number of melanocytes in them. Then, what makes the difference is only the distribution and location of melanosomes[1].

In lighter skin people, keratinocytes of both the thigh and volar skin exhibit complexed melanosomes while the remaining skin usually processes singly dispersed melanosomes. In contratry to that keratinocytes from the thighs of dark-skinned individuals display singly dispersed melanosomes. But invariably keratinocytes from the lighter volar skin have complexed melanosomes. Interestingly it is amazing to know that the melanosomes in the minimally pigmented volar skin of dark-skinned individuals closely resemble the melanosomes of lighter-skinned individuals. Such findings reiterate the fact that the skin color has direct correlation with the distribution of melanosomes[1].

Table 1. Popular Skin lightening ingredients currently in the market

Active Ingredient	Source	Mode of action
Pre-melanin synthesis		
Tretinoin (all-trans retinoic acid)	Synthetic (acid form of vitamin A)	Unknown
During melanin synthesis		
Hydroquinone	Synthetic	Cytotoxic to melanocytes
Glycyrrhizin	*Glycyrrhiza glabra*	Tyrosinase inhibitor
Beta-Arbutin	Uva ursi (bearberry) extract, Morus bombycis (mulberry), Morus alba (white mulberry), and Broussonetia papyrifera (paper mulberry)	Tyrosinase inhibitor
Kojic Acid	By product in the manufacturing of 'Sake' (Japanese rice wine)	Makes melanocytes nondendritic and decreases melanin content
Glabridin	Licorice (*Glycyrrhiza glabra*)	Tyrosinase inhibitor
Emblica	Phyllanthus emblica	Tyrosinase inhibitor
Tyrostat	Rumex occidentalis extract	Tyrosinase inhibitor
Azelaic acid	Wheat, Rye, Barley, *Malassezia* spp.	Tyrosinase inhibitor
Alpha-Arbutin	Bio-synthetic	Tyrosinase inhibitor
Vitamin C (Magnesium ascorbyl phosphate, L-ascorbic acid, ascorbyl glucosamine, and ascorbic acid)	Synthetic	Acts as reducing agent on melanin pathway intermediates
Melanostat	Synthetic (peptide obtained by amino acid synthesis)	Tyrosinase inhibitor
Paper mulberry extract	*Broussonetia kazinoki*	Tyrosinase inhibitor
Post melanin synthesis		
Niacinamide	Synthetic (amide of nicotinic acid (vitamin B_3 / niacin)	Inhibition of melanosome transfer
Alpha hydroxyl acids (lactic/ glycolic acid)	Synthetic	Remove hyperpigmented cells by exfoliation
Monobenzone	Synthetic (Monobenzyl ether of hydroquinone)	Destruction of melanocytes
Mequinol	Synthetic (Monomethyl ether of hydroquinone)	Destruction of melanocytes
Soy extract	Soya bean	Interaction with PAR-2 of keratinocytes
Pycnogenol	*Pinus pinaster* (French maritime pine	Removes existing melanin
Septiwhite MSH®	Undecylenoyl phenylalanine	Alpha MSH(melanotropin) antagonist

Further, the investigators found that the skin complexion was affected both by epidermal melanin concentration and to a smaller extent by the deoxyhemoglobin residing in the superficial venous plexus. Skin color can be mildly manipulated by use of fairness creams with skin lightening/ whitening ingredients. Several skin lightening ingredients of synthetic/herbal origin [4,5,6] are widely used in fairness/skin lightening creams, underarm lightening creams/ facial and body massage creams (Table 1).

Sometimes extracts of the plants are also used in these formulations. Some of the skin lightening ingredients are reported to be harmful to skin and health due to their deleterious effects. Yet the 'quest for fairness' is global and that puts the research on safe skin lightening products as one of the pinnacles in the billion dollar cosmetic industry.

Tyrosine is the precursor in the sequels of biochemical pathways that lead to the formation of melanin pigment. Tyrosinase is the key enzyme that mediates two steps in the biochemical conversion of tyrosine to melanin (Figure 1).

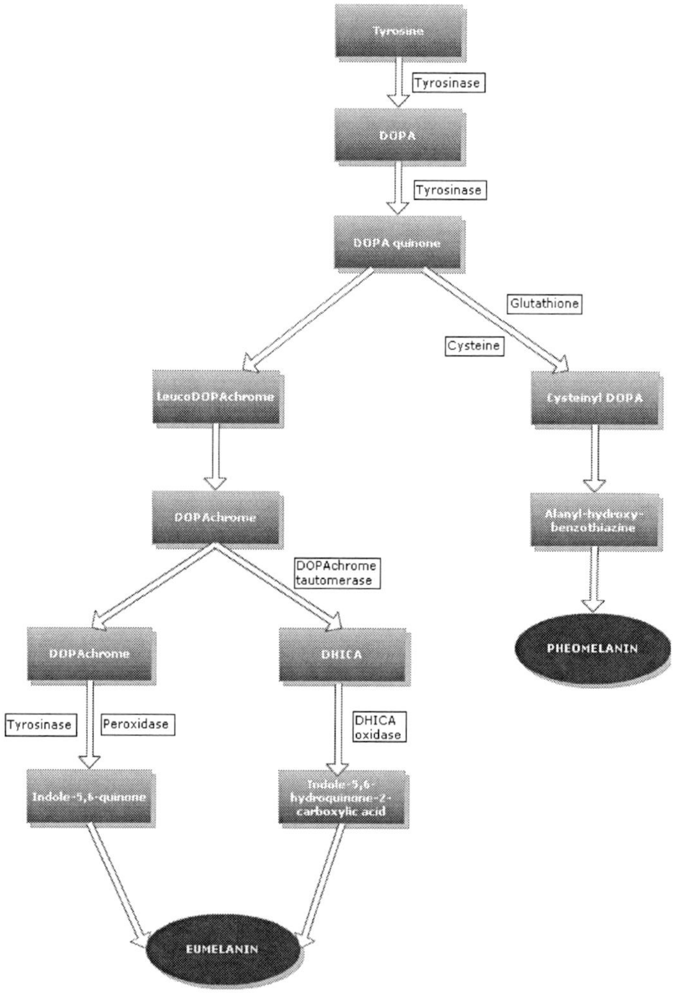

Figure 1. Pathway of melanin synthesis.

Hence most skin lightening ingredients exhibit their mode of action by tyrosinase inhibition (Table 1). Extracts of several plants belonging to different geographical locations have been screened and reported to have anti-tyrosinase activity (Table 2). Further, the anti-tyrosinase activity depends on the plant parts, the solvents used for the extraction and the process of extraction.

Hence, anti-tyrosinase compunds that acts as a tyrosinase inhibitor either by inhibiting the conversion of tyrosine to DOPA or DOPA to Dopaquione and eventually into melanin. So far, a number of anti-tyrosinase compounds are identified, manufactured/extracted and used in the cosmetic formulations. Some are synthetically produced while some are isolated from the plants. Agents such as hydroquinone, salicylhydroxaminc acid, azealic acid, retinoids, arbutin, glabaridin are synthetically manufactured tyrosinase inhibitors whereas kojic acid, quercetin, extracts of several plants such as bearberry, cranberry, mulberry or blueberry are natural tyrosinase inhibitors.

Table 2. Plants screened and reported to have anti-tyrosinase activity from different countries

Country	*Name of the plant*
Malaysia	*Anacardium occidentale, Etlingera eliator, Etlingera fulgens, Etlingera littoralis, Etlingera maingayi, Etlingera rubrostriata, Garcinia mangostana, Hibiscus mutabilis, Hibiscus rosa-sinensis, Hibiscus sabdarifa, Hibiscus tliaceus, Macaranga gigantea, Macaranga pruinosa, Macaranga tanarius, Macaranga triloba, Psidium guaava, Pulchea indica, Quercus infectoria*
Thailand	*Aloe vera, Aspidisra sutepensis, Boesenbergia pandurata, Blumea balsamifera, Coriandrum sativus,Cucumis sativum, Curcuma aromatica, Cymbopogon citratus, Daucus carota* ssp.*sativus, Duguetia uniflora, Eurycoma longifolia, Garcinia mangostana, Herperethusa cernulata, Hibiscus esculentus, Hibiscus sabdariffa, Lycopersicon esculentum, Mabea nitida, Mentha cordifolia, Momordica charantia, Nelumbo nucifera,, Ocimum basilicum, Piper longum, Piranhea trifolia,Psophocarpus tetragonolobus, Rapanea parviflor, Raphanus sativus, Ruprechtia sp.,Schefflera leucantha, Sesbania grandiflora, Trigonostemon reideoides*
Korea	*Cornus walteri, Cudrania tricuspidata,Distylium racemosum, Ficus erecta var.sieboldii, Limonium tetragonum, Maackia faurier, Morus bombycis, Morus alba,Myrica rubra, Phormium tenax, Rhus javanica, Rumex crispus, Toxicodendron succedaneum, Veratrum patulum*
Japan	*Allophylus timorensis, Asparagus cochinchinensis, Bidens pilosa var. radiate, Calophyllum inophyllum, Carex pumila, Cassytha filiformis, Cerbera manghas, Clerodendrum inerme, Crinum asiaticum var. japonicum, Crossostephium chinense, Exocoecaria agallocha, Flagellaria indica, Garcinia subelliptica, Hernandia nymphaefolia, Hibiscus tiliaceus, Ipomoea pes-caprae subsp. Brasiliensis, Ishchaemum muticum, Ixeris lanceota, Lactuca formosana, Limonium wrightii var. arbusculum, Liriope spicata, Lysimachia mauritiana, Maytenus diversifolia, Morus australis var. glabara, Pandanus tectorius var. tectorius, Pemphis acidula, Peucedanum japonicum, Pongamia pinnata, Scaevola taccada, Sesuvium portulacastrum, Sophora tomentosa, Spinifex littoreus, Stenotaphorum secundatum, Terminalia catappa, Thespesia populnea, Tournefotia argentea, Vigna marina, Vitex trifolia var. Trifolia, Wedelia biflora*
India	*Aloe vera, Asparagus racemosus, Curcuma zedoaria, Holarrhena antidysenterica, Lippia nodiflora, Pachygone ovata*
China	*Gentiana macrophylla, Glycyrrhiza uralensis, Lithospermum erythrorhizon, Morus alba, Pharbitis nil, Sophora japonica, Spatholobus suberectus*
Taiwan	*Camellia sinensis, Citrus grandis, Koelreuteria henryi, Malus doumeri var. formosana, Rhodiola rosea*
Thailand	*Cymbopogon citrates, Piper longum, Raphanus sativus, Aloe vera, Sesbania grandiflora , Ocimum basilicum, Momordica charantia, Hibiscus esculentus, Abelmoschus esculentus , Boesenbergia pandurata, Psophocarpus tetragonolobus, Lycopersicon esculentum, Coriandrum sativum, Cucumis sativus, Ocimum sanctum, Mentha cordifolia, Daucus carota* ssp.*sativus*
Pakistan	*Vitex negundo* Linn.

The natural tyrosinase inhibitors are believed to be relatively safer and known as mild agents for treating hyper pigmentation disorders and used extensively as cosmetic agents for skin whitening effect. Synthetic compounds like hydroxyquinone are completely eliminated in modern cosmetics as they can cause allergic reactions, cytotoxicity and mutagenicity.

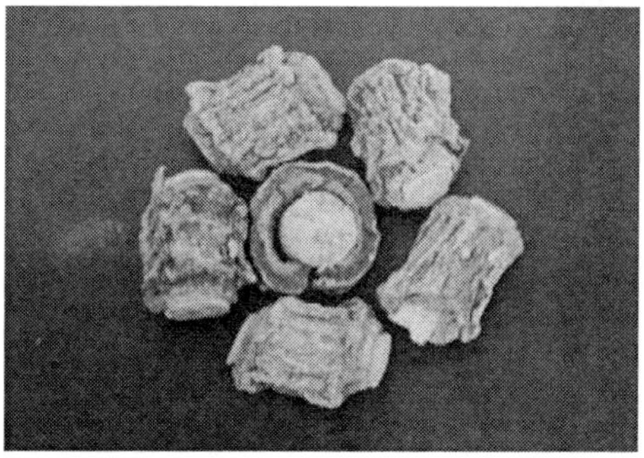

Figure 2. *Decalepis hamiltonii* – Root.

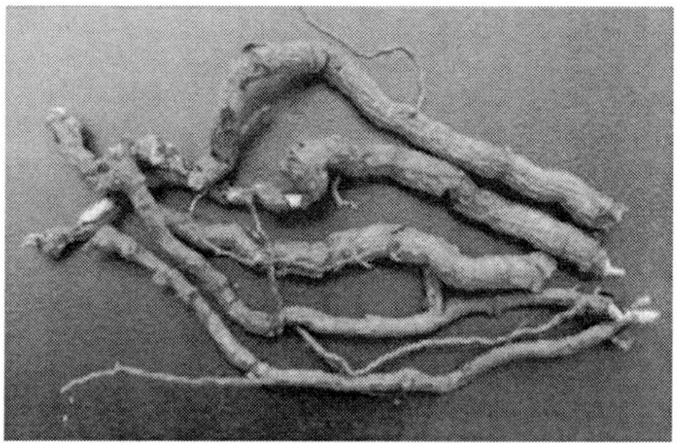

Figure 3. *Hemidesmus indicus* – Root.

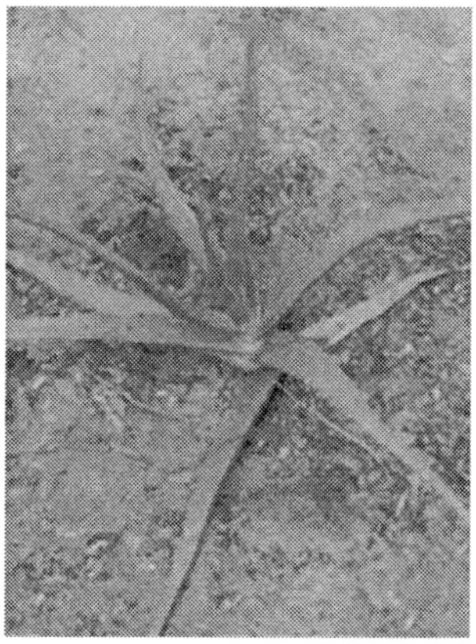

Figure 4. *Aloe vera* – Whole plant.

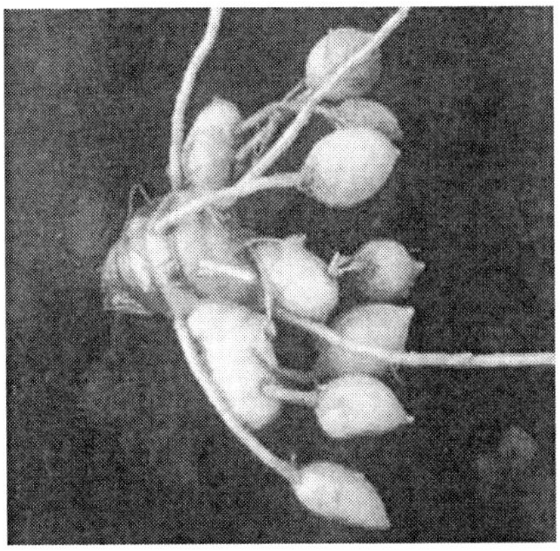

Figure 5. *Curcuma zedoria* – Rhizome.

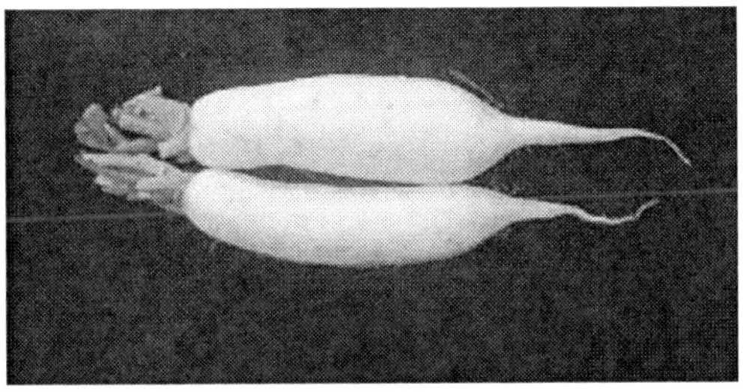

Figure 6. *Raphanus sativus* (white) – Root.

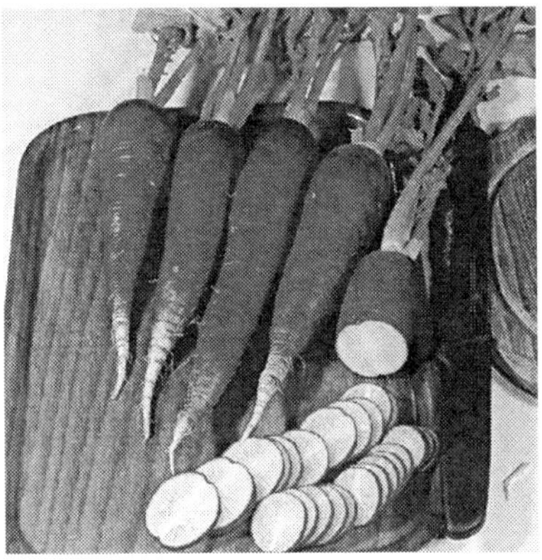

Figure 7. *Raphanus sativus* (Red) – Root.

Melanocytes are dendritic cells and they are involved in the transfer of melanosomes to the keratinocytes. This process is aided by the dendrites in the melanocytes. Any qualitative and or quantitative changes to the dendrites in the melanocytes would affect the transfer and thereby the melanization of the skin. Besides understanding the tyrosinase modulating activity, it is also necessary to study the effect of the skin lightening agent on the dendrites in the melanocytes. Six plants commonly grown/ cultivated in India (*Hemidesmus indicus, Decalepis hamiltonii, Raphanus sativus* var. longipinnatus (white), *Raphanus sativus* var.

sativus (Red), *Curcuma zedoaria* and *Aloe vera)* were identified for the present study(Figures 2-7) and investigated for their effect on melanin synthesis and transfer. The extracts of these plants/plant parts were tested both individually and in different combinations.

Decalepis hamiltonii Wight and Arn. (Asclepiadaceae)

Vernacular names – *Sanskrit* – Svetasariva; *Tamil* – Mavilikizhangu, Mahalikizhangu.

Habit - Climbing shrub with aromatics roots. Leaves elliptic-obovate. Flowers whitish-brown, in paniculate cymes. Follicles stout, short.

Distribution in India– Peninsular India, Tamilnadu and Andhra Pradesh.

Chemical constituents – Roots contains aldehyde inositol, saponins, tannins, crystalline resin acid, sterols.

Hemidesmus indicus (L.) Schult. (Periplocaceae)

Vernacular names: *Sanskrit* – Sariva; *English* - Indian Sarsaparilla- *Tamil* – Nannari.

Habit – Twining or prostrate or semi-erect laticiferous herbs. Leaves linear-lanceolate, often with white streaks above. Flowers yellow to brownish, in cymes. Follicles slender, divaricate.

Distribution – India (Upper to Gangetic plains eastwards to Bengal and from Madhya Pradesh to South India), Srilanka.

Chemical constituents – Roots contain hexatriacotanes, lupeol,α-amyrin, β-amyrin, sitosterol, *p*-methoxysalicylic aldehyde as the major constituents.

Aloe vera (L.) Burm.F. (Liliaceae)

Vernacular names: *Sanskrit* – Kumari; *English* - Aloe ; *Tamil* – Katrazhai.

Habit – Perennial herbs with fleshy ensiform leaves. Flowers reddish-yellow, in long scapes.

Distribution – Native to West Indies and is now naturalized in India.

Chemical constituents – Plant contains aloesone and aloesin. Leaves contain barbuloin, glycoside and isobarbaloin and β –barbaloin, free anthraquinone like aloe emodin, iso-emodin.

Curcuma zedoria (Berg.) Rosc. (Zingiberaceae)

Vernacular names: *Sanskrit* – Kumari; *English* - Zedoray ; *Tamil* – Kachora, Kicchilikizhangu.

Habit – Herbs with rhizome bearing palmately branched sessile cylindric tubers. Leaves with long petiole, oblanceolate. Flowers yellow, in spikes; flowering bracts cymbiform, green tinged with red.

Distribution – Cultivated throughout India.

Chemical constituents – Rhizome contains sesquiterpenoids – curcumol, zederone, fyranodiene, cumolone, curcumenone, zedoarol etc.

Raphanus sativus Linn. (Brassicaceae)

Habit – Annual herb with fleshy fusiform tap root. Roots 22-25 cm long, 3-5cm dia., cylindrical, skin pure white and smooth; flesh snow white crisp, solid and mild in flavour. Leaves in rosette, radical, lyrate. Flowers pink, in racemes. Fruit cylindrical, gibbous at base.

Distribution – Uttar Pradesh, Punjab, Maharastra and Baroda (India).

Chemical constituents – Roots contains Vit-A,C and proteins.

Table 3. Details of plants and parts used for extraction

Botanical name	Common English name	Part used
Hemidesmus indicus	Indian Sarsaparilla	Root
Decalepis hamiltonii	Swallow root	Root
Raphanus sativus var. *longipinnatus*	Radish (White)	Root
Raphanus sativus var. sativus	Radish (Red)	Root
Curcuma zedoaria	Zedoary (White turmeric)	Rhizome
Aloe vera	Aloe, Burn plant	Leaves

Cell Culture

B16F10 murine melanoma cells were cultured in Eagles minimal essential medium supplemented with 10% heat inactivated fetal bovine serum and 2mM L-glutamine at 37°C in a humidified atmosphere containing 5% CO_2. Different concentrations of the extracts of the herbs were used for the study on as is basis and in different permutation combinations. Extracts ranging from 1-5 μl were added to the culture after the cells were seeded. The cells were incubated for 24, 48 or 72 hrs. After incubation the cell numbers were determined by counting using a haemocytometer chamber. Melanin contents and Tyrosinase activities were also determined[7] in triplicate for each treatment as detailed below.

Melanin Measurement

Melanin content was measured as per the method described below. Approximately 10 [7] cells were pelleted by centrifugation at 1000 g for 5 minutes and then washed twice with phosphate buffered saline.

After further centrifugation, the supernatant was decanted, the precipitated cells were suspended in 200 μl of distilled water, and 1 ml of ethanol- ether 1:1 was added to remove opaque substances other than melanin. The mixture was then stored and suspended at room temperature for 15 minutes.

After further centrifugation at 3000 g for 5 minutes, the precipitate was solubilized by treatment with 1 ml 1N NaOH/10% dimethyl sulfoxide at 80°C for 30 minutes in a capped tube. The absorbance was measured at 400 nm and the melanin content per cell was calculated and expressed as percentage of control (=100%) using standard procedure[7].

Tyrosinase Assay

Tyrosinase activity was assayed as DOPA oxidase activity [7]. Approximately 107 cells were pelleted and then washed twice with phosphate buffered saline. After centrifugation, the supernatant was decanted. The cell pellet was dissolved in 1.0 ml of 0.5% sodium deoxycholate in distilled water and allowed to stand at 0°C for 15 minutes.

Tyrosinase activity was assayed spectrophotometrically by following the oxidation of DOPA to dopachrome at 475 nm. The reaction mixture consisting of 3 ml of 0.1% L-DOPA in 0.1 M phosphate buffer, pH6.8 was mixed with cell lysate.

Assay was performed at 37°C in a spectrophotometer. The reaction rate was measured during the first 10 minutes of the reaction while it was linear. Corrections for auto oxidation of L DOPA in controls were made. Specific activity was defined as the amount of DOPAchrome formed per 10 min per cell, and is expressed as percentage control (=100).

Dendrite Length and Number Measurement

The extracts treated melanocytes were examined under microscope and the number and relative length of dendrites in each melanocytes were recorded at random and compared with untreated control[7].

A New Breakthrough in Skin Lightening Benefit: Synergy of Poly Herbal Combination in Inhibiting Melanin Synthesis and Transfer

1) *Curcuma zedoaria* recorded the highest anti-tyrosinase activity followed by *Decalepis hamiltonii* (Table 4)
2) Based on the above findings the following combinations were made with three herbal extracts (in 1:1:1 ratio) keeping *Curcuma zedoaria* and *Decalepis hamiltonii* in all the four combinations.

   a) *Aloe vera*, *Curcuma zedoaria* and *Decalepis hamiltonii*
   b) *Raphanus sativus* var. *longipinnatus*, *Curcuma zedoaria* and *Decalepis hamiltonii*
   c) *Raphanus sativus* var. *sativus*, *Curcuma zedoaria* and *Decalepis hamiltonii*
   d) *Hemidesmus indicus*, *Curcuma zedoaria* and *Decalepis hamiltonii*

Aloe Vera was found to be synergistic with the combined poly herbal extract of *Curcuma zedoaria* and *Decalepis hamiltonii* in exhibiting anti-tyrosinase activity and inhibiting the dentrite length and numbers in the melanocytes which indirectly affects the melanin transfer to the keratinocytes. A similar synergistic activity was also recorded with the poly hebal combination of *Hemidesmus indicus, Curcuma zedoaria* and *Decalepis hamiltonii* (Table 5).

Table 4. Effect of individual plant extracts on Tyrosinase inhibition, dendrite length and number

Plants	Tyrosinase inhibition %	Dendrite length (μm)	Dendrite number
Hemidesmus indicus	51	70 ±2	12 ±3
Decalepis hamiltonii	64	68 ±4	7 ±2
Raphanus sativus var. longipinnatus	40	85 ±3	15 ±3
Raphanus sativus var. sativus	41	96 ±3	15 ±2
Curcuma zedoaria	68	65 ±4	8 ±2
Aloe vera	49	87 ±3	11 ±3
Control	-	108 ±4	17 ±3

Table 5. Effect of polyherbal extracts on Tyrosinase inhibition, dendrite length and number

Extract combinations	Tyrosinase inhibition %	Dendrite length (μm)	Dendrite number
Control	-	108 ±4	17 ±3
Aloe vera, Curcuma zedoaria and *Decalepis hamiltonii*	73	61 ±2	6 ±2
Raphanus sativus var. longipinnatus, *Curcuma zedoaria* and *Decalepis hamiltonii*	68	75 ±3	10 ±3
Raphanus sativus var. sativus, *Curcuma zedoaria* and *Decalepis hamiltonii*	65	80 ±3	11 ±2
Hemidesmus indicus, Curcuma zedoaria and *Decalepis hamiltonii*	70	60 ±2	7 ± 2

3) The dendrite length (μm) of the control was 108 ±6 while the best of the polyherbal combinations showed a reduction in the length to a level of 60-61 ±4. A similar reduction of the dendrite number 6-7±2 was observed as against the control which recorded 17±3.
4) *Aloe vera, Curcuma zedoaria* and *Decalepis hamiltonii* polyherbal extract combination recorded a maximum reduction of 71% in the melanin content assay

5) Hakozaki et al[8] have reported that niacinamide reduces cutaneous pigmentation by suppression of melanosome transfer. Such an effect can occur because of reduced number of dendrites on melanoctyes or reduction in their length. Krishnamoorthy et al[7] are the first to record that poly herbal extracts can bring about reduction in the dendrite length and number. In our present study we have reestablished the fact that poly herbal extracts combination can bring about suppression of melanosome transfer effectively. A schematic representation of the reduction in dendrite length and number in extract treated melanocyte in comparison to the control is represented in Fig 8 and 9.

Table 6. Effect of polyyherbal extracts on melanin content

Plants	Melanin inhibition (%)
Aloe vera, Curcuma zedoaria and *Decalepis hamiltonii*	71
Raphanus sativus var. longipinnatus, *Curcuma zedoaria* and *Decalepis hamiltonii*	64
Raphanus sativus var. sativus, *Curcuma zedoaria* and *Decalepis hamiltonii*	56
Hemidesmus indicus, Curcuma zedoaria and *Decalepis hamiltonii*	69

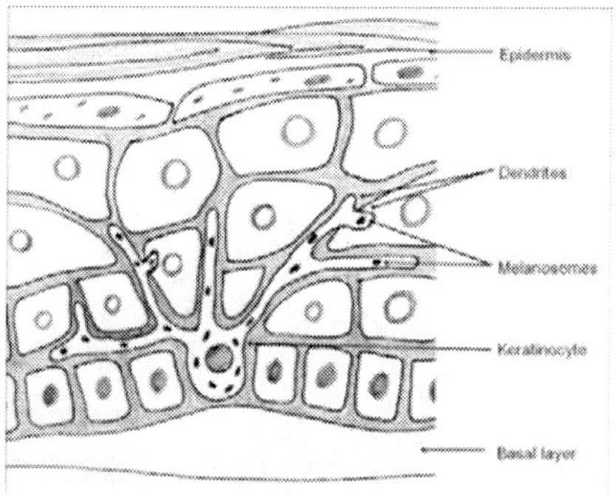

Figure 8. Schematic representation of Melanocyte with normal dendrites and melanosmoes – Control.

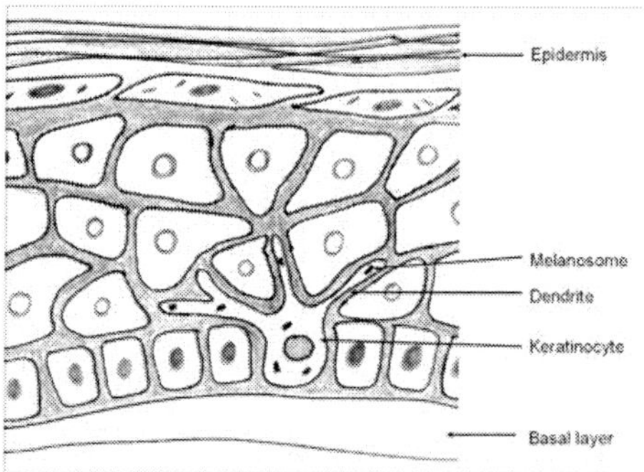

Figure 9. Schematic representation of Melanocyte with reduced number of dendrites with shortened length- treated with polyherbal extract.

Conclusion

Beauty is a qualitative element that boosts the self esteem of a person and is a joy for the eyes of the beholder. Aesthetic appearance is indeed the pleasure to the senses and the esteemed status that beauty offered to people is commendable since the primordial times [9] Cosmetology, the science of alteration of appearance has gained popularity with time. In countries like India, the art of beautifications finds its origin from the traditional fields of medical science like Siddha and Ayurveda. The secrets of the glorious medicinal herbs were confidentially written on palm leaves and were carefully handed over for ages from Guru (teacher) to Shishya (taught) in a closed circuit. Hence the age of herbal cosmetics is much older than the modern cosmetics. In recent years there is a rediscovery of this traditional knowledge and the market research shows the growing interest on herbal cosmetics and natural beauty among consumers world wide [10]. The current study in fact highlighted the cosmetic potential of poly herbal extracts especially in skin care management. There are several herbal formulations/ingredients available in the market that confers skin lightening benefit by inhibiting melanin synthesis at different stages. One of the most obvious cellular targets for depigmenting agents is the enzyme tyrosinase[11]. Since a huge number of tyrosinase inhibitors have been developed [12-15], clarifying the validation of these inhibitors in skin-whitening efficiency has become more relevant and important [16]. The current study reveals the need to adopt the following approaches for better and effective results on skin lightening benefit and highlights the possibility of exploring polyherbal extracts as skin lightening ingredients in cosmetic formulations

a) It is important to screen the time tested herbs of the traditional system of Medicine like Siddha and Ayurveda through modern research methods and establish their cosmetic claims through *in vitro* substantiation studies and thereby rediscover the secrets of the traditional knowledge in modern cosmetology.
b) It is better to use a combination of poly herbal extracts that act at different stages of melanin synthesis than using a stand alone herbal extract in a skin lightening formulation with a single mode of action viz not only in effective tyrosinase inhibition (during the process of melanin synthesis) but also in preventing the melanin transfer to the keratinocytes (post melanin synthesis)
c) It is necessary to screen and study the poly herbal extract for a combined synergistic effect for effective functional benefits in cosmetics.
d) It is ideal to screen the anti-tyrosinase activity/melanin synthesis inhibition activity of plant products extracted using non- toxic solvents like water and propylene glycol as used in the present investigation. Such extraction enables easy miscibility of the poly herbal extract in the same solvents used for extraction during formulation of cosmetics which makes the cosmetic more skin and eco-friendly.
e) Poly herbal extracts of *Aloe vera*, *Curcuma zedoaria* and *Decalepis hamiltonii or Hemidesmus indicus*, *Curcuma zedoaria* and *Decalepis hamiltonii* were found to be effective in inhibiting the melanin synthesis and may also have a suggestive role in preventing the melanin transfer to the keratinocytes thereby could bring about the desired skin lightening benefit. The reduction in melanin synthesis is evident from

tyrosinase inhibition assay and the melanin measurement done on the treated and control cells

f) Poly herbal extracts of *Aloe vera, Curcuma zedoaria* and *Decalepis hamiltonii or Hemidesmus indicus, Curcuma zedoaria* and *Decalepis hamiltonii* can be further evaluated for skin lightening benefits by formulating these synergistic herbal extracts in cosmetic formulations and tested for the functional claims through clinical trials.

References

[1] Leslie Baumann, Sogol Saghari (2009), Skin Pigmentation and Pigmentation Disorders Leslie Baumann eds. Cosmetic Dermatology: Principles and Practice, ISBN: 978-0-07-164128-9 McGraw-Hill.

[2] Hearing, V. J. (1997) The regulation of melanin production. Hori, W. eds. *Drug Discovery Approaches for Developing Cosmeceuticals, Advanced Skin Care and Cosmetic Products*, 3.1.1-3.1.21 IBC Library Series Southborough, Massachusetts.

[3] Fitzpatrick, T. B., Breathnach, A. S. (1963) The epidermal melanin unit system. *Dermatol. Wochenschr.,* 147:481-489.

[4] Kim, Y.J.; Uyama, H. Tyrosinase inhibitors from natural and synthetic sources: structure, inhibition mechanism and perspective for the future. *Cell. Mol. Life Sci.,* 2005, *62*, 1707-1723.

[5] Parvez, S.; Kang, M.; Chung, H.S.; Bae, H. Naturally occurring tyrosinase inhibitors: mechanism and applications in skin health, cosmetics and agriculture industries. *Phytother. Res.,* 2007, *21*, 805-816.

[6] Rendon, M.I.; Gaviria, J.I. Review of skin-lightening agents. *Dermatol. Surg.*, 2005, *31*, 886-889.

[7] Krishnamoorthy J.R., Ranjith M.S., Gokulshankar S (2010) Extract combinations of Curcuma zedoaria and Aloe vera inhibit melanin synthesis and dendrite formation in murine melanoma cells *Journal of Applied Cosmetology*:25:95-100.

[8] Hakozaki T, Minwalla L, Zhuang J, et al. (2002). "The effect of niacinamide on reducing cutaneous pigmentation and suppression of melanosome transfer". Br. J. Dermatol., 147 (1): 20–31. doi:10.1046/j.1365-2133.2002.04834.x. PMID 12100180.

[9] Prashant LK, Hemant RJ, Prasad T, et al. (2005) Cosmetics potential of herbal extracts. *Natural Product radiance*, 4(4): 315-321.

[10] Ashawat M.S., Madhuri Banchhor, Shailendra Saraf, Swarnlata Saraf, (2009) Herbal Cosmetics "Trends in Skin Care Formulation" *Pharmacognosy Review*, 3(5), 82-89.

[11] Nico Smit, Jana Vicanova and Stan Pavel (2009) The Hunt for Natural Skin Whitening Agents International *Journal of Molecular Sciences*, 10,5326-5349.

[12] Kuo-Hsien Wang, Rong-Dih Lin , Feng-Lin Hsu et al (2006) Cosmetic applications of selected traditional Chinese herbal medicines *Journal of Ethnopharmacology*.106,353–359.

[13] Vuthy TY, Natalia Drouart, Mathieu Leti et al. (2011) Screening of anti-tyrosinase activity of Cambodian plants. Mekong Health Congress, University of Health Sciences of Cambodia.

[14] Nithya Narayanaswamy, Arun Duraisamy, Balakrishnan KP (2011) Screening of some Medicinal Plants for their Antityrosinase and Antioxidant activities International *Journal of PharmTech Research*, 3(2) 1107-1112.

[15] Ji-Young Moon, Eun-Young Yim, Gwanpil Song et al (2010) Screening of elastase and tyrosinase inhibitory activity from Jeju Island plants. *Eur.Asian Journal of Bio. Sciences*.,,4, 41-53.

[16] Te-Sheng Chang (2009) An Updated Review of Tyrosinase Inhibitors *International Journal of Molecular Sciences. Mol. Sci.*, *10*, 2440-2475; doi:10.3390/ijms10062440 .

Index

A

B

C

D

E

F

G

Q

R

S

T

U

V

W

X

Y